FOREWORD

T his remarkable and informative book blends the perspectives of patients with breast cancer and the physicians who treat them. In contrast to many other diseases affecting women, breast cancer requires treatment decisions that involve not only the physical malady but the quality of life as well. These quality-of-life issues are influenced by familial, social, cultural, emotional, and spiritual variables that are very personal and unique to each woman. In view of this, medical and surgical decisions must integrate the perspectives of both the patient and her physicians. Thus listening skills, empathy, sensitivity, and a willingness to accept the patient as a partner in treatment planning are a must for physicians. The patient, in turn, needs to be familiar with medical terminology and be well informed about treatment options and their potential impact on her life, both physically and emotionally. The bottom line in the decision-making process is this: do the benefits outweigh the risks for a given combination and sequence of treatments after taking into account all the available options?

This invaluable book should be read by every physician who sees women with breast diseases. It provides unique and valuable insights into women's perspectives about breast cancer, including their fears, emotional needs, and desire for the information that is critical to assuming a responsible decision-making role in their own treatment and rehabilitation. Every woman who has breast disease or who is at risk for developing breast cancer will benefit greatly by reading this informative and well-illustrated book. The voices of women and their loved ones that permeate these pages will help others face the trauma associated with this disease and cope with the decisions that must be made knowing that they do not face this crisis alone. These pages offer a woman a better understanding of the complex choices she faces and thus reduce her anxieties. She can also learn about the option of breast reconstruction, the different operations available for breast restoration, and the associated risks and benefits. Such a factual, realistic, and no-nonsense information base is the best way to deal with these issues, for it allows a woman to act knowledgeably in selecting her physicians and in making the treatment decisions that are right for her.

I want to compliment Karen Berger and John Bostwick on their significant and unique contribution to the literature. Karen Berger is a leading medical publisher and writer who has devoted years to working with women with breast cancer. This book reflects her desire "to educate women about the treatment alternatives available to them so that they can more effectively influence their own destinies and play an active role in their own health care." Dr. John Bostwick is one of the foremost breast reconstructive surgeons whose extensive experience working with breast cancer patients is well known. His care and compassion for patients are evident throughout this book. These authors have written a meaningful and easily understood text to help women deal with the fear and reality of breast cancer by enabling them to become informed participants in the treatment-planning process. They have succeeded admirably. This book will enhance the understanding and trust between those who are afflicted with breast diseases and those who care for them.

Charles M. Balch, M.D.
Head, Division of Surgery and Anesthesiology
The University of Texas
M.D. Anderson Cancer Center
Houston, Texas

When I undressed I would go in the bathroom and slip my nightgown on. I would never turn toward my husband when I put on my bra. I was reluctant to let him see me unclothed. That was my stigma. Mentally I felt that I was not a total woman because part of me was missing.

Now, when I get up in the morning and put on my bra, I feel wonderful. I don't worry anymore. I don't think cancer. I am whole again. Breast reconstruction has changed my life. At night, God forgive me, when I take off my bra, I find myself just standing there and looking at myself and thinking, "Is this really me?" I love the way I look.

> **— Denise,**
> who had a mastectomy and breast
> reconstruction 13 years later, is one of
> "Thirteen Women Who Tell Their Stories" in
> A WOMAN'S DECISION

A WOMAN'S DECISION

Breast Care, Treatment, & Reconstruction

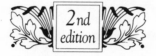

2nd edition

Karen Berger and
John Bostwick III, M.D.

Illustrations by William Winn

QUALITY MEDICAL PUBLISHING, INC

ST. LOUIS, MISSOURI
1994

Printed in the United States of America.

Quality Medical Publishing, Inc.
11970 Borman Drive, Suite 222
St. Louis, Missouri 63146

LIBRARY OF CONGRESS CATALOGING-IN-PUBLICATION DATA

Berger, Karen
    A woman's decision : breast care, treatment, and reconstruction /
Karen Berger and John Bostwick III ; illustrations by William Winn.
— 2nd ed.
        p.   cm.
    Includes bibliographical references and index.
    ISBN 0-942219-04-X
    1. Breast—Cancer—Surgery.   2. Breast—Care and hygiene.
3. Mammaplasty.   4. Breast—Cancer—Psychological aspects.
I. Bostwick, John.
RD667.5.B47   1993
616.99' 449059—dc20   93-5544
                                                                     CIP

TH/R/R
5   4   3   2   1

CONTENTS

Appendices

NOTE:
THE GENDER PROBLEM

In writing this book, we were confronted with the
dilemma of which gender pronouns to use to refer to the
surgeons and plastic surgeons we discussed. Because all of the
patients in the book are female and are referred to as she,
we decided to avoid confusion and use the male
pronoun for all the doctors in this book.

ACKNOWLEDGMENTS

A book progresses through many stages and numerous revisions during its evolution. Initially the authors struggle in isolation committing their thoughts to paper. Transforming their rough manuscript into a published book, however, requires the assistance of others. Our book was no exception. Although this is a second edition, the writing process was as intense as if it were a new creation. All aspects of the book were carefully reexamined and most chapters were rewritten to incorporate the latest information in a field that has become increasingly complex and dynamic.

For a time, we felt that our book was a moving target that shifted its direction at every turn. The breast implant controversy and subsequent developments made last-minute changes a chronic necessity, as did a series of exciting discoveries in breast cancer research. We saw no end in sight. These ongoing changes more than doubled the size of this edition. Ultimately, as all authors must, we relinquished the manuscript, ever hopeful that it was as current as the publishing process allows. Most likely we would still be reworking the manuscript if it had not been for the assistance of numerous experts who contributed their time and knowledge to help finalize this writing project. We were fortunate to have the advice of medical experts, skilled editors, and sensitive friends and associates. With their guidance and encouragement, we worked through our problems and maintained our perspective. Therefore we have many people to acknowledge and to thank.

A debt of special gratitude is due to Audrey Lenharth, whose influence and assistance are pervasive throughout this book. It was Audrey who helped launch this second edition. She is one of those dedicated, talented, and organized individuals who willingly gives of her time and talent with no expectation of reward. Her assistance was integral to our writing effort. She helped to develop, produce, and distribute 950 surveys to breast cancer patients throughout the United States. It is this survey that forms the basis for much of the material presented. She also was instrumental in assembling the Appendix, contacting different agencies and organizations for resources and information. Because of Audrey we have a book that reflects the needs, hopes, and desires of a broad spectrum of women throughout the United States.

We would especially like to thank the many women who responded to our surveys. These women took time out of their lives to answer our questions because they desired to help other women and because they had a statement to make about their experiences. We received hundreds of letters and phone calls from them. Their response was both gratifying and helpful in formulating our ideas. Their words not only inspired us but taught us how to improve this edition to better meet their needs.

Additionally, we are grateful to Vicki Castleberry of Bosom Buddies Breast Cancer Support Group, Atlanta; Barbara A. DuCharme of Bosom Buddies Breast Cancer Support Group, Phoenix; Sharon Green of Y-ME National Organization for Breast Cancer Information and Support Inc., Chicago; Michele Nobs of St. John's Mercy Medical Center Breast Cancer Support Group, St. Louis; Lynn Stadnyk of Focus Breast Cancer Support Group, St. Luke's Hospital, St. Louis; and the American Cancer Society for soliciting the cooperation of breast cancer patients throughout the country to participate in this survey. Their assistance is deeply appreciated.

Much of the tone and focus of this book was a natural outgrowth of the emotion-packed interviews we had with the women and men who allowed us to record their feelings about and experiences with breast cancer and breast reconstruction. Particular thanks are reserved for the 14 women and three men whose stories are recorded within these pages. They allow us to relive their experiences with them and in so doing to learn from them. Even though the names and personal details of these individuals have been changed to protect their privacy, their feelings and experiences reflect their real-life encounter with breast cancer and breast reconstruction.

Several chapters contain major contributions from others, and we would like to acknowledge these experts here. Our contributors include the following:

Kenneth J. Arnold, M.D.
Clinical Assistant Professor of
Surgery, Washington University
School of Medicine, and Staff
Surgeon, Barnes and St. Luke's
Hospitals, St. Louis

John M. Bedwinek, M.D.
Director, Cancer Care Center,
St. Joseph Hospital, St. Louis

Benjamin A. Borowsky, M.D.
Associate Professor of Internal
Medicine, Washington University
School of Medicine, St. Louis

Roger S. Foster, Jr., M.D.
Chief of Surgical Services,
Crawford Long Hospital and
Wadley Glenn Professor of Surgery,
Emory University School of
Medicine, Atlanta

Mary Ellen Hawf, R.N., O.C.N.
Private practice, St. Louis

Jacob Klein, M.D.
Assistant Professor of Clinical
Obstetrics and Gynecology,
Washington University School of
Medicine, St. Louis

Lynne A. McCain, B.S.N., R.N.
Emory Clinic, Atlanta

John S. Meyer, M.D.
Chief Pathologist and Director of
Laboratories, St. Luke's Hospital,
St. Louis

Barbara S. Monsees, M.D.
Associate Professor of Radiology
and Section Chief, Breast Imaging,
Mallinckrodt Institute of Radiology,
Washington University School of
Medicine, St. Louis

Gary A. Ratkin, M.D.
Clinical Associate Professor of
Medicine, Washington University
School of Medicine, Medical
Oncologist In Practice, Barnes and
Jewish Hospitals, St. Louis

William C. Wood, M.D.
Joseph Brown Whitehead Professor
and Chairman, Department of
Surgery, Emory University School
of Medicine, Atlanta

These experts wrote the sections on what they do in their respective roles as internist, gynecologist, radiologist, general surgeon, radiation oncologist, medical oncologist, oncology nurse, and plastic surgery nurse and also reviewed, revised, and even rewrote the information presented on these topics in Chapter 5, "Breast Lumps and Other Breast Conditions," and Chapter 6, "Breast Cancer Facts and Treatment Options." Recognition is also due to Mimi Greenberg who allowed us to reprint information on the patient's responsibilities from her book *Invisible Scars*. The contributions from these experts provide a comprehensive update on current breast cancer therapy and breast reconstruction technique that is unavailable elsewhere in a single book for the general public.

Some of our contributors merit special recognition for their assistance in critiquing the entire manuscript, writing or revising sections as requested, and obtaining much-needed resource material. Dr. Gary A. Ratkin was one of these individuals; he always made time to help. No request was too much. Never did he make us feel that we were intruding on his time, despite his hectic schedule and overwhelming patient load. He critically reviewed the book and offered many helpful suggestions for expansion and revision. He also wrote new sections on support services, chemotherapy drugs and expected side effects, follow-up care, tests, and staging.

Despite having just relocated to Atlanta from Vermont, Dr. Roger S. Foster still took the time to thoroughly review the book and offer suggestions that influenced our writing. He carefully read and critiqued the previous edition and our current revision, making valuable recommendations and providing us with answers to significant questions. Whenever we realized that some topic had not been covered, it was Roger whom we called on to provide the missing data or write the needed material. He also checked our statistics and wrote sections on the breast cancer trials with tamoxifen, bone marrow transplantation and cell seeding techniques, staging, follow-up, and the doctor-patient relationship. He always found time to assist us, no matter how inconvenient the request.

We are equally grateful to Dr. John S. Meyer, who was enormously helpful in explaining the latest in breast cancer research. The female author's frequent calls to him requesting explanations of oncogenes, *erb B-2/neu*, ploidy, and *BRCA1* were always met with a patient explanation in understandable terms. His translation of a complex topic gives our readers the benefit of this highly scientific knowledge that is so crucial to their lives. He not only updated his job description as a pathologist but provided us with exciting material on new areas of breast cancer research.

Dr. Barbara S. Monsees contributed an entire chapter on mammography and also critiqued and revised the information on new imaging methods and diagnostic techniques. Dr. John M. Bedwinek totally reworked his sections on breast-conserving surgery and irradiation and on the role of the radiation oncologist in treating the breast cancer patient. He also reviewed the information on mammography. Dr. William C. Wood, as the new Chairman of Surgery at Emory University School of Medicine, still found time to write two sections:

one on follow-up after breast cancer treatment and the other on immediate breast reconstruction.

We also want to thank Mary Ellen Hawf, R.N., O.C.N., who prepared the section on what the oncology nurse does and how she helps the patient, and Lynne A. McCain, B.S.N., R.N., who described the role of the plastic surgery nurse in ministering to the breast reconstruction patient's physical and emotional needs. These nursing professionals provided a major service for breast cancer patients and their families by informing them of the excellent nursing resources that are available to support them through this trying experience.

In addition to the experts who contributed to our book, a number of professionals in this field reviewed the manuscript, provided input, and assisted us in gathering resource materials. In particular, they reviewed the new information on breast cancer research, breast cancer diagnosis and treatment, breast implants, and breast reconstruction. We would like to acknowledge the encouragement and assistance of Dr. Wendy Schain, Dr. Neal Handel, Rosemary Locke, Sharon Green, Dr. Garry Brody, Dr. Charles Balch, Dr. Bahman Teimourian, Dr. Ian T. Jackson, and Dr. Stephen Mathes.

Drs. William C. Wood and the surgical oncology group at Emory, including Drs. Toncred Styblo, Douglas Murray, Grant Carlson, and George Danneker, set a standard for us; they represent the type of quality care that this book is all about. Drs. Foad Nahai, Jack Culbertson, Grant Carlson, and Glyn Jones have also been helpful through their willing efforts to assist their partner while he struggled to finish his writing. Dr. Nahai took time from his own writing and plastic surgery practice to review the chapter on surgical options, rework the section on microsurgery, and contribute insightful comments to improve our descriptions of the various surgical techniques and devices used for reconstruction. Thanks are also due to the plastic surgery residents, physician assistants, and dedicated nursing staff of the Emory University Affiliated Hospitals and the Plastic Surgery Section of the Emory Clinic.

The editing skills of Carolita Deter were an invaluable asset. She polished our prose and offered critical suggestions for shaping and reworking our manuscript. Although too busy to take on another project, Carolita accepted this assignment because the female author prevailed on her friendship. She read our chapters, making valuable editorial and stylistic suggestions and bringing her incredible skill to bear on our writing. We are both grateful for the care she lavished on our book. Her efforts on our behalf have greatly enhanced this writing effort.

This manuscript would never have been completed had it not been for the efforts of Karen Kierath, Suzanne Murat, Kay Ehsani, and Amanda Griffith, who tirelessly transcribed tapes from the interviews and typed and retyped the manuscript because they cared about the project. Daniel Kopolow enthusiastically participated in this effort by searching the literature and helping to update the references, while Kay Ehsani and Beth Campbell-Blethroad checked sources and gathered other information. Mary Stueck laid out the pages of the book so that the information was presented in the most artistic and informative manner possible, Susan Trail skillfully styled the book's special elements, and Billie Forshee arranged for the book's scheduling and manufacture. Other staff members of Quality Medical Publishing, Inc., also provided support and expertise throughout this endeavor. Their assistance and encouragement were deeply appreciated as was the cooperation and assistance of Melba Mullins and Cathy McCrary, who effectively coordinated the Atlanta half of this endeavor.

William Winn sensitively rendered the drawings for this book, and his artistic contributions have added immensely to this edition. Diane Beasley's cover and book interior design have given this second edition a new look. As always her designs manage to capture the essence of a book. Appreciation is also due to Lester Robertson for his excellent photography.

Our friends and associates were an ongoing source of support as they shared in our concerns and assisted us with our problems. Anitra Sheen and Dr. Jack Sheen were always positive and encouraging. Anitra took time from her own writing to review chapters and offer insightful comments. Jeff Friedman, a poet and skilled editor, reviewed the manuscript and provided editing suggestions. Harriet Kopolow was the true friend that the female half of our writing team has always valued; her support was pervasive, as was that of Anne Smith Carr, Diane Feldman, Dr. Joel Feldman, Joan Foster, Johnna Hart Matthews, and Marjorie Jackson. Dr. Jessica Lewis was one of the reasons the book was written; it meant a great deal to know that she believed in the project and in the authors. Marilyn Ratkin, Pat Simons, Colleen Randall, and Vicki Friedman were a source of needed encouragement.

Our final appreciation belongs to our families: our spouses, Phil and Jane; our children, David and Andrew, Mary and John; and our parents, Bobbie and Dorothy, who understood our feelings about this subject, allowed us freedom to explore them, and encouraged us in the process.

Karen Berger
John Bostwick III

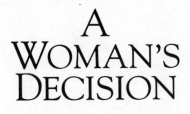

A
WOMAN'S
DECISION

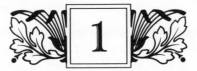

OUR PURPOSE IN WRITING

"C ancer" and "surgery" are words that we all have come to fear.
For the woman who develops a breast malignancy, these two
fears often merge when the treatment of her cancer results in
the surgical removal of part or all of her breast. The idea of this operation or any operation terrifies most of us, and yet with increasing frequency, more and more women who have had mastectomies are now
opting for additional, elective surgery to restore their missing breasts.

Breast reconstruction represents a notable advance in the rehabilitation of women with breast cancer and an example of the expanding treatment horizons now available to women confronting this life-
threatening disease. Today, women stricken with breast cancer have
significantly better options from which to choose—lumpectomy with
irradiation and mastectomy with breast reconstruction promise optimal cancer treatment without physical disfigurement. A woman no
longer must choose between her life and her breast. For women whose
condition mandates mastectomy or for those who select this operation,
knowledge that breast restoration is a possibility is enormously reassuring.

With increasing emphasis on informed consent, many women diagnosed with breast cancer now learn of reconstruction as an acknowledged component of their total treatment program. This was not always
the case. Although techniques for rebuilding breasts have existed for
many years, they were not always accepted by surgeons or known to
patients. Furthermore, the results of early reconstructive efforts often
did not offer sufficient aesthetic improvement to the mastectomy
patient aware of this operation to interest her in further surgery. Only
recently, with the development of new procedures enabling plastic
surgeons to create fuller, more lifelike breasts and to fill in major chest
wall deformities, have these results improved significantly.

Despite growing acceptance of reconstruction among mastectomy
patients and members of the medical community, the general public is
still largely unaware of the physical and psychological transformation

that is possible through reconstructive breast surgery. Our book, now in its second edition, is meant to fill this void by offering a comprehensive, but easily understandable account of this topic. Intended as a source of current and reliable information on breast reconstruction and its role in the rehabilitation of the breast cancer patient, it also focuses on a woman's options for breast care and includes routine self-inspection tips, descriptions of commonly occurring breast problems, and recent therapeutic approaches to breast cancer.

Although breast reconstruction is central to our discussion, it is not all encompassing. Not all women will have mastectomies. Some will choose lumpectomy and irradiation, and we do not want to neglect their needs. Nor will all women having mastectomies want the additional procedures involved in breast reconstruction. Some will choose an external prosthesis and then get on with their recovery. Our hope is that this book will educate women about the spectrum of therapeutic alternatives available to them. Equipped with this information, women can more effectively influence their own destinies and play an active role in their own health care.

Ours is not a medical text. We are speaking as professionals, but the scope of our book extends far beyond statistical analysis or technical descriptions of tumor behavior. Rather, we address the concerns of women in confronting their fears of breast malignancy and in monitoring their breasts. Our book evolved from the need for a common-sense approach to issues that women with breast problems face in dealing with physicians and issues physicians face in treating these patients. As co-authors, we try to provide a personal, but medically accurate account.

Readers will observe that these pages are liberally sprinkled with medical terms. Care has been taken to define these words, not to eliminate them. We are not proponents of medical jargon, just realists who respect the intelligence of our readers. Despite doctors' best efforts to provide understandable explanations to their patients, it is only natural for these medical experts to rely heavily on the communication tools that they routinely use. For a woman to feel fully in control, she must familiarize herself with this terminology so that she is not frustrated in her efforts to learn more about her condition. We strongly believe that it is important to use the language that women will encounter as they seek treatment.

Clearly, our audience for this book is a broad one, as it should be, because breast cancer touches many people. Since the first edition was published in 1984, breast cancer has afflicted over one million women. Now the alarming news is that it will strike one out of eight women* during her lifetime. For the female half of our writing team, these statistics have come home. She notes with each passing year that breast cancer is an intimate reality for more and more relatives and friends. She feels that she is writing this book for herself, to answer all of those questions that have always worried and haunted her. The physician half of our writing team sees the need for such a book to help answer patient questions. Over the years he is seeing significantly greater numbers of women in search of breast reconstruction; alarmingly, many of these women are in their thirties and forties, far younger than the patient population he was treating a mere 10 years ago. Both of us wish to reach more than two million women in the United States today who have had mastectomies or lumpectomies and the 180,000 American women each year who develop breast cancer. We want these women to know about the option of breast reconstruction. Then women who have had mastectomies can consider this possibility and women who develop breast cancer can choose a mastectomy (still the most frequent therapy) knowing that they can have their breasts restored. This book is also directed at women who are disease free. If they know that reconstructive breast surgery and lumpectomy and irradiation are available, they might be less prone to procrastinate seeking medical attention for suspected breast problems. We are also writing for men, not because they will suffer from breast cancer (the incidence of breast cancer among men is 1% that of women), but because they will know, love, work with, and live among women who have had this experience. Perhaps this knowledge will sensitize them to the psychological and physical concerns that this disease creates.

Much of the information contained within the pages of this book is drawn from 10 years of research, over 1000 questionnaires, hundreds of letters and comments received from our readers, and numerous interviews with men and women. We principally surveyed women who had mastectomies and lumpectomies for breast cancer and asked them to describe their feelings and experiences not only with this disease, but also with their subsequent therapy and rehabilitation. Of particular interest to us was information on breast reconstruction, and we posed a number of questions about this operation to determine

---

*This assumes a lifetime beyond age 85. The one out of nine statistic still applies, assuming a lifetime of 85 years.

what women knew about it and their resulting concerns and expectations. We asked women to supply us with questions that they wanted answered and issues that they wanted addressed.

The women who responded to our surveys invested considerable time pondering our questions and thoughtfully answering them. They painstakingly recorded their thoughts on the backs of pages, typed extra sheets, wrote letters, and attached articles and reading lists that they thought would assist us. Some women even took the time to phone the female half of our writing team (who had listed her phone number on the survey) to ask questions and offer recommendations. Especially gratifying for us were communications received from women who had read the first edition of this book; they graciously described the book's impact on their lives and provided suggestions for revision. As a group, these women engendered critical changes in the tone and direction of our book. Because of them, we have added new chapters on mammography, implants (the controversy erupted in the midst of our research), and doctor-patient communication, a topic all agreed merited further exploration. We have also greatly expanded the Appendix to include comprehensive information on support services, patient education resources, and informed consent.

Some provocative trends emerged from our recent canvassing efforts. Whereas only 15% of women with mastectomies opted for breast reconstruction 10 years ago, our most recent questionnaires revealed a striking increase in interest and acceptance of this source of rehabilitation. In our personal series of 500 women surveyed in the 1990s, 46% had chosen to have breast restoration. Of those who had not had breast reconstruction, 31% indicated that they would like to reserve this possibility for a future date. We also noted that the average age of women responding had shifted from the late fifties to the middle forties, with a disturbing increase in the number of women in their thirties reporting that they had contracted breast cancer, often in the absence of a family history of this disease.

We also carefully reexamined all of the information contained in existing chapters, rewriting and amplifying as we went along and significantly updating this material. Since our last literary excursion, many new developments have occurred in breast cancer research and therapy. These have been incorporated in this edition. Of particular interest are expanded sections on new tests and therapies for diagnosing and treating breast cancer, methods for breast cancer staging, criteria for choosing lumpectomy with irradiation, and the latest chemotherapy and hormonal therapy regimens. Additionally, we have included information on the clinical trials under way to assess the value of tamoxifen for possible breast cancer prevention in women at high risk. In our previous edition the nurse's role in working with breast cancer patients and their families was not given the attention that it rightfully deserves. To rectify this omission we have added input from the nursing profession to the chapter entitled "What Your Doctors Can Do For You" (now appropriately renamed "What Your Doctors and Nurses Can Do For You"). Finally, we have totally rewritten the sections on breast reconstruction to incorporate the numerous advances that have taken place in the past 10 years and to respond to women's questions about breast restoration. All of the currently available reconstructive techniques, from the simplest to the most complex, are described in detail and accompanied by numerous photographs and drawings of the procedures and their expected results, as our readers proposed. To reflect the mounting demand for immediate breast reconstruction, this topic has been explored in depth.

The concluding chapter of the first edition was cited by most of our readers as particularly valuable to them in understanding the possibilities and limitations of breast reconstruction. It captured conversations we conducted with breast reconstruction patients throughout the country. In this edition totally new interviews have been included to reflect the latest reconstructive techniques. Thirteen women poignantly explain their motivations for seeking breast reconstruction. All of these women freely shared the details of their surgery as well as their intense feelings about it.

Although the primary focus of our book is not on breast disease and breast cancer, these issues are closely related to the subject of breast reconstruction. Despite the existence of numerous books and articles on the general health issues of breast disease, our surveys indicate that many women remain woefully ignorant of them. Therefore we have interwoven basic information on these subjects throughout.

Still, most of our book concentrates on breast reconstruction. Why do women seek breast restoration? Who is a candidate? What is the correct timing for this surgery? What is the best operation for breast reconstruction? What are the risks and benefits? What are the facts about breast implants? Answers to these frequently asked questions and many others are combined with the personal accounts of women who have had their breasts restored. Pain, recuperation, and expense are issues of primary concern to any woman contemplating elective surgery, and these have been dealt with in great detail. We itemize the costs, risks, and benefits and describe and illustrate the different reconstructive techniques available. We try to present all sides of this topic.

Clearly, breast reconstruction is not for every woman. Many will not wish to undergo further surgery, pain, or expense. But for those with a potential interest, we provide information to enable them to make an educated decision.

BREAST ANATOMY AND PHYSIOLOGY

How much do most women really know about their breasts? Most likely very little. Unless they develop breast problems, they usually are not motivated to learn about the inner structure of this intimate female body part. Yet women need to be more familiar with the normal anatomy and physiology (function) of their breasts if they are going to be able to recognize the earliest and most treatable signs of breast cancer. With this knowledge, they will not be so frightened every time they notice a breast change. This chapter provides that information in a simple and straightforward manner. It offers women a baseline for evaluating their own health care requirements. Additionally, it provides assistance for women interested in performing breast self-examination, a crucial routine for proper breast surveillance.

The breast is a mound of glandular, fatty, and fibrous tissue located over the pectoralis muscles of the chest wall and attached to these muscles by fibrous strands (Cooper's ligaments). The breast itself has no muscle tissue, which is why exercises (often vigorously engaged in by teenagers intent on enlarging their breasts) will not build up the breasts. A layer of fat surrounds the breast glands and extends throughout the breast. This fatty tissue gives the breast a soft consistency and gentle, flowing contour. The actual breast is composed of fat, glands (with the capacity for milk production when stimulated by special hormones), blood vessels, milk ducts to transfer the milk from the glands to the nipples, and sensory nerves that give feeling to the breast. These nerves extend upward from the muscle layer through the breast and are highly sensitive, especially in the regions of the nipple and areola, which accounts for the sexual responsiveness of some women's breasts. Because the breast is made up of tissues with different textures, it may not have a smooth surface and often feels lumpy. This

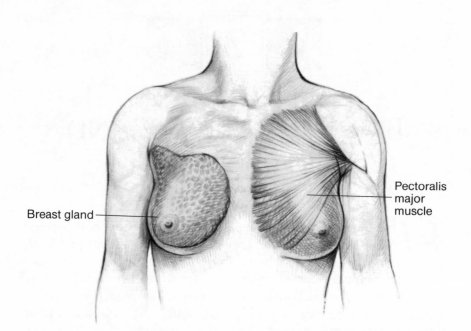

Breast gland

Pectoralis
major
muscle

irregularity is especially noticeable when a woman is thin and has little breast fat to soften the contours; it becomes less obvious after menopause, when the cyclic changes and endocrine stimulation of the breast have ceased and the glandular tissue softens. Estrogen supplements after menopause can cause continued lumpiness. The breast glands drain into a collecting system of ducts that go to the base of the nipple. The ducts then extend through the nipple and open on its outer surface. In addition to serving as a channel for milk, these ducts are often the source of breast problems. Experts now believe that most breast cancer begins in the lining of the ducts and sometimes the milk glands. Benign fibrocystic changes also originate from these ducts.

The ducts end in the nipple, which projects from the surface of the breast, and are a conduit for the milk secreted by the glands and suckled by a baby during breast feeding. There is considerable variation in women's nipples. In some the nipple is constantly erect; in others it only becomes erect when stimulated by cold, physical contact, or sexual activity. Still other women have inverted nipples. Surrounding the nipple is a slightly raised circle of pigmented skin called the areola. The nipple and areola contain specialized muscle fibers that make the nipple erect and give the areola its firm texture. The areola also contains Montgomery's glands, which may appear as small, raised

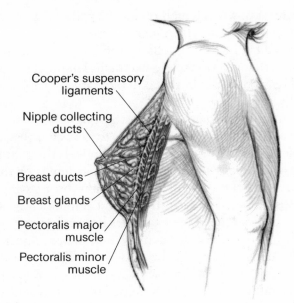

Cooper's suspensory
ligaments

Nipple collecting
ducts

Breast ducts

Breast glands

Pectoralis major
muscle

Pectoralis minor
muscle

lumps on the surface of the areola. These glands lubricate the areola and are not symptoms of an abnormal condition.

Beneath the breast is a large muscle, the pectoralis major, which assists in arm movement; the breast rests on this muscle. (Portions of three other muscles are also found under the lower and outer portions of the breast.) Originating on the chest wall, the pectoralis major extends from deep under the breast to attach on the upper arm. It also helps form the axillary fold, created where the arm and chest wall meet. The axilla (armpit) is the depression behind this fold. Removal of the pectoralis major muscle, as was formerly done during a radical mastectomy (an operation rarely performed anymore), left a considerable deformity: the chest had a hollowed-out appearance under the collarbone, the skin was tight and drawn over the rib cage, and the axillary fold and axilla were missing.

A rich system of blood vessels transport and supply nutrients and hormones to the breast. Because blood flow is increased during the menstrual cycle, pregnancy, and sexual stimulation, the breasts become engorged.

Fluid leaves the breast through the venous part of the bloodstream and the lymphatic channels. The lymphatics are small vessels that carry tissue fluid away from the breast, where it passes through a system of filters known as lymph nodes. As part of the body's immune system, the lymph nodes can enlarge in response to local infection or tumor. Trapped breast cancer cells multiplying in these lymph nodes also can cause them to swell. The two main lymph drainage areas are under the breastbone and in the axilla. Enlarged lymph nodes in the axilla usually can be felt.

In examining a woman's breasts the physician first checks the appearance of the skin and nipple-areola for any changes such as dimpling, nipple inversion, or crusting. He then feels the glandular tissue of the breast to detect suspicious or unusual lumps or thickenings. (Despite the beneficial value of mammograms [breast x-ray films], the physical breast examination is still the most common way of detecting breast masses.) In addition, he examines her underarm to determine if there is lymph node enlargement. When breast cancer spreads, it often can be detected first in the underarm. Thus a patient who is being treated for breast cancer usually has some of these lymph nodes from the underarm removed and examined by a pathologist to see if the cancer has spread to them and if so to what extent. Removal of the lymph nodes can accentuate the depth or hollow appearance of the armpit.

Each woman's breasts are shaped differently. Individual breast appearance is influenced by the volume of a woman's breast tissue and fat, her age, a history of previous pregnancies and lactation, her heredity, the quality and elasticity of her breast skin, and the influence of breast hormones.

The breast is responsive to a complex interplay of hormones that cause the breast tissue to develop, enlarge, and produce milk. The three major hormones affecting the breast are estrogen, progesterone, and prolactin, which cause glandular tissue in both the breast and uterus to change during a woman's menstrual cycle. Because of reduced hormonal levels the breasts are less full for 1 to 2 weeks after menstrual flow; therefore it may be easier to detect breast lumps during this time. Reduction of hormonal levels is also responsible for the breast's return to its prepregnant state after breast feeding is concluded.

Some women have a large amount of breast tissue and/or breast fat and thus have large breasts. Others have a small, but normal amount of breast tissue with little breast fat and thus have small breasts. After weight loss, pregnancy, or menopause many women experience a decrease in breast size and volume. If the skin does not have sufficient elasticity, the breasts also can appear to droop or sag. The size of a woman's breasts often influences whether they will sag. The larger the breasts are, the more likely they are to succumb to the constant force of gravity. This sagging appearance (ptosis) often accompanies the aging process, particularly if the breast size decreases.

Few women have completely balanced breasts; one side is often larger or smaller, higher or lower, or shaped differently from the other side. The underlying chest wall may also be asymmetric. Breast asymmetry is normal, even though some women are not aware of it unless it is pointed out to them.

Breast shape and appearance change as a woman ages. In the young woman the breast skin is stretched and expanded by the developing breasts. The breast in the adolescent is usually hemispherical, rounded, and equally full in all areas. As a woman gets older, the top side of the breast tissue settles to a lower position, the skin stretches, and the shape of the breast changes. After menopause, with the decrease of hormonal activity, the composition of the breast changes: the amount of glandular tissue decreases and fat and ductal tissue become the predominant components of the breast. Reduction in glandular volume can result in further looseness of the breast skin.

Skin quality influences breast shape. Even though breast skin contains special elastic fibers, there is much natural and hereditary variation in the amount of elasticity and thickness of each individual's breast skin. Some women have thicker skin with considerable elasticity or stretch. They tend to have tighter and firmer breasts longer than women who have thinner skin with less elasticity. Women with very thin skin may even develop stretch marks, or striae. These marks are actual tears of the deeper layers of the thin skin and usually indicate a lack of elasticity.

Few women realize the large area of their chest that is actually covered by breast tissue; it may extend from just below the collarbone to the level of the sixth rib and from the edge of the breastbone to the underarm area. A portion of the breast even reaches into the armpit region. The breast also has mobility on the chest wall because of loose fibrous (fascial) attachments to the underlying muscles. This breast motion is limited and the breasts are given support by special ligaments known as Cooper's ligaments. When a breast is removed, these ligaments, their fascial attachments, some lymph nodes from the armpit area, and sometimes even the underlying muscles are removed. Thus the deformity created encompasses much more than a missing breast, and for breast reconstruction to be successful, it must fill in or restore all of these areas.

BREAST SELF-EXAMINATION

Breast self-examination (BSE) can save a woman's life. Many women fear finding a breast lump and therefore avoid checking their breasts; this neglect can prove to be foolishly dangerous. It may even allow cancer to go undetected and spread outside the local breast tissue, thus lessening a woman's chances for cure and long-term survival. Periodic breast examinations are important to the early detection of breast cancer, which ranks second to lung cancer as the most frequent cause of cancer death in women. Statistics reveal that most breast cancers are actually discovered by women themselves. If more women practiced routine BSE, the incidence of death from breast cancer might be reduced by as much as 18% because BSE-detected tumors usually are discovered when the tumor is in its early, more curable stages. In addition to checking her own breasts, a woman should have her gynecologist, internist, or family physician examine them at least once a year.

BSE is clearly an essential part of a woman's health care. It is easy to learn and perform, does not require a special setting, and can be incorporated into any woman's normal routine. BSE helps acquaint a woman with the look and feel of her breasts and their normal cyclic changes, making it easier for her to detect breast changes early, when treatment is most likely to be effective. As a result of early detection of breast cancer, a woman may be able to have a less extensive operation.

Many women are puzzled by their breasts' natural lumpy texture and question their ability to find a small lump within this irregular breast tissue. Initially it may be difficult to differentiate between normal and abnormal breast tissue during BSE. A woman may even want to ask her doctor to go through the procedure with her the first time. He can examine her breasts, tell her what he feels and why, and help her to understand what she is looking for. Eventually, with monthly inspection, she will feel more comfortable and knowledgeable about this process.

Some women have fibrocystic changes that give their breasts a lumpy texture and confound their attempts at BSE. These lumps frequently shrink and swell with the menstrual cycle. Women with fibrocystic breasts should identify the ordinary bumpy areas of their breasts so that they can monitor cyclic changes and thus discover any new, distinct lumps.

Ideally, BSE should be conducted once a month. If a woman is still menstruating, she should inspect her breasts approximately 7 to 10 days after the beginning of menstruation, when they are not swollen and tender. If she is no longer menstruating, she should still perform regular monthly examinations; the first day of each month is often a good, easy-to-remember schedule. Monthly BSE should also remain a part of a woman's routine after she has had a mastectomy or lumpectomy or after breast reconstruction.

HOW TO DO BSE

BSE consists of visual inspection and palpation (feeling).

Visual Inspection

To examine your breasts visually, stand in front of a mirror in a well-lighted room and carefully observe all sides of your breasts for unusual characteristics. Any differences in the size or shape of your breasts should be noted. You are looking for discharge from your nipples, sudden nipple inversion (if your nipples were previously erect), a skin rash, scaling, redness, puckering, or dimpling. Some women may notice that they have prominent veins in their breasts. This condition, in itself, is not cause for alarm if it is the normal state of a woman's breasts. Changes in the appearance of these veins are important. If you notice any of these variations in your breast appearance, you should immediately report them to your doctor.

To identify any changes in the shape of your breasts, observe yourself in three positions: (1) straightforward with your hands at your sides, (2) hands raised and clasped behind your head with hands pressed forward, and (3) hands pressed firmly on your hips with shoulders and elbows pulled forward. As you assume the last two positions, you should be able to feel your chest muscles tense. The outline of your breasts should have a smooth curve in all positions.

If you have had a mastectomy or lumpectomy or breast reconstruction, you must also observe the breast scar for any sign of new swelling,

Visual Inspection

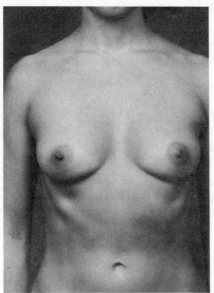

Stand straightforward with your
hands at your sides.

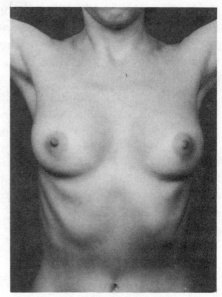

Raise your hands and clasp
them behind your head with your
hands pressed forward.

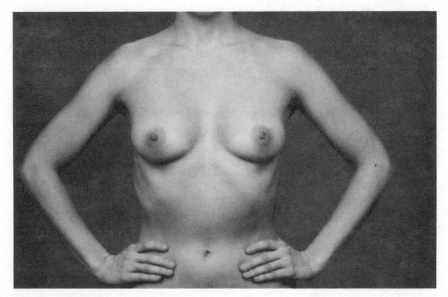

Press your hands firmly on your hips with your shoulders and elbows pulled forward.

lumps, redness, or color change. Although redness may be caused by chafing from your undergarments or your prosthesis, it should be reported to your doctor.

Palpation (Feeling)

The most important part of the examination, feeling your breasts, can be done while you are standing or lying down. There is no need to be embarrassed about feeling your breasts; this is a normal part of a woman's health care.

Many women prefer the privacy of the shower for this inspection. The soap and water make their skin feel slippery and their fingers smoothly glide over their breasts, making it easier for them to detect any textural changes underneath.

If palpation is performed while standing, begin the inspection by raising your left arm and using the flat, cushioned part of your fingers of your right hand (not the fingertips) to feel your left breast. Place your fingers at the outer edge of your breast and slowly press or compress the breast tissue gently down to the chest wall beneath.

There are several patterns that you can use for examining your breasts. With one, the strip pattern, you start at the top of your chest and palpate your breasts in a vertical pattern, carefully compressing the breast tissue, strip by strip, until all breast tissue has been inspected. With another pattern, you examine your breasts by moving your fingers in small circles around your breast, gradually working toward the nipple. Still another pattern approaches the breast as if it were a circle divided into wedges (sometimes referred to as the "wedge" pattern). Then you examine your breast wedge by wedge, working from the outer portion of your breast toward the nipple until the whole breast is examined. Which pattern you choose is not important. What is important is selecting one, using it consistently, and allowing yourself enough time for a thorough and deliberate examination. With all of these patterns, be sure to palpate the entire breast region, the areas above the breast and under the collarbone and the underarm, including the armpit itself. Sometimes lumps are discovered in this area. You are looking for any thickening, masses, swollen lymph nodes, or unusual lumps under the skin and especially a change from any previous examinations. They might feel like firm, distinct bumps. Repeat this examination on your right side.

Palpation

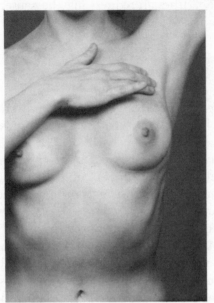

Place your fingers at the outer edge of your breast and slowly compress the breast tissue.

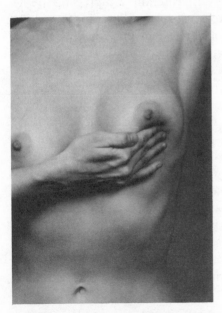

Move your fingers in small circles, working toward the nipple.

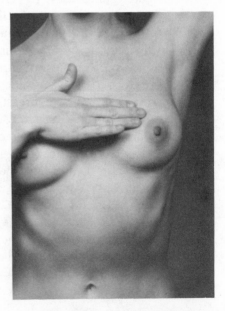

Check the entire breast and underarm, including the armpit.

Palpation Patterns

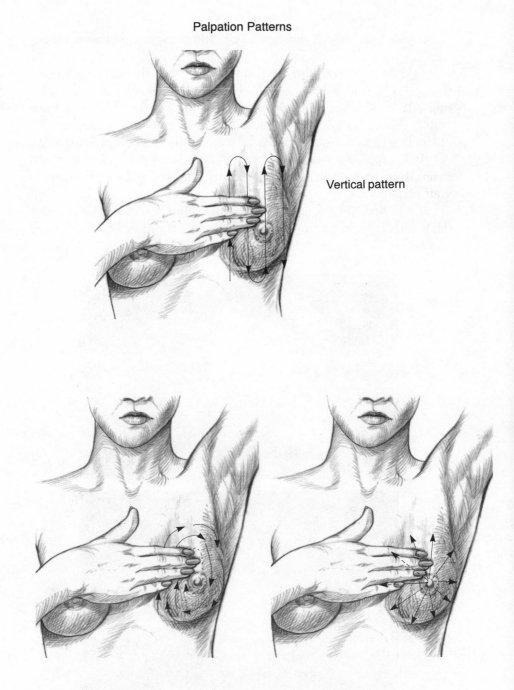

Vertical pattern

Circular pattern

Wedge pattern

If you have had a mastectomy, a lumpectomy, or breast reconstruction, you should feel your chest area, paying close attention to the scar and tissue surrounding it. Raise your arm on the unoperated side (or opposite side if you have had bilateral surgery) and using your opposite hand place three or four fingers at the top of the scar. Press gently using the circular motion described previously. Inspect the entire length of the scar. You are looking for lumps, bumps, hard spots, or thickenings. As with your breasts, familiarity with your scar will make it easier for you to recognize any changes and report them to your physician.

If you perform the inspection while lying down, lie flat on your back with your left arm over your head and a pillow or rolled towel

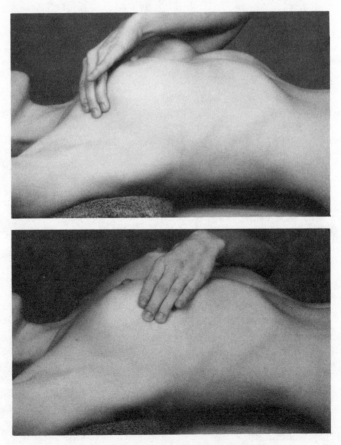

Breast self-examination while lying down

under your left shoulder. This position flattens your breasts and makes it easier for you to examine them. Use the same strip, circular, or wedge pattern described previously and repeat the procedure on your right breast.

Remember, most women's breasts have a bumpy texture and the upper, outer portion is usually the lumpiest. The best way to discover abnormal breast lumps is to know what is normal for your breasts; then if a problem develops, you can spot it immediately. Essentially what you are looking for are persistent lumps that do not disappear or change size after menstrual cycles. These are dominant lumps, appearing suddenly and remaining. Abnormal breast lumps will vary in size, firmness, and sensitivity. They may be hard or irregular with sharp edges. Still others appear as thickened areas with no distinct outlines. Some lumps are painful and tender. Pain is not ordinarily a sign of breast cancer, however, and may just indicate the development of a breast cyst. Sometimes natural underlying anatomic structures such as breast glands, breastbone, or ribs can be mistaken for lumps. A firm ridge in the lower curve of each breast is normal. Don't worry about making a mistake. Suspected lumps always should be reported to your doctor. It never hurts to be wrong, but it can definitely be damaging and even fatal to ignore a cancer.

Whether you perform BSE while standing or lying down, the important point is to make the decision to do a self-inspection each month. Any breast changes, unusual pain or tenderness, or lumps you discover should be investigated further by your doctor. Along with your monthly BSE, you should have regular checkups by your family physician, internist, or gynecologist. A breast examination should be a routine part of this yearly office visit.

Most breast lumps are benign, but for those that are malignant, mammography, BSE, and physician surveillance will ensure early detection and a significantly higher cure rate.

MAMMOGRAPHY AND
EARLY DETECTION
BARBARA S. MONSEES, M.D.

M ammography (x-ray examination of the breast) is the single most sensitive method for early detection of breast cancer. Yet, surprisingly, many women fail to take advantage of this lifesaving diagnostic tool. Fear of finding that their worst suspicion is confirmed and apprehension that radiation exposure from mammography may cause the very breast cancer it seeks to detect often deter women from having their breasts x-rayed. These irrational fears may prove to be a woman's worst enemy. Many well-documented studies have demonstrated that women who have routine mammography have a lower death rate from breast cancer than those who do not. When properly performed and interpreted, mammography has the potential to disclose approximately 90% of breast cancers. The fact is that most masses detected on mammograms are benign. Of the cancerous tumors detected by mammograms before they are large enough to be felt, approximately 90% can be cured. Furthermore, the radiation delivered during mammography is so small that the benefits of diagnosing a possible tumor far outweigh the theoretical risk of developing breast cancer.

Basically there are two types of mammograms: screening mammograms and diagnostic mammograms.

SCREENING MAMMOGRAMS

Screening is the process of evaluating healthy people with no symptoms to detect early signs of disease. A baseline screening mammogram provides a record of normal breast tissue appearance against which later changes can be compared. Once a baseline has been established, annual or semiannual screening mammograms are used to find possible abnormalities. Further workups may then be necessary to determine the significance of the findings. Although mammograms are extremely effective in finding most breast cancers, they cannot provide a definitive diagnosis; that can only be done by a biopsy (see Chapter 5).

Mammography is a very sensitive method for detecting breast cancer, but it is not perfect. For this reason, a woman should not request a screening examination if she suspects that she has a breast lump or other signs suggestive of breast cancer. A mammogram interpreted as normal in that circumstance may offer false assurance that breast cancer is not present. Therefore, if a lump or area of breast thickening is present, a woman should seek the advice of her personal physician and a diagnostic mammogram is warranted.

DIAGNOSTIC MAMMOGRAMS

A diagnostic mammogram is used to evaluate a woman with symptoms indicative of breast cancer. A diagnostic mammogram is performed when a lump or thickening has been felt or a screening mammogram reveals a problem (such as a shadow) that requires further investigation. Physical examination of the breast performed as part of this examination can be correlated with the findings on the mammogram. Specially tailored additional views may better assess an area of abnormality found on mammography or physical examination. Preferably, the diagnostic examination should be monitored by a radiologist, which adds to this cost.

The diagnostic mammogram may demonstrate that a palpable abnormality, one that can be felt, is a characteristically benign or malignant lesion and therefore determine whether a biopsy is warranted. The mammogram may also detect another abnormality at a different location in the same breast or in the opposite one. Therefore women over the age of 35 scheduled to have a biopsy should first have a mammogram to determine if another suspicious area requires attention.

The location, character, and extent of disease seen on a mammogram can often be helpful in determining if a woman is a good candidate for lumpectomy. If a biopsy is positive, a postoperative mammogram may be ordered to spot other tumors in the breast whose presence would dictate mastectomy rather than breast-conserving therapy.

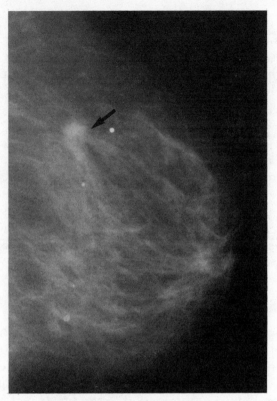

Mammogram showing irregular mass
that is breast cancer

RECOMMENDATIONS

When should a woman have her first mammogram and how often should she repeat this process? The American Cancer Society recommends a mammogram before age 40 as a baseline by which to judge any future changes and then one every 1 to 2 years until the age of 50. At age 50 and after a woman should have yearly mammograms. Mammograms are most effective for women over age 50 since their breasts are not as dense and abnormalities can be readily identified. A woman's gynecologist or family physician usually arranges for this test to help monitor her health care. Between the ages of 50 and 74 the incidence of breast cancer rises, and screening mammograms are especially important. For women with a previous breast cancer or a family history of breast cancer (a mother or sister with breast cancer), yearly mammography is suggested. Like any test, however, mammography should be used with caution and regular mammograms are not routinely advised for young women under the age of 35 who are not at high risk. Girls and teenagers have the highest risk of developing a radiation-induced breast tumor. Also, younger women's breasts are denser, making it more difficult to distinguish a mass or dense spot on a mammogram.

THE EXAM

A mammogram unit has compression plates to thin and flatten the breast to a uniform thickness. Adequate compression not only improves the quality of the breast pictures, but also lowers the x-ray dose to the breast. During a typical examination two or three views are taken of each breast: one with the breast squeezed between two vertical plates and one more with the breast squeezed between two horizontal plates. More than one view of each breast is necessary to unfold the overlapping breast densities seen on the film.

Some women complain of discomfort from the squeezing necessary to pull the breast tissue away from the chest wall and compress it between the plates for the x-ray pictures. However, this process takes only a few seconds for each exposure. The entire examination usually takes less than 5 minutes. Many women have no problem at all. Women who complain of breast tenderness at menstruation should consider delaying the test until after their period or early in the monthly cycle. As with any test or procedure, a person's ability to tolerate pain and discomfort may vary. Most admit, however, that any pain associated with mammography is short-lived and the benefits far outweigh the momentary discomfort.

WHERE TO GET YOUR MAMMOGRAM

Many women wonder where to go to have a high-quality mammogram. Screening mammography may be performed in a breast diagnostic center, at the physician's office, or on a mobile mammography unit. Before making a decision about where to go, a woman should inquire if the facility is accredited by the American College of Radiologists (ACR). This is a voluntary accreditation and means that the equipment, personnel, and procedures of that hospital or clinic have been evaluated and approved. Facilities applying for unit accreditation are judged on film quality and patient dose. Accredited facilities have radiation technologists who are specially trained to take the breast x-ray pictures and radiologists who are trained to interpret the results. They use modern equipment that provides high-quality breast x-ray films with an acceptable amount of radiation exposure.

The ACR evaluates individual units rather than the entire facility; many facilities have multiple units. Therefore, when visiting a particular facility, ask if the particular unit to be used is accredited. The ACR now provides a sticker with an expiration date that should be affixed to the accredited units. A listing of facilities with ACR-accredited units is available through the American Cancer Society.

Because accreditation is voluntary not all facilities of high quality are accredited by the ACR. If you are considering a facility that has not been accredited, the following questions can help you determine whether the facility is of high quality:

Does the facility use machines specifically designed for mammography? Does the facility have a film processor expressly for developing mammograms or does it develop other x-ray films in the same processor?

All mammograms should be performed on dedicated x-ray equipment made expressly for that purpose. Film processors used for chest or bone x-ray films are not likely to result in top-quality mammograms.

How many mammograms are taken each day?

If 20 or more procedures are performed per day, there is a higher likelihood that the technologist and radiologist will be experienced.

Is the person who takes the mammograms a registered technologist?

Only registered radiation technologists (certified by the American Registry of Radiologic Technicians or licensed by the state in which they work) should perform mammography to ensure correct breast positioning and exposure and to get the best image.

Is the radiologist who reads the mammograms specially trained to do so?

The radiologist should be board certified and should have taken specific training courses in mammography. The more experienced the radiologist, the better he or she will be in interpreting the findings.

How often is the mammography machine calibrated?

The machine should be of recent vintage and should be calibrated at least once a year to ensure that its measurements and doses are correct.

•   •   •

Be wary of mammogram units installed in doctor's offices that are owned and operated by a group of physicians. A medical center or a breast diagnostic center usually has better quality control. If you have found a good facility, return there year after year; that strategy will make it easier to compare current and older films. If you switch facilities, try to bring copies of your old films for comparison.

WHAT ARE THE COSTS?

Because of widespread recognition of the importance of breast x-ray films, many hospitals, clinics, and medical centers are offering low-cost screening mammograms ranging from $50 to $150, and many states are requiring insurance carriers to cover the expenses of this test. Additionally, as of January 1, 1991, Medicare now pays for screening mammography, and the Omnibus Budget Reconciliation Act sets forth quality standards for facilities billing Medicare for screening mammography. Insurance carriers and Medicare should reimburse for both screening and diagnostic mammography when it is indicated. To find the least expensive source for mammograms, a woman can compare prices by calling the American Cancer Society's national toll-free number, 800/ACS-2345, to request a list of low-cost, quality mammography facilities in her local area.

MAMMOGRAPHY IN SPECIAL CIRCUMSTANCES
Augmentation Mammaplasty

Breast implants can affect the quality of the mammogram and the radiologist's ability to detect breast cancer. Because the implant is opaque to x-rays, any breast tissue overlying the implant cannot be seen on the films. If a woman is at higher risk for developing breast cancer because of her family history, she should discuss this matter with her plastic surgeon prior to undergoing augmentation.

Extra views can be obtained to compensate for the inability to "see through" the implant. Most helpful are the so-called implant displacement views that allow visualization of the breast after the breast tissue has been gently pulled in front of the implant. Implant displacement views provide better visualization if the implant has been placed under rather than over the chest wall muscle (submuscular position), if a smaller implant has been used, and if the breast has remained soft. Women should routinely notify the technologist that they have breast implants before having a mammogram taken. If the

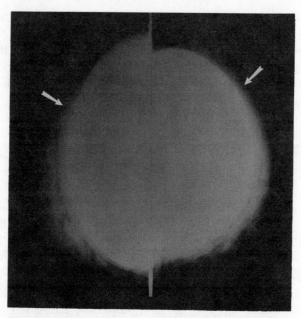

Standard mammographic view of breast with implant

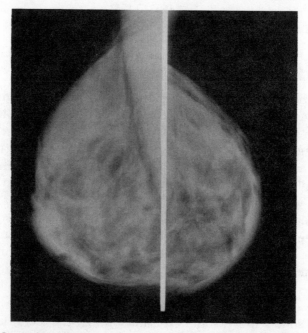

Special implant displacement view of breast with implant

facility does not routinely obtain displacement views in all women with implants, the woman should go elsewhere for her mammogram.

Reduction Mammaplasty

Women who have had breast reduction should also inform the radiation technologist and radiologist of this before a mammogram is taken. Scarring exhibited by a reduced breast does not ordinarily present a problem for radiographic interpretation. Unless an implant has been placed in the breast at the time of reduction, no special views are necessary. Routine screening mammography as suggested by the American Cancer Society is recommended. If an implant has been placed at the time of reduction, then the woman should have implant displacement views appropriate for mammography in women with breast implants.

If a woman is contemplating having reduction or augmentation mammaplasty, a preoperative mammogram should be performed to screen for breast cancer if the woman is over the age of 30. A follow-up mammogram should be taken 1 year after the procedure. If the woman has a family history of carcinoma of the breast, screening might be warranted at an even earlier age. Again, this should be discussed with the plastic surgeon prior to the surgery.

After Mastectomy

A woman who has had a mastectomy for breast cancer needs routine surveillance of the opposite breast to screen for breast cancer. Mammography should be performed every year following the initial diagnosis, regardless of the patient's age. Women often ask if they need mammograms taken on the mastectomy side. Some facilities obtain special chest wall views to examine for recurrence in the skin or muscle of the chest wall. There is no evidence that such views can change the outcome by earlier detection of recurrences on the chest wall. However, if a woman or her physician can feel a nodule on the chest wall, views of that area can be helpful in evaluation and may determine the need for a biopsy. If a woman has had a mastectomy and subsequent reconstruction, yearly mammography of the opposite breast is warranted to screen for breast cancer. However, as in the case of a woman who has had a mastectomy without reconstruction, mammography of the reconstructed breast is not necessary because no breast tissue remains on the mastectomy side. If a problem develops in the reconstructed breast, detailed views of the region can be obtained and are often useful in evaluation.

After Breast-Conserving Surgery and Irradiation

A woman who has undergone lumpectomy and radiation therapy must have meticulous follow-up mammograms of the treated breast. Yearly screening of the opposite breast is adequate, but mammographic follow-up of the treated breast should be done at 6-month intervals for the first year and then annually thereafter. If a new mass or area of microcalcifications is found on the mammogram, then biopsy may be necessary to determine if there is a recurrence in the treated breast.

OTHER IMAGING MODALITIES

Ultrasonography

Ultrasonography is a useful adjunct to mammography, but it is not a match for mammography in detecting small cancers. Its ability to differentiate a breast mass containing fluid (a cyst) from a solid mass (a benign or malignant tumor) offers distinct benefits. If a mammogram discloses the presence of a rounded mass in the breast that cannot be felt, an ultrasound scan is often obtained. If the mass is a simple cyst containing fluid, then biopsy is not necessary. However, if the cyst is not typical and contains a solid area, then biopsy may be necessary. With the use of ultrasound guidance the fluid can be drained from a breast cyst if desired. In most instances, however, unless the cyst is painful or large (greater than 2 cm), aspiration is usually not warranted.

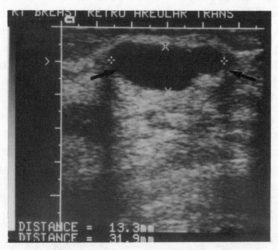

Ultrasound scan showing breast cyst

Techniques With Occasional Application

Computed tomography (CT), positron emission tomography (PET), magnetic resonance imaging (MRI), transillumination light scanning, and thermography have all been tested as methods of breast imaging. None of these techniques has proved effective for breast imaging, especially in screening for breast cancer. Thermography and transillumination light scanning have such a poor track record for the detection of breast cancer that very little research continues in these fields. CT has been used to evaluate areas of the chest wall too deep to be imaged on a mammogram. Examples of its use might include evaluation of the ribs that underlie a breast cancer positioned deep within the breast or evaluation of the chest wall under a reconstructed breast where a recurrence is suspect. PET scanning is another imaging modality that is still considered experimental. It is being evaluated in some centers for its usefulness in assessing the axillary lymph nodes and the extent of metastatic disease. MRI has some promise for the evaluation of patients with extremely dense breasts, for women who have had an abnormality detected on a mammogram and who need further evaluation, and for women with breast implants. Applications for this technology are evolving and expanding. Research into other technologies is ongoing.

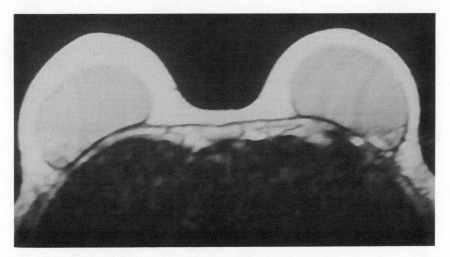

MRI scan of the chest of a woman with bilateral breast implants

• • •

The growing magnitude of the breast cancer problem demands women's attention. Breast cancer currently accounts for 32% of new cancers and 19% of cancer deaths among women in the United States. Any test that can facilitate early detection and improve the chance of surviving this disease merits consideration. Mammography is such a test; it gives us the capability to detect breast cancer 2 to 4 years before it can be felt on physical examination. However, as with most tests, mammography is not infallible, particularly in younger women, underscoring the complementary role of mammography and breast physical examination. Routine breast physical examination by a skilled examiner, breast self-examination, and routine screening mammography currently represent the most effective way to monitor women for breast cancer and to ensure detection in its earliest stages with the best chance for cure or long-term survival.

BREAST LUMPS AND OTHER BREAST CONDITIONS

When a woman discovers a breast lump, she naturally fears that she has breast cancer. Fortunately, most breast lumps are benign and are not related to breast cancer. Nevertheless, these conditions can cause a woman and her family considerable anxiety. Because of breast engorgement or inflammation, her breasts also may be painfully uncomfortable. Although many women immediately equate breast pain with cancer, most tender lumps are not malignant. Lumpy breasts, however, can be a problem and may make it difficult for a woman or her doctor to detect possible breast tumors. Awareness of commonly occurring benign breast conditions is therefore extremely valuable information for alleviating unwarranted fears and assisting a woman in early detection of a cancer if it does occur.

Although breast cancer occurs in women of all ages and the incidence among younger women has risen, one of the important factors in predicting whether an isolated breast lump is a cancer is the person's age. Less than 3% of breast cancers occur in women under the age of 35. Most breast cancers develop after menopause. When a woman in her thirties or forties finds a lump, it is more likely to be a simple cyst filled with fluid than a cancer. Less than one third of breast cancers occur in women under the age of 50. After menopause, benign breast conditions occur less frequently and the incidence of breast cancer rises; thus any lump is viewed with more concern.

BENIGN BREAST CONDITIONS
Fibroadenomas

When lumps are found in the breasts of teenagers and women in their twenties, they are almost always benign. The most common benign breast lump found in this age group is a firm, rounded, rubbery tumor known as a fibroadenoma. Fibroadenomas are not related to and are not precursors of breast cancer. Surgical removal is recommended for these tumors.

Fibrocystic Breasts

It is normal for many women in their childbearing years to notice that their breasts swell and become painfully tender before their menstrual periods. Along with this swelling the breasts often develop a lumpy texture that in some cases might become a permanent breast characteristic. Although this lumpy condition reflects normal changes within the glandular tissue and milk ducts of the breast, it is commonly described as *fibrocystic disease*. Calling this condition a *disease* is inappropriate and unnecessarily frightening to women since these physiologic changes occur in at least half of all North American women and are particularly common in women from age 20 to menopause. Because they occur during a time when a woman has a high level of female hormones, they are believed to be related to the response of the breast to those hormones. After menopause, fibrocystic activity usually subsides because of a woman's reduced hormonal level. Women taking hormones after menopause may note a persistence of fibrocystic activity and breast fullness.

The symptoms of fibrocystic change frequently vary with a woman's monthly cycle and are often associated with breast pain, which may be constant or may be accentuated when her breasts are swollen. Breast tenderness further increases a woman's anxiety that a tumor may be present in her breast. The soreness also can prevent a careful breast examination by the woman herself or by her physician.

Fibrocystic breasts usually feel "bumpy" because of cysts, irregularities, or thickened areas; some of these lumps are indistinguishable from tumors. These fibrocystic changes are not believed to be precancerous, but they may produce noticeable breast lumps that can be confused with cancer or even obscure the diagnosis of a small cancer.

Fibrocystic change is usually managed without an operation if the doctor confirms that no other breast condition is present. Because it is a chronic condition, it may require surveillance over a long period by both the woman and her doctor, including regular breast self-examination, physician follow-up and examination, mammograms, ultrasound tests, aspiration of cysts, and biopsies of lumps that persist after aspiration.

In addition, some experts believe that caffeine can accentuate the symptoms of fibrocystic breasts and recommend that women with this problem try to avoid caffeine-containing substances such as colas, coffees, teas, and chocolates. Some women notice a significant improvement in breast tenderness after abstinence from these foods, whereas others notice no change in their breasts. Vitamin E in a daily dosage of 800 IU (international units) is believed by some to lessen the symptoms of fibrocystic change in some women, but controlled studies have demonstrated no benefit from vitamin E. In exceptionally severe cases the doctor can prescribe danazol (Danocrine) or tamoxifen (Nolvadex) to control the pain and swelling. These drugs are rarely indicated, however, because of undesirable side effects, expense, and lack of efficacy.

Nipple Drainage

Nipple discharge is usually not caused by cancer. The only nipple discharges of significance are those that occur spontaneously without manipulation or squeezing of the nipple. A discharge of blood or serum, however, can indicate the presence of cancer and should never be ignored. The doctor can study a sample of the nipple discharge by spreading a thin layer of fluid on a glass slide and sending it to the pathologist for examination under the microscope.

Small benign tumors within the nipple ducts (ductal papillomas) as well as fibrocystic changes or inflammation can be the source of drainage. Sometimes a localized infection within a duct can cause persistent drainage. Treatment occasionally involves removal of the source of the drainage within the ductal system. The doctor also may order some hormonal studies of the blood to identify other benign causes of the nipple discharge.

Calcifications

Calcifications are calcium deposits in the breast that can only be detected by mammography. These deposits are common in the breasts of women over the age of 50 and in a smaller percentage of younger women. Calcifications are associated with benign or noncancerous conditions and most likely represent degenerative changes in a woman's breasts subsequent to aging of the breast arteries, old injuries, inflammations, or common benign conditions such as fibrocystic changes. Calcifications may be large and coarse (macrocalcifications) or tiny (microcalcifications).

Sometimes minute particles of calcium are discovered on a woman's mammograms. Although these microcalcifications can be an indication of precancerous changes or of breast cancer itself, this is not usually the case and a woman should not panic if these are diagnosed. Microcalcifications are common in breast tissue and most, over 80%, are benign and are not markers of breast cancer.

A woman who has numerous microcalcifications in both breasts is less likely to have cancer. Of more concern is a cluster of microcalcifications in one breast, especially if it is new; this may be the earliest finding indicating intraductal cancer. Grouped or clustered microcalcifications are perhaps the most significant secondary sign of malignancy, frequently suggesting the presence of a breast cancer. The probability of malignant disease increases with the degree of irregularity in the shapes of the microcalcifications as well as their size variations.

Currently, mammography cannot accurately distinguish between benign and malignant microcalcifications; therefore, in most cases, biopsy is needed for a definitive diagnosis and to rule out the possibility of breast cancer. A new density in the breast visible on two mammographic views should also be investigated. If calcifications are discovered on a woman's first mammogram, the doctor may sometimes delay biopsy for several months and then take another mammogram to see if this is a normal breast problem or if the calcifications have changed. Usually, however, these calcifications need to be positively identified by the pathologist after a biopsy.

DIAGNOSIS AND MANAGEMENT

Assuming that a breast problem is detected on a mammogram or that a woman finds a lump in her breast, what can she expect when she visits her doctor? The procedure varies, depending on her symptoms and her doctor's preferences. Some physicians will refer her to a surgeon immediately, whereas others might prefer to examine her first. A medical history is always taken.

It is important to understand that referral to a general surgeon does not necessarily mean that a biopsy will be done. Surgeons do not just operate; they are skilled in examining breast lumps, discussing and advising women about commonly occurring breast conditions and breast disease, and helping to detect and treat cancer at an early stage.

As a preliminary step, when a lump is first detected, the physician can use several noninvasive (nonsurgical) diagnostic tools. The doctor may suggest that the woman have diagnostic mammography or ultrasonography, in which sound waves are used to evaluate lumps. Ultrasound is a less specific and less dependable technique for detecting breast abnormalities than mammography and therefore is not as effective for screening. Unlike mammography, ultrasound does not consistently detect microcalcifications or identify very small cancers. However, ultrasonography is particularly useful for distinguishing a simple cyst from a solid lump. It is also useful for examining younger women who have normally glandular breasts. The most frequently used and reliable nonoperative diagnostic test is mammography. Magnetic resonance imaging (MRI), a technique that does not use radiation, may be useful in some diagnostic situations. Its applications are evolving. (More detailed information on mammograms and other imaging modalities is provided in Chapter 4.)

Breast examination and mammography are complementary diagnostic tools. Mammography alone without breast examination is inadequate. Sometimes even obvious breast lumps will not show up on x-ray examination; this is more often the case when the woman is under 50 years old and her breasts are relatively dense. A mammogram is a very valuable diagnostic tool, however, because it can indicate a breast abnormality at a very early stage before it can be felt and while it is still small and curable. It cannot, however, positively identify a calcification or a mass as cancerous; this can only be done through a biopsy of the area for examination under a microscope. A biopsy is done after all appropriate diagnostic tests have been completed.

Needle Aspiration

When there is a palpable lump in the breast and it feels like a cyst, it is usually drained (aspirated) with a thin needle. Occasionally the doctor may tell the patient to return to his office after her next menstrual cycle so that he can reexamine her breast before doing needle aspiration. Tissue that shrinks and then swells again before her next cycle could indicate a cyst or an area of fibrocystic change (both are benign and not related to cancer).

Needle aspiration is a method for determining if a breast mass is cystic or solid. It is a simple and relatively painless procedure that can be done in the surgeon's office. A biopsy may be avoided if the lump disappears after the fluid has been withdrawn from the suspected cyst. The doctor may want to send the fluid for analysis to a pathologist, especially if it is bloodstained. If no fluid is aspirated, the lump could be a fibroadenoma, a fibrocystic change, or a cancer. Most cysts are benign; breast cancer is usually a solid tumor.

If the fluid is bloody or if a mass persists that cannot be aspirated, further investigation is warranted to rule out the possibility of breast cancer regardless of the findings on mammography. In these cases the surgeon needs to remove the lump or sample a portion of the lump so that a specific diagnosis of the tissue can be made by a pathologist. This sampling is called a biopsy and can be performed by needle aspiration and/or surgery.

Fine-Needle Aspiration Biopsy
JOHN S. MEYER, M.D.

Fine-needle aspiration biopsy (FNAB) is a method for making a definitive diagnosis of breast carcinoma without an incision or surgical procedure. This approach uses a narrow-gauge needle (similar to or smaller than the type employed to draw blood) that is attached to a syringe. The mass is localized (located) by touch, and the needle is introduced into it as the syringe plunger is drawn back to produce negative pressure, thereby drawing cells and fluid into the needle. Several repeat passes of the needle are necessary to obtain a satisfactory sample. A local anesthetic may be used during the procedure to prevent discomfort. From a few to over 100,000 cells may be obtained in a drop or two of fluid. The cells are deposited on glass slides, stained, and examined microscopically. Interpretation is similar to that for Papanicolaou (Pap) smears. Malignant cells are recognized by their large abnormal nuclei (centers) and disorderly relationships one to another.

Aspiration biopsy in lieu of formal surgical biopsy can be done in the doctor's office, often without the need for anesthesia, and the results can be available so that a decision on therapy can be reached prior to surgery. A number of studies have shown accuracy to be very high when cancer is diagnosed with FNAB; only about 1 in 1000 such diagnoses have been in error. Fibroadenoma (a benign tumor discussed earlier in this chapter) may rarely be indistinguishable from carcinoma in needle aspiration biopsies, and premalignant changes accompanying fibrocystic breasts can at times be confusing to the cytopathologist. For the most part, however, a *positive* aspiration cytologic diagnosis of cancer can be considered equivalent to a diagnosis by formal biopsy.

FNAB is not as accurate, however, when the results are *negative*, indicating that no cancer is present. There are several reasons for this diminished reliability. One is the possibility of missing the tumor with the needle. This risk increases as the tumor size becomes smaller. The other reason is that some breast carcinomas have small nuclei with minimal abnormalities, and these cells are difficult to distinguish from cells of fibroadenomas or other benign conditions. Therefore cyto-pathologists err on the side of caution in diagnosing carcinoma and in certain cases may withhold diagnosis, recommending surgical biopsy for further clarification. If a suspicious lump persists after a negative needle biopsy, a surgical biopsy is necessary for definitive diagnosis.

FNAB may also be used when the physician is uncertain about the existence of a breast mass or a mammogram shows a focus of uncertain significance. In this situation the suspicious area can be examined by FNAB to help exclude the possibility of carcinoma. If the FNAB is positive, a diagnosis may be made at an early stage in the evolution of the disease.

Investigational studies are currently under way to test the efficacy of using preoperative chemotherapy after a FNAB diagnosis of cancer. In this situation the patient undergoes chemotherapy and then a mastectomy or conservative surgical operation may be done.

Core-Needle Biopsy

Core-needle biopsy uses a cutting-type needle (somewhat larger than the needle used for FNAB) to remove a sample of the breast mass for microscopic examination. The piece of tissue excised is not large enough for identification of biochemical receptors, but is big enough for the pathologist to make a diagnosis. The role of this type of needle biopsy is to make a reasonably definitive diagnosis without a formal operation on a fairly large breast tumor. In medical centers where breast surgery is routinely performed, core-needle biopsy is increas-ingly being replaced with FNAB, which is reliable for positive cancer diagnosis, less painful for the patient, and produces less bleeding.

Closed-Needle Biopsy of Nonpalpable Breast Lesions

One of the newer methods for biopsying suspicious areas that can be seen on mammograms but cannot be felt is called closed-needle biopsy. This technique combines FNAB or core-needle biopsy with computer imaging (stereotactic guidance) or with ultrasonography. This nonoperative or closed technique does not require an incision and is performed under local anesthesia by a diagnostic radiologist who removes a sample of tissue (core-needle biopsy) or a sample of cells (FNAB). Although both biopsy methods are used in some centers, the core-needle biopsy method is becoming a more common approach because specific diagnoses can be made from exact tissue samples that can be evaluated by standard methods in most pathology departments. Multiple samples (four or five cores) maximize the accuracy of this procedure.

Ultrasonography can only be used if the abnormality can be seen on the ultrasound scan. Usually areas of microcalcification cannot be visualized. When stereotactic guidance is used, computer-assisted mammography equipment maps the precise location of the lesion or suspicious area. Then the needle can be inserted through the skin and into the lesion, which is accurately pinpointed on the x-ray film. Either cells or samples of tissue are removed through the needle and sent to the pathologist for evaluation. This technique, however, requires expensive specialized machinery and the skilled use of this equipment by a radiologist to position the needle and collect the samples.

As mentioned in the previous discussion on fine-needle and core-needle biopsy, false negative results may occur since the needle may miss malignant cells, the lesion itself (that is why multiple samples are suggested to improve accuracy), or may not yield sufficient tissue or cells for a diagnosis. This technique is becoming more widely used and is available in most major cities and large teaching hospitals.

Surgical Biopsy

A more specific and definitive procedure is known as a surgical biopsy. This method requires a small incision in the skin; the surgeon then directly identifies the lump and either removes the entire lump (excisional biopsy) or a representative sample (incisional biopsy). This *open* biopsy is the most reliable method for obtaining a specific diagnosis of a breast lump or of a suspicious area that is discovered on mammography. It can be done under local anesthesia; however, some surgeons and patients prefer general anesthesia.

When calcifications or suspicious abnormalities are seen on a mammogram but are not palpable, an open biopsy is often done after preoperative *needle localization* (also known as mammographic localization). Needle localization is usually performed under local anesthesia by a radiologist who uses the film image for guidance to locate the suspicious area and to insert a small needle into the breast pointing toward the lesion. Then a wire with a hook on the end is passed through the needle and positioned so that it rests where the calcification, density, or suspicious area has been seen. The wire is left in the breast when the patient goes to the operating room to guide the general surgeon when he performs the open biopsy. Sometimes, rather than inserting a needle, the mammographer places some dye on the suspicious area to help the surgeon localize the area. This is called dye localization. After the incision is made for the biopsy, the surgeon follows the wire and removes the area of tissue surrounding the wire or the area containing the dye. The tissue is then sent to the radiology department, where it is x-rayed to determine that the correct area has been removed. Once the accuracy is confirmed, the specimen is sent to pathology for evaluation. In some cases, to be sure that all of the calcifications or suspicious areas have been removed, the patient may need a follow-up mammogram 3 to 6 months later.

When a surgical biopsy is recommended, the surgeon is concerned that the suspicious area or lump may be malignant. Plans must be made before the biopsy to consider the options for treatment if the lump proves cancerous. It is possible to diagnose the lump and do a lumpectomy or mastectomy in one operation (a one-step procedure) or remove the lump and delay treatment to allow the patient time to consider her options (a two-step procedure).

If her doctor recommends a surgical biopsy to clarify the diagnosis of her lump, a woman should ask questions about this procedure in advance so that she fully understands what is involved. She should also ask her doctor if he recommends a one-step or two-step procedure.

One-step procedures are requested by some women who have already decided that if they have breast cancer they prefer a mastectomy or lumpectomy and axillary dissection. These women, having already made a decision for therapy, may select a one-step procedure to avoid the anxiety-filled interval between the diagnosis of cancer and the surgery to treat that disease. They should also consider immediate breast reconstruction as part of this one-stage procedure. One-step procedures are usually done under general anesthesia after the biopsy. The woman remains on the operating table while the tissue specimen is sent to the pathologist for a *frozen section analysis*. The pathologist slices the tissue, quick freezes it, and stains it to permit the specific characteristics of the tissue to be identified. Through this technique the pathologist is able to make an immediate determination as to whether the lump is benign or malignant. This technique has the advantage of speedy diagnosis, but it is expensive and not as reliable. Occasionally the pathologist cannot make a specific diagnosis based on these findings. If the report indicates that the lump is benign, the incision is closed and the woman is returned to the recovery room. If malignancy is diagnosed in the one-step approach, the doctor will proceed with the mastectomy or lumpectomy with lymph node removal during this one-step procedure.

The *two-step procedure* allows a woman with breast cancer time to investigate her options and make an informed decision. She may wish to obtain a second opinion and explore the different types of therapy available for treating her cancer and for possible breast reconstruction. In a two-step procedure the biopsy and treatment are done at separate times. The biopsy usually can be done on an outpatient basis under local anesthesia or even by fine-needle aspiration in the office. The pathologist then performs a "permanent section," which takes longer but the results are easier to read than a frozen section. This permanent section process takes approximately 24 hours. At this time the pathologist is able to make his final report.

A woman should also ask about the length and location of the biopsy scar. Many times these scars are short and can be hidden around the outer edge of the areola, placed in inconspicuous areas of the breast, or planned to facilitate a future incision for lumpectomy or mastectomy and reconstruction. Such scars often are practically invisible once they have faded, but the final appearance depends on how a person heals.

A woman who detects a breast lump either during self-inspection or after physician examination should constantly keep in mind the most significant fact that countless women overlook: not all lumps are cancerous. *Eighty percent of all breast lumps are benign.* If a calcification or suspicious area is detected on a mammogram, she should not panic. Again, most of these problems are *not* associated with cancer. She should not hesitate to have her doctor examine her and determine what needs to be done. Early detection and conclusive identification can ensure a better chance for cure if a cancer is present and can quickly alleviate a woman's needless fears if the breast condition is benign.

BREAST CANCER FACTS
AND TREATMENT OPTIONS

B reast cancer typically invades healthy women in their prime
years. Disbelief and shock are natural responses of women faced
with this shattering experience. Frequently they are as worried
about the loss of a breast as about the presence of cancer. To them
"cancer" is a word, a general medical entity that strikes other people,
whereas a breast is a personal and intimate body part and its loss directly threatens them in many ways.

Breast cancer is the most common cancer occurring in U.S. women today. The American Cancer Society reports that one out of
every eight women* in the United States will develop breast cancer in
her lifetime, and it is the second most common cause of death from
cancer for women in the United States between the ages of 15 and 75.
(Because of smoking, lung cancer, a much less treatable form of cancer,
has become the most common cause of cancer death.) This year alone
over 180,000 U.S. women will develop breast cancer. For many of
these women, attempts to treat their disease and save their lives will
also result in the loss of their breasts. Information about cancer, its
prognosis, and the options for therapy is necessary before they can
make informed and enlightened decisions about their future.

NATURAL HISTORY OF BREAST CANCER

Breast cancer most often develops in the drainage ducts of the mammary glands and is called ductal carcinoma. This is the most common
type of breast cancer and occurs in 70% to 80% of all cases. In most
other instances it develops in the mammary or milk glands (called

*Assuming a life span beyond 85 years. The one out of nine figure is based on a lifetime
of 85 years.

breast lobules) and is called lobular carcinoma. Lobular cancers involve both breasts more frequently than other types of breast cancer. A special type of ductal cancer, known as Paget's disease of the nipple, is characterized by a rash on the nipple and an underlying small ductal cancer.

A type of breast cancer previously considered uncommon, intra-ductal carcinoma or ductal carcinoma in situ, has been diagnosed with increasing frequency with more widespread use of mammography for screening. Recent reports indicate that 15% to 20% of all breast cancers being diagnosed now are intraductal; these cancers are usually very small, often less than 1 cm (or less than ½ inch), and may be too soft and small to be felt. They usually are found by mammography, thus underscoring the importance of this test for early detection. Intraductal cancers are not invasive when they are found at this early stage and thus the prognosis for cure and long-term survival is excellent.

Breast cancer does not appear overnight. It is not precipitated by injury or a bump to the breast. Instead, it is thought to be a gradual process in which certain cells lining the ducts (the epithelial cells) change from normal cells showing an abnormal amount of growth (hy-

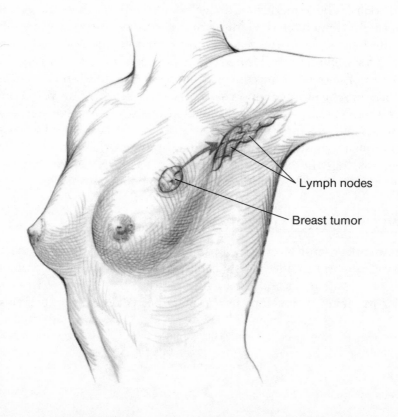

Lymph nodes

Breast tumor

perplasia) to cells that are noticeably different from normal breast cells (atypical) but are not cancerous by definition. These atypical cells eventually begin to regenerate themselves (autonomous growth), an uncontrolled growth that can extend through the cells lining the breast ducts. Thus breast cancer begins when a change in a breast duct cell gives that cell a growth advantage over other breast duct cells. The advantage may be a faster rate of cell division or a lower probability of cell death.

These cancerous cells initially grow in the breast ducts (intraductal cancer) before they spread. It is best to discover cancer in the intraductal phase (or in situ) since it has not yet spread outside the duct lining and potentially throughout the body. When the cells of the intraductal carcinoma break through the lining outside the breast ducts, the cancer is then described as *invasive*. Once the cells become invasive they can be picked up in the small lymph vessels of the breast and transported to the lymph nodes surrounding the breast, especially those present in the armpit or beneath the breastbone. The potential also exists for invasive tumor cells to be picked up by the bloodstream and carried to other parts of the body. When tumor cells migrate outside the breast to other parts of the body and continue to grow, the process is known as *metastasis*.

Since breast cancer develops from extremely small, microscopic cells, some experts believe that it is often 1 to 10 years before the cancer has grown large enough to be felt as a mass or tumor. (Breast imaging helps to identify breast cancers in their earliest stages.) These tiny cancer cells have the potential to become invasive and spread to other parts of the body before the tumor can be felt, accounting for the high mortality from breast cancer and the serious nature of this disease. This invasive potential is also the reason it is so important to identify the patient at high risk so that her breast cancer can be found in its earliest stages, before it has a chance to spread.

NEW DEVELOPMENTS IN BREAST CANCER RESEARCH

JOHN S. MEYER, M.D.

Research in breast cancer genetics offers hope for new treatments aimed at blocking the process that makes cells cancerous. Investigation of the mechanisms by which cells become cancerous has identified the existence of growth-regulating genes that are normally present in all cells. These genes appear to play an important role during the years of growth and development but are normally dormant or relatively inactive once a person reaches adulthood. If these genes become activated, tumors can result. Because these genes play a role in producing cancers, they are called *oncogenes* ("onco" comes from the Latin root meaning *tumor*). Several of these oncogenes have been identified as factors causing breast cancer. The activity of some of these genes can now be measured in the clinical laboratory. For instance, breast carcinomas with overactivity of the *erb B-2/neu* (also known as *HER-2/neu*) or epidermal growth factor receptor (EGFR) genes are known to have high growth rates.

Increased knowledge in this area has also led to a better understanding of how a tendency toward breast carcinoma can be passed from one generation to another in certain families. Families in which more than one woman develops breast cancer are not uncommon, but in most instances probably do not represent inherited tendencies toward breast cancer. The disease is sufficiently common to account for multiple instances in families by chance. For example, one would not think that a family with two or three members developing arthritis in later years necessarily had an inherited tendency toward that disease because arthritis also is common. If arthritis developed in childhood or the twenties or thirties in several members, one's suspicions of hereditary disease would be raised. The same applies to breast cancer. Whereas a mother and child or two sisters might develop breast cancer after age 50 by chance, if they developed the disease before age 50, inherited genetic transmission of a breast cancer tendency would be much more suspect. Recent studies of inherited breast cancer have begun to establish that the disease tends to occur at younger ages, even in the twenties, when breast cancer ordinarily is quite rare.

The current challenge is to recognize women who carry inherited breast cancer tendencies (breast cancer genes). Encouraging progress has been reported recently in localizing a breast cancer gene named *BRCA1* on a particular chromosome, the long arm of chromosome 17 (*17q*). Hereditary breast cancer researcher Mary Claire King has shown the approximate position of the *BRCA1* gene on the chromosome, and studies of nearby genes on the same chromosome now permit people who have the *BRCA1* gene to be identified with a good deal of certainty by a process called *linkage analysis*. This testing is not yet available outside a few research laboratories. If progress proceeds on schedule, researchers hope to localize and identify the *BRCA1* gene within a short time. Then a reliable test to determine its presence should become available for general application.

The *BRCA1* gene is thought to belong to a class of cancer-related genes known as suppressor oncogenes. These genes, rather than directly causing cancer, produce substances that prevent cells from becoming cancerous. When both copies of a suppressor oncogene are missing or defective, cancer may occur. If a person has, by heredity, only one rather than the normal two copies of a suppressor oncogene, damage to or loss of the remaining gene in a particular cell can cause cancer. A number of suppressor oncogenes are currently known, and many more will likely be discovered. Consequently, other genetic causes of a familial breast cancer tendency probably will be discovered in addition to the *BRCA1* gene. This new knowledge can be valuable in targeting surveillance of women for detection of breast cancer to the groups with highest risk.

More than 50 oncogenes have been identified, and at least several of them play roles in breast carcinoma, indicating that there is more than one pathway whereby a breast duct cell can become cancerous. Therefore it is not surprising that there are also different types of breast cancers and that these cancers vary in their growth rates and in their ability to invade and metastasize (grow in other parts of the body). Certain types have an excellent prognosis, even without chemotherapy or hormonal therapy, and others are more aggressive and have a poorer prognosis. Histologic assessment (microscopic analysis of cells and tissues) of breast cancer cell characteristics is helpful in determining whether the cancer might have spread. Growth rate measurements are also helpful in prognosis. Cancers with high rates of growth are more likely to produce recurrences within a few years of treatment than those with slow growth rates. (These new tests are discussed later in this chapter under prognostic factors and in Chapter 7.)

RISK FACTORS

Some women are at higher risk of developing breast cancer than others. Age, a family history, and previous breast cancer are three factors associated with high risk. (More information on risk factors is included in Chapter 15.)

Age

A woman's age strongly influences her risk of developing cancer. Breast cancer is unusual before age 30. The largest number of breast cancers are detected in postmenopausal women between the ages of 50 and 70 years. A third of the cases occur in patients under the age of 50 and 25% in women over 65.

During the past 15 years, however, the breast cancer rate among women age 25 to 44 has increased, as it has in women of all ages. Our surveys and interviews confirm these findings. Many of the women we have canvassed during the last 5 years were in their thirties and early forties with no previous family history of breast cancer. This increase in young women with breast cancer excludes the statistical increase resulting from better detection through mammography. Experts cite various reasons for the rise. Some point to late childbearing, fat in the diet, toxins in the environment, or some other unknown cause. Whatever the cause, it is crucially important that breast lumps in young women be thoroughly evaluated to rule out the possibility of cancer. This disease does occur in young women, and if a suspicious lump persists, it should be biopsied for definitive diagnosis.

Family History

Having first-degree maternal relatives (mothers and sisters) who developed breast cancer increases a woman's risk by two or three times, with a lifetime risk of about 20%. When these relatives have cancer in two breasts (bilateral) or cancer develops before menopause, the risk is even greater (six to eight times or up to a 50% chance of developing breast cancer).

Previous Breast Cancer

When breast cancer occurs in one breast, the cumulative risk of a cancer in the other breast is about 14% for women younger than 50 years old with a first cancer. It is less, approximately 4%, for women older than 50. If the first was lobular carcinoma or if lobular carcinoma in situ is present, the risk is somewhat greater. The risk of a second breast cancer is also greater if the first cancer is diagnosed before age 50.

Relative Risk Factors

Women in the following categories have a slightly increased risk of developing breast cancer:
• History of breast cancer in maternal or paternal grandmother, father's sister, or mother's sister.

- Excessive exposure to radiation, particularly before age 20. Currently used diagnostic x-ray examinations (even cumulatively) do not reach these levels.
- Early menarche (beginning of menstruation).
- Birth of first baby after age 30.
- Never having borne children (nulliparity).
- Late menopause.
- Obesity.
- History of some types of fibrocystic change.
- High fat diet. A high fat diet has long been suspected as a risk factor for breast cancer. Although the connection has not been proved, the National Academy of Sciences and many experts recommend reducing total fat intake from 40% of calories (average U.S. consumption) to 30% to try to reduce the incidence of cancers. Alcohol has also been implicated; many experts recommend limited or no consumption.
- Estrogen supplements or replacement. Because estrogen stimulates the growth of breast tumors, controversy exists over the advisability of taking estrogen in pill form, either as an oral contraceptive or for estrogen replacement therapy (ERT). Some studies suggest that women who started taking the pill in their teens may be at greater risk than women who started later or not at all. This may be because pills contained more estrogen when they were first marketed. Studies also indicate a slightly increased risk of breast cancer after 5 years of estrogen replacement therapy. This risk becomes even greater after 15 years. However, because estrogen replacement therapy also reduces the risk of heart disease and osteoporosis, women who take estrogen live longer than those who don't. Newer low-dose estrogen supplements are thought not to add to the risk.

BREAST CANCER STAGES

Once the diagnosis of breast cancer has been made, the stage of the breast cancer is determined to aid in making treatment decisions. Physicians classify the localization and spread of cancer in terms of stages. A basic element of staging is classifying the cancer as invasive, meaning it has the potential to metastasize (grow in other parts of the body), or noninvasive. Invasive breast cancer is graded from stage I to stage IV, and both treatment and prognosis are directly related to the stage of the cancer when detected. Unquestionably, it is best to discover the breast cancer before it becomes stage I (in its preinvasive form) and before it has spread beyond the breast ducts. Breast cancer in this preinvasive form is known as *in situ* cancer (in situ means in place), and if a woman's breast tissue is removed at this stage, invasive cancer can be prevented. If no treatment is undertaken, up to 40% of these women may develop a more serious invasive cancer.

Staging is determined by the size of the tumor, local extension to the chest wall or skin, the number and location of lymph nodes involved, and whether there are metastases in other areas of the body. To provide a more precise and standardized approach to staging, the TNM system has been developed: T stands for tumor size, N stands for nodal spread, and M stands for distant metastases. The TNM staging system ranks patients as stage group TIS (tumor in situ, or noninvasive cancer) or (as mentioned earlier) stages I through IV, with stage IV indicating known distant metastases. Although there are various staging methods, the system devised by the American Joint Commission on Cancer Staging is now considered the standard method (see Appendix E for this classification system).

Special Tests for Breast Cancer Staging
ROGER S. FOSTER, Jr., M.D.

Opinion differs as to what tests should be done before surgery to help stage breast cancer when the patient has no signs or symptoms that the cancer has spread beyond the breast and axilla. Experts agree that appropriate studies should be carried out for specific symptoms or any abnormal findings discovered on physical examination. There is also general agreement that patients with invasive cancer should have a chest x-ray film, a complete blood count, and a liver enzyme assay. Selected patients may need additional studies such as bone scans to rule out evidence of tumor spread to bone. At one time liver scans were commonly obtained, but experience has shown that they contribute very little to the care of most patients, and special scans of the liver usually are now done only if liver enzymes are abnormal or specific physical symptoms are present.

PROGNOSIS OF CANCER

The outcome, or prognosis, for a woman with breast cancer is related to the extent or spread of the disease at the time of diagnosis. Some experts believe that survival is directly related to the size of the tumor at the time of diagnosis. Those with small cancers (less than 1 cm, or less than ½ inch, in diameter) have a 10-year survival rate of over 95%.

Large tumors with direct extension to the chest wall or with skin involvement have a significantly worse prognosis.

The lymph nodes removed during an axillary dissection provide the best prediction of the course of the disease and outcome of the patient. The number of lymph nodes in each armpit (axillary) area varies. During an axillary dissection usually more than half of the existing nodes are removed by the surgeon and examined by the pathologist to determine if the breast cancer has spread to this area. Patients with no involved or cancerous lymph nodes in their axilla (stage I) have a 65% to 75% likelihood of survival for 10 years. If one to three nodes are found to be cancer bearing (stage II), a 40% to 60% chance exists for 10-year survival. If more than four nodes are involved, there is less than a 25% possibility of survival for the next 10-year period. If any axillary nodes are involved, chemotherapy usually is recommended in an attempt to improve the chances of survival.

After pathologic identification of the tumor type, other microscopic studies of the cells can be conducted to determine whether they are likely to be aggressive. Additional information can be obtained by examining the tumor to determine histologic type. For instance, some cancers are of special histologic types, for example, tubular carcinomas and papillary carcinomas, and have a more favorable prognosis. Cell differentiation is also an indicator. Cancer cells that closely resemble normal mature breast cells are considered well differentiated and are associated with a better prognosis than poorly differentiated cancer cells that are less normal, or atypical, in appearance and have a less favorable prognosis because they are thought to be more aggressive. The prognosis is also less promising when tumor necrosis (areas of dead cells) is identified or when there is evidence of tumor invasion into the blood vessels or lymphatic vessels.

Measurement of the estrogen and progesterone hormone receptors on the tumor cells is also helpful in predicting prognosis and response to hormonal therapy. If laboratory evaluation shows the mass to be cancerous, hormone receptor tests will be run to determine if proteins that are called receptors are present. Estrogen and progesterone are female hormones that can affect breast cancer cell growth. When breast cancer cells have higher levels of receptors for these hormones (estrogen receptor positive, or ER+), that often indicates the tumor is slower growing and the prognosis is slightly better. It also suggests that this patient's tumor will probably respond favorably to hormonal manipulation. Hormone receptor tests help your doctors determine whether cancer cells might be destroyed or slowed by administering anti-estrogen or other anti-hormones or if chemotherapy will be more effective.

A major thrust of breast cancer research seeks new markers that will improve the ability to predict a patient's prognosis and more important the outcome after specific therapy. A good deal of this research is focusing on growth rate measurements. Scientists have identified growth factors that are important in the transformation of hyperplastic cells to those with atypical features to frank cancer cells. With such unlikely names as S-phase, ploidy, erb B-2/neu oncogene, epidermal growth factor receptor, and cathepsin-D, these markers can tell physicians how the malignant cells are growing and how likely the cancer is to spread or recur. In other words, measurement of the genetic material (DNA) in tumor cells enables the physician to determine the growth rate of cells (S-phase fraction) and how they behave based on whether or not the tumor cells contain abnormal quantities of DNA (ploidy). Other potential markers are related to the genes on cells that influence cell behavior (the oncogenes mentioned earlier). Current studies of families with multiple cases of bilateral breast cancer are focusing on analyzing their DNA for evidence of cancer-causing genes. In particular, scientists are studying the erb B-2/neu oncogene, a breast cancer gene that may be involved in 40% of all hereditary breast cancer. Especially promising are the recent breakthroughs in localizing a breast cancer gene dubbed BRCA1 on chromosome 17 (17q). Now women with a familial history of breast cancer can be tested with success with linkage analysis to identify the presence of the BRCA1 gene.

Today a panel of tests in addition to the microscopic description of the tumor and lymph nodes is compiled to estimate a woman's risk of future cancer and to identify those individuals who might benefit from preventive treatment with chemotherapeutic or anti-estrogen drugs. The role of these and other new tests is not yet well established, but promising advances are being made in understanding the nature of changes in cells that make them cancerous.

Breast cancer remains a threat because of unpredictable growth and its potential to invade and spread to other parts of the body before the tumor can be detected. Death from breast cancer and virtually all symptoms are due to spread to other organs of the body such as the liver, lungs, bone, or brain. Research continues to seek the answer to why cancers invade and metastasize. Early detection is critical today, but an understanding of the basic nature of cancer will allow innovative treatments to prevent invasion or spread.

• • •

Even though cancer statistics can be quite frightening and information on oncogenes, DNA, and cell growth factors intimidating, it is important to remember that progress is being made. Primary treatment does influence survival rates. The length and quality of life also are influenced by adjunctive treatment such as chemotherapy and hormonal therapy. The use of chemotherapy and/or hormonal therapy for the patient with involved axillary nodes represents a significant advance in the care of cancer patients and is one method for trying to improve the prospects of those women at high risk by preventing further spread or recurrence of their breast cancer. Selected women also benefit from the adjunctive use of radiation to prevent recurrence in the chest wall.

PRIMARY THERAPY

Mastectomy

Today a mastectomy is still the most frequently applied treatment for breast cancer. The goal of this operation is to surgically remove a woman's breast while the tumor is still confined to the breast area and before it has spread to other parts of her body. A mastectomy is advocated by many surgeons who believe that breast cancer is a multifocal disease in which microscopic cancers may coexist in other areas of a woman's breast along with her already identified cancerous tumor. They recommend total breast removal as necessary to protect against these minute cancer cells that may remain in a woman's breast if only the invasive tumor is removed.

Several different types of surgical treatment are used for removing a woman's breast. With a radical mastectomy, the breast, underlying chest wall muscles (pectoralis major and minor muscles), and lymph glands of the armpit (axillary lymph nodes) are removed. The Halsted radical mastectomy, which was introduced 100 years ago, was the first effective operation for local control of breast cancer. Although this procedure effectively removed the breast cancer, it left the woman with a large deformity. A radical mastectomy created a hollowed-out area on the chest just below the collarbone, and the ribs were prominent because they were covered by a very thin layer of skin.

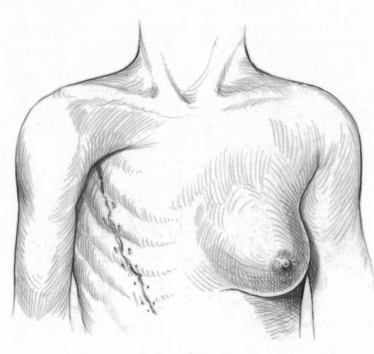

Radical mastectomy

The mutilating aspects of radical mastectomy and the early diag-nosis of smaller breast cancers led to the development of the modified radical mastectomy. Today the radical mastectomy is rarely performed; the modified radical mastectomy (also called total mastectomy with axillary dissection) is the method for total breast removal chosen by most surgeons for operable breast cancer. It has been shown that this operation is as effective as radical mastectomy for local control of the breast tumor.

With this procedure, the surgeon removes the breast, nipple-areola, and lymph nodes in the axilla. The lymph nodes provide fur-ther information about the spread or extent of the cancer so that the course of the tumor can be predicted. If tumor spread is evident, then appropriate adjunctive treatments such as chemotherapy, hormonal therapy, or radiation therapy can be chosen. The largest chest wall mus-cle, the pectoralis major, remains intact. This muscle is located in the front of the chest and helps to support the breasts; preservation of this muscle greatly reduces the deformity resulting from the mastectomy.

After a modified radical mastectomy, the chest wall will not have a hollowed-out appearance, and the ribs will still be covered by muscle

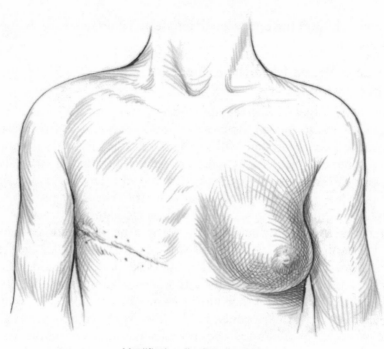

Modified radical mastectomy

and therefore will not seem overly prominent. The loss of the breast and nipple will result in a flatness to the chest. A scar will extend horizontally or diagonally across the chest. In addition, the area of the mastectomy is usually numb because the nerves that supply sensation to the chest and breast were threaded through the breast tissue, which is now gone. The inside of the upper arm can also be numb because the nerves to this area that go through the axillary region may have to be removed with the axillary dissection. After the mastectomy, the armpit is usually deeper and harder to shave, and many women notice less perspiration on that side than on the other normal side. Because the operation extends beneath the upper arm into the axilla, the woman may experience temporary pain after the operation when she moves her arm. The general surgeon usually will recommend postoperative exercises to ensure the return of full use and function of the arm.

Some women also report experiencing a phenomenon called *phantom pain* in the area of the missing breast. They may feel throbbing, tingling, numbness, or stabbing pains. These sensations are probably caused by the nerve endings that were cut during surgery and regrow incompletely after the operation. Exercise and pain medication might alleviate this discomfort.

Immediate Breast Reconstruction
WILLIAM C. WOOD, M.D.

Today many surgeons who recommend a mastectomy for women with breast cancer also inform them of the option of breast reconstruction to rebuild their breasts and fill in the defects left from their cancer surgery. Immediate breast reconstruction has become an appealing option for women undergoing mastectomy, and they are choosing it with increasing frequency because it combines the most proven and accepted treatment for breast cancer with immediate breast restoration. With this approach, the general surgeon and the plastic surgeon must closely coordinate their efforts and work as a team since the mastectomy and the breast reconstruction are done during one operation, which means the patient will have to undergo anesthesia only once. Since there is only one procedure, a woman will not have to wear a breast prosthesis or experience breast loss. Most women prefer this more extensive procedure to two shorter surgeries. Depending on the reconstructive procedure chosen, the patient may need a blood transfusion. Therefore, as a precaution, most patients undergoing immediate breast reconstruction donate their own blood in advance (autologous donation) to avoid the risk involved in receiving another's blood.

Immediate breast reconstruction often permits less skin removal with shorter scars. By removing the breast and replacing the volume immediately the skin that is not excised as a part of the cancer operation can then be used for the reconstruction. If the mastectomy is performed separately, more breast skin must be removed initially to create a smooth skin surface over the chest wall and to avoid leaving redundant folds of breast skin that would thicken and toughen over time. Later, when breast reconstruction is performed, the missing breast skin must be replaced either by transferring new skin from another part of the body on a muscle-skin (musculocutaneous) flap or by stretching the skin at the mastectomy site (tissue expansion) to make it expand to the desired size.

In the past some have expressed concern that breast reconstruction, particularly when done immediately, would make it difficult to examine the chest wall for recurrent disease. This has not proved to be the case. In most instances there is no contraindication to immediate reconstruction for patients with stage I or II breast cancer. However, women with stage III breast cancer (locally advanced) must have a combination of surgery, chemotherapy, and chest wall radiation therapy; therefore, for these patients, it may be prudent to complete all therapy before pursuing breast reconstruction. Treatment should be the first priority, and any complication of reconstruction that would delay therapy should be avoided. For the majority of women facing mastectomy, however, immediate reconstruction is a welcome option that permits them to receive optimal treatment of their breast cancer without suffering the trauma of breast loss.

Breast-Conserving Surgery and Irradiation
JOHN M. BEDWINEK, M.D.

An alternative to mastectomy that is in widespread use today is a procedure called breast-conserving surgery and irradiation. As its name implies, the chief advantage of this treatment approach in comparison with mastectomy is that the woman's own natural breast is preserved. The surgeon removes only the cancerous lump along with a small margin of normal breast tissue. This procedure is referred to as a *lumpectomy*. It is also called *tumorectomy* or *tylectomy*.

In addition to removing the lump, the surgeon also removes some of the lymph nodes under the arm in a procedure called an *axillary*

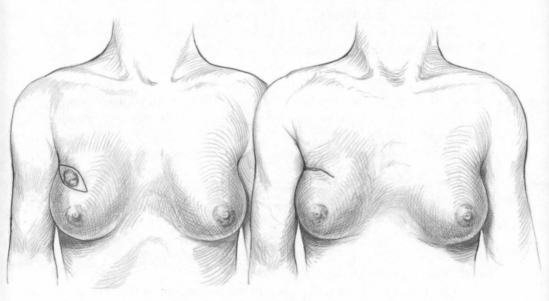

Lumpectomy

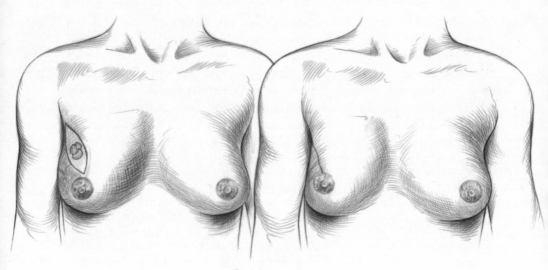

Quadrantectomy

dissection to determine if the cancer has spread to the axillary lymph nodes and to get information for staging. Knowing whether these nodes contain cancer helps the medical oncologist decide whether to recommend systemic therapy (chemotherapy and/or hormone therapy) and, if so, what kind of systemic therapy.

After the lumpectomy and axillary node dissection, the entire breast is treated with radiation to kill any residual cancer cells. The radiation therapy consists of one treatment, every day, 5 days a week, for a total of 25 to 28 treatments (5 to 6 weeks of therapy). A total radiation dose of approximately 5000 rad is delivered to the entire breast (rad refers to a unit of radiation dose; the term "rad" is being replaced today with a newer term, "centiGray," abbreviated cGy). After irradiation of the entire breast is completed, an additional radiation dose of approximately 1000 to 2000 cGy is applied only to the site from which the tumor was removed. This additional dose to the tumor site is referred to as the "boost" and is given to ensure that all residual cancer in that area is eradicated. The boost will either be administered with electron beams of appropriate energy externally or with hollow needles containing implants of radioactive material, which are internally placed in the breast.

The radiation treatment used in breast conservation does not cause hair loss, nausea, or any significant loss of energy. It will, however, cause a temporary reddening of the breast skin, similar to a mild sunburn. This reddening usually occurs 3 to 4 weeks after radiation therapy is started and completely disappears 2 weeks after its completion. The goal of this treatment is for the irradiated breast to appear and feel normal, just like the opposite breast, provided there is proper patient selection and both the radiation therapy and surgery have been properly carried out. Slight thickening of the skin of the breast can occasionally occur because of increased fluid in the skin (edema). This results from the axillary node dissection, which cuts the small lymph vessels through which breast fluid normally escapes. In 18 to 24 months these vessels regenerate, and the skin thickening disappears.

Breast-conserving surgery and irradiation were considered controversial 10 years ago, but there is no longer doubt regarding the safety of this treatment approach. Large randomized studies have proved that the cure rate achieved with breast-conserving surgery and irradiation is identical to that obtained with mastectomy. In 1990 the National Institutes of Health (NIH) issued a consensus statement on breast-conserving surgery and irradiation stating that "breast conservation treatment is an appropriate method of primary therapy for the majority of women with Stage I and II breast cancer" and that it "provides survival equivalent to total mastectomy and axillary dissection while preserving the breast." Women for whom this breast-sparing approach is appropriate (that includes most women with breast cancer) will have the same chance of cure with this method of treatment as they would with mastectomy.

When Breast-Conserving Surgery Is Not the Right Choice

Breast-conserving surgery and irradiation, however, *is not always appropriate*. For some, it may produce a poor cosmetic result. For others, it may result in a higher than normal risk of tumor recurrence in the breast. For still others, those few women who do not feel strongly about breast loss, conservation surgery may be unnecessary since they would be just as satisfied with mastectomy, which is a quicker and easier method of treatment. Because of personal logistics some women choose not to commute to the nearest radiation therapy facility for 6 weeks of daily treatment and opt for mastectomy. Finally, there are some women for whom breast conservation would be psychologically inappropriate. The women who fall into one or more of the above categories comprise only a small minority of all women with breast cancer; nonetheless, it is very important that these women know who

they are and even more important that they know why breast conservation is inappropriate for them. Armed with this knowledge, they
can then consider whether mastectomy, with or without reconstruction,
is preferable to breast-conserving surgery and irradiation. The responsibility of recognizing, advising, and educating these women falls to
the radiation oncologist and surgeon. It is therefore important that all
women considering breast conservation see both of these specialists
before making a decision. If either of them thinks that mastectomy
with reconstruction should be considered, then the plastic surgeon
joins the team.

The major factors that determine whether a woman is or is not a
good candidate for breast-conserving surgery and irradiation are described
below.

Tumor size. The tumor should be smaller than 5 cm (2 inches).
Also, it should be small enough compared with the size of the breast so
that complete excision (removal) will not leave a surgical defect that
will mar the aesthetic result. If the surgeon thinks that to remove the
entire tumor he will have to remove such a large segment of the breast
that a significant deformity will result, then the cosmetic outcome
with breast conservation may be poor. In this situation, mastectomy
and subsequent reconstruction may produce a better cosmetic result.
The woman with a tumor that is large relative to the size of the breast
should have a team consisting of a surgeon, radiation oncologist, and
plastic surgeon to advise her as to whether mastectomy with reconstruction or breast-conserving surgery with irradiation would yield the
better cosmetic result. In some instances a combined approach may be
recommended. Recent advances in reconstructive surgery now allow
larger tumors to be excised and immediate partial breast reconstruction done.

Breast size. If the breast is so small that complete removal of even
a small tumor would leave a significant deformity, then the woman
should be advised that breast conservation may produce a poor cosmetic result. In this case she might want to consider the option of
mastectomy with reconstruction.

The opposite extreme, a very large breast, is also a factor in the
cosmetic outcome. An extremely large, pendulous breast will tend to
exhibit more shrinkage following irradiation than a small or moderate-
sized breast, and some asymmetry between the treated and the untreated
breast may result. This degree of asymmetry is usually mild and is
certainly less than the asymmetry produced by mastectomy. Special

techniques can be used to minimize the shrinkage that can occur with radiation therapy of an extremely large breast. Thus women with large, pendulous breasts should not be discouraged from having breast-conserving surgery and irradiation, but they should be aware of possible limitations. For some patients, the lumpectomy can be incorporated into a reduction mammaplasty, thus providing local treatment of the cancer combined with breast reduction.

Two cancers in the same breast. Although it is a rare occurrence, occasionally a woman will have two separate cancers in one breast. The usual scenario is that a woman or her doctor feels a breast lump. A mammogram then discloses an undetected abnormality in addition to the lump that was felt. Biopsy shows that both the lump and the mammographically detected abnormality are malignant, two separate cancers. When there are two cancers within the same breast, the risk of recurrence, even if both cancers can be removed, is extremely high, approximately 40%. Most radiation oncologists feel that this risk is too high for breast-conserving surgery and irradiation to be a reasonable option; therefore women who have two cancers within the same breast should be advised to have mastectomy.

Ensuring that there are not two cancers in the same breast is one very important reason for obtaining a mammogram before deciding whether to have breast-conserving surgery or mastectomy. In fact, the mammogram should be obtained even before the biopsy since the biopsy can produce an artificial density on the mammogram that can obscure subtle densities or microcalcifications that might indicate a second cancer.

Tumor location. Two tumor locations can cause problems following breast-conserving surgery and irradiation. The first is when a tumor lies against the chest wall in an area of the breast where there is more than 5 cm (roughly 2 inches) of overlying breast tissue. In this situation, delivering an adequate boost dose to the deeply located tumor site means that the large volume of overlying breast tissue will receive a high dose. This high dose to a large volume can produce thickening (referred to as fibrosis), which can detract from the cosmetic result.

The second problematic location is just under the armpit. If a tumor lies so high in the breast that it is almost in the armpit, then it may be impossible for the surgeon to remove the tumor through an incision that is separate from the incision used for the axillary node dissection. When the axillary node dissection and the tumor removal are not done through two separate incisions, the surgically dissected axillary area receives the same high radiation dose (5000 cGy plus 1000 to 2000 cGy from the boost) that is delivered to the tumor area. This high radiation dose causes tissue thickening, or fibrosis, to form in the armpit area. The cumulative effect of the fibrosis caused by the high radiation dose and the fibrosis already produced by the node dissection can result in swelling of the breast, swelling of the arm, and/or lateral deviation of the breast.

For the woman with a tumor in one of the two locations described above, the ultimate cosmetic outcome with breast conservation may be significantly less than optimum. It is therefore important that she be thoroughly counseled regarding the potential aesthetic problems that may apply to her particular situation so that she understands the severity of these problems. For the tumor locations noted above, mastectomy and reconstruction may provide a better aesthetic outcome than breast-conserving surgery and irradiation. The process to determine which is the better option starts with an evaluation by the radiation oncologist and the surgeon. If either the radiation oncologist or surgeon thinks that the cosmetic outcome may be poor, then the plastic surgeon's input is needed. As previously noted in the section describing a tumor that is too large to be cosmetically excised, a team approach involving the radiation oncologist, surgeon, and plastic surgeon is the best method to help the woman decide which would be the better option for her.

Type of cancer

Intraductal carcinoma. If cancer is detected before it penetrates the wall of the duct, it is said to be noninvasive or intraductal. These noninvasive (or intraductal) cancers seldom spread to lymph nodes or to other parts of the body, and the cure rate with mastectomy is therefore close to 100%. If breast-conserving surgery and irradiation can be used successfully and safely for invasive cancer, why can't it also be used for noninvasive cancer? The answer is that it can be if the intraductal cancer is limited to one area of the breast. Unfortunately, this is not always the case. Some of them grow for great distances throughout ducts of the breast, somewhat like squeezing toothpaste through the tube. Thus these extensive intraductal cancers, even though they are noninvasive, may consist of a large amount of cancer, sometimes spreading throughout a quarter or even half of the breast tissue. When the intraductal cancer is extensive, many cancer cells can be left behind in the breast following tumor excision. Sometimes the amount of residual (remaining) cancer in the breast is too great to be eradicated by radiation. For this reason, when breast-conserving surgery and irradiation are used to treat extensive intraductal cancer, the risk of cancer recurring in the breast can be as high as 25% to 30%. This risk of recurrence is much higher than the recurrence risk when conservation surgery is used for invasive cancer (approximately 5%). An even greater cause for concern is that approximately 50% of the recurrences following conservation treatment of intraductal cancer will be invasive. The recurrence, if invasive, has the potential to spread to lymph nodes or other parts of the body, whereas the original intraductal cancer did not have this potential. It is therefore hard to justify breast-conserving surgery and irradiation for an extensive intraductal cancer when the cure rate with mastectomy is close to 100%.

Only the limited form of intraductal cancer should be treated with breast conservation. If there is any evidence that the intraductal cancer is extensive, then mastectomy should be recommended. Distinguishing between the limited and extensive forms of intraductal cancer is ultimately the responsibility of the radiation oncologist. It is sometimes a difficult distinction to make, and it always requires special help and input from the radiologist, surgeon, and pathologist.

Extensive intraductal component. Occasionally an invasive breast cancer will be accompanied by a large amount of noninvasive cancer. This noninvasive portion, if it comprises more than 25% of the entire cancer and if it extends out beyond the main cancer, is said to be an extensive intraductal component (EIC). An invasive cancer with EIC is probably nothing more than the previously described extensive intraductal cancer that has finally invaded through the walls of the ducts. Investigators at Harvard University have shown that invasive cancer with EIC has a higher rate of recurrence than invasive cancer without EIC. It would appear, however, that this higher rate of relapse with EIC may not occur if all of the cancer is in the middle of the removed piece of breast tissue and is well away from the edge or margin of the tissue.

By marking the margin of the removed breast tissue with India ink the pathologist can determine whether or not there is any cancer near or at the margin. When there is cancer near or at the margin, it is said that the margin is positive. For invasive cancer without EIC, whether the margin is negative or positive may not be all that important, but it is very important for a cancer with EIC. With EIC, if the margin is positive, additional tissue must be removed until the margin becomes negative. Occasionally removing enough additional tissue to achieve a negative margin will create a significant breast deformity, particularly in a small breast. If achieving a negative margin would produce such a deformity, then mastectomy with reconstruction should be discussed as a possible option, again using the team approach.

Diffuse calcifications. Women with diffuse calcifications on their mammograms are also better served with a mastectomy than with breast-conserving surgery with irradiation; these calcifications may indicate the presence of extensive intraductal carcinoma.

Patient attitude. The woman's personal feeling about breast loss constitutes one of the most important factors in deciding whether mastectomy or breast conservation is the better option. Some women do not have a strong desire for breast preservation but seek alternatives to mastectomy for other reasons. Some do so because of external pressure from a friend, daughter, or spouse. Others ask about breast conservation only because they want to explore and understand all possibilities before making a decision. Still others want breast conservation because of misconceptions such as the notion that it will eliminate the need for major surgery or that it is a newer and therefore better form of treatment. None of these reasons is the appropriate motivation for having breast conservation and irradiation. The only acceptable motivation is the woman's strong desire to preserve her own natural breast. Otherwise mastectomy and immediate breast reconstruction may be a better choice since it is simpler and quicker than breast conservation and irradiation. It is therefore important for the radiation oncologist to help the woman discern her true motive for wanting breast conservation.

Some women worry about the late effects of radiation. Careful discussion and understanding of the very minimal nature of these effects can usually allay such concerns. Although there is a theoretical risk that radiation may produce cancer in either the treated breast or in the opposite breast, long-term studies of women receiving radiation to the breast (or chest wall) after mastectomy show no increase in cancer of the opposite breast. Nevertheless the fear of radiation-induced cancer looms large for an occasional patient. For such patients, the ease of mastectomy and reconstruction is a great comfort. Other women view the affected breast as a cancer-forming organ and would have continued anxiety unless they were rid of it. Obviously, for psychological reasons, mastectomy is the better option for these women.

...uccessful breast-conserving surgery and irra-
...ilability of a surgeon and radiation oncolo-
...l in performing this procedure. Both the
...tic aspects of breast-conserving surgery and
...ise; serious mistakes can be made if the
...ologist do not know how to avoid some of
...oman may be better off to have a mastec-
...t-conserving surgery and irradiation by a
...ologist who have only limited experience
...t reconstruction after conservative surgery
...but somewhat more difficult than with
...h immediate breast reconstruction.

A Woman's Options

Today women with breast cancer have several viable options to
choose from for primary treatment of their disease. Their preferences
may be genuinely respected without compromising their chance for
survival. Mastectomies followed by breast reconstruction and breast-
conserving surgery with irradiation are both positive therapeutic responses to women's requests for cancer treatment without permanent
breast loss.

ADJUVANT THERAPY
Adjuvant Chemotherapy
GARY A. RATKIN, M.D.

Chemotherapy is the use of drugs to kill or damage cancer cells.
Healthy tissues can be temporarily affected, thereby causing side
effects, but usually recover and normal function returns. Although
chemotherapy was first employed in patients with widespread metastatic cancer, a major advance in breast cancer management has been
the use of chemotherapy to prevent the recurrence or spread of breast
cancer. Adjuvant chemotherapy uses drugs to destroy cancer cells
when they are present in a microscopic form.

Much attention has been paid to defining patients who are at high
risk for spread or recurrence of breast cancer after surgery. An advanced

stage (II or above) or microscopic features of the cancer cells on the biopsy indicate a greater chance of cancer recurrence or spread at some future time. Specialized tests to measure the cancer growth rate can also assist in detecting those with an increased chance of recurrence. Chemotherapy or hormonal therapy is indicated for patients who are found to have this higher risk of metastasis.

Most chemotherapy is administered by intravenous injection. Few agents are available in pill form. Combinations of chemotherapeutic drugs have become standard for adjuvant therapy. These drugs are administered in brief courses (6 months or less is typical) every 3 to 4 weeks, depending on the specific program. Some of the most frequently used medications include methotrexate, 5-fluorouracil, cyclophosphamide, vincristine, doxorubicin, and prednisone. Three or more of these medications may be used in combination. Some of the chemotherapeutic drugs used in breast cancer are as follows:

Adjuvant Therapy	Hormonal Therapy
Cyclophosphamide (Cytoxan)	Tamoxifen (Nolvadex)
Methotrexate (often with calcium leucovorin)	Megestrol acetate (Megace)
	Estrogen (dietheylstilbestrol)
5-Fluorouracil (5-FU)	Androgen (Halotestin)
Vincristine (Oncovin)	Aminogluthemide (Cytadren)
Prednisone	Ketoconazole (Nizoral)
Doxorubicin (Adriamycin)	Luteinizing hormone–releasing
L-Phenylalanine mustard (L-PAM)	hormone (LH-RH) agonist
Vinblastine (Velban)	
Thiotepa	
Mitoxantrone (Novantrone)	
Mitomycin-C (Mutamycin)	

Combination Chemotherapy	
CAF (also called FAC)	Cytoxan, Adriamycin, 5-FU
VATH	Velban, Adriamycin, Thiotepa, Halotestin
Cooper regimen	Cytoxan, Oncovin, methotrexate, 5-FU, prednisone
CMF	Cytoxan, methotrexate, 5-FU

It is important to start adjunctive chemotherapy as soon as possible after the patient has healed from surgery (usually within 4 to 6 weeks). More intensive treatment programs for shorter periods of time are under study. In general, oncologists try to administer as much chemotherapy as safely possible to get the best results with adjunctive regimens.

COMMON SIDE EFFECTS OF CHEMOTHERAPY DRUGS

Drug	Hematologic	Nausea	Oral	Diarrhea	Cardiac	Neurologic	Skin	Hair Loss
Cyclophosphamine	++	++	+		+		+	+
Methotrexate	++	+	++	+		+	++	+
5-Fluorouracil	+	+	++	++		+	++	+
Doxorubicin	++	++	++	+	++		++	+++
Vincristine	+	+				++		+
Vinblastine	++	+	+			++		+
Thiotepa	++	++					+	+
Mitomycin-C	++	++	+				+	+
Novantrone	++	++	+		+		+	++

Patients with large tumors and many positive nodes are being considered for intensive treatments using lethal doses of chemotherapy and also radiation therapy. Those receiving the very aggressive forms of therapy are supported with bone marrow transplantation or a technique called *peripheral stem cell support* to protect them from the life-threatening side effects of treatment. (See p. 73 for more detailed information on this topic.)

Although chemotherapy is used to try to improve a woman's prognosis, the drugs can cause temporary side effects. Four of the most common are nausea, vomiting, hair loss, and low blood counts. Other symptoms due to chemotherapy might include interruption of the menstrual cycle, fatigue, mouth sores, tingling in the fingers and toes, and rarely diarrhea.

Much progress has been made in controlling the more serious or bothersome of these side effects. It is common to administer anti-nausea medications at the same time as chemotherapy to prevent this side effect. Even hair loss, which is a widely publicized side effect of chemotherapy, does not occur with every drug and can be avoided in many patients who receive a drug such as doxorubicin (Adriamycin). Careful attention must be paid to blood counts to avoid excessively lowering the white blood count or platelet count. Patients with a low white blood count (leukopenia) are at increased risk of bacterial and fungous infection. Those with a low platelet count (thrombocytopenia) can bleed or bruise easily. Therefore blood counts are monitored before and frequently between courses of chemotherapy to ensure the safety of a regimen. Patients are examined regularly to be certain that uncommon side effects such as bladder irritation or heart scarring are not occurring. Doxorubicin can cause heart scarring if used in cumulative doses that go beyond a "safe" limit.

Uncommon toxicities of chemotherapeutic drugs include:

Drug	Uncommon Complications
Cyclophosphamide	Bladder
Doxorubicin, cyclophosphamide, mitomycin-C, methotrexate	Pulmonary
Mitomycin-C	Renal
Mitomycin-C, doxorubicin	Skin infiltrates
Methotrexate, mitomycin-C	Liver

The specific symptoms of each chemotherapy program should be explained to the patient before treatment so she is aware of the risks and practical steps to take to help herself.

Since many of the medications used can irritate the veins, great care must be exercised in starting an intravenous infusion for chemotherapy administration. A semipermanent venous access device can be implanted under the skin and attached to a catheter placed directly in a large vein. This infusion device, or port, can facilitate chemotherapy administration in selected patients and can often also be used for blood drawing, transfusion, or even the administration of pain medications.

Adjuvant Hormonal Therapy

Another drug that may improve the prognosis of breast cancer is an anti-estrogen, tamoxifen (Nolvadex). Tamoxifen is now recommended in both postmenopausal and premenopausal patients who are at risk of recurrence of breast cancer after surgery and who have positive estrogen receptors measured in the cancer tissue.

Estrogen and progesterone receptors should be measured in every patient with a new diagnosis of breast cancer. The test may help in predicting the risk of recurrence, but more important, it allows the selection of patients who might benefit from hormonal therapy. Approximately 50% of patients with positive estrogen receptors will respond to some hormonal treatment, especially tamoxifen, whereas less than 10% with negative receptors react favorably. The estrogen receptor assay along with other pathologic tests allows physicians to prescribe tamoxifen as a preventive measure in those patients who might benefit. Current recommendations are for the long-term administration of tamoxifen (at least 5 years and possibly indefinitely).

Tamoxifen usually has few side effects. Hot flashes similar to those many women experience during menopause are the most common reaction. Patients who are on long-term tamoxifen (over 2 years) should be screened for uterine cancer, a rare complication. Other unusual risks include thrombophlebitis (blood clots), vaginal bleeding or discharge, eye problems, low blood count, nausea, weight gain, skin rash, and an elevated blood calcium level. Some patients may have an increase in bone pain or discomfort in an area of a tumor mass after the start of tamoxifen therapy, which usually abates with time. Contrary to many women's concerns, the use of an anti-estrogen actually strengthens the bones in postmenopausal women and can lower serum cholesterol and other lipids. The risk of breast cancer metastasis may be far greater than the rare toxicities listed here. In addition, there is evidence that there is a lower incidence of cancer of the opposite breast in patients who are taking tamoxifen. New clinical trials are being designed to evaluate the usefulness of tamoxifen in preventing breast cancer in the high-risk individual. (See p. 76 of this chapter for more information on these trials.)

Other hormonal treatments such as progesterone derivatives or oophorectomy (surgery to remove the ovaries) have been used as preventive measures after breast cancer surgery. There are now data to suggest that oophorectomy increases survival. Some experts feel that estrogen replacement drugs should be avoided after breast cancer is detected and treated since they might accelerate cancer growth. (See p. 47 for more information on estrogen replacement therapy.)

Adjuvant Irradiation
JOHN M. BEDWINEK, M.D.

In the past, women who had mastectomies and were found to have positive axillary lymph nodes were given radiation therapy after surgery. The radiation was directed to the chest wall and to the lymph nodes above the collarbone and beneath the breastbone. It was thought that this postoperative radiation therapy would improve survival by killing any cancer cells not removed by the mastectomy. Radiation does, indeed, drastically reduce the likelihood of a local recurrence, that is, the reappearance of cancer on the chest wall or in the nearby lymph nodes. This prevention of a local recurrence does *not* seem to improve the chances of cure, however, since most patients who have a local recurrence of cancer after a mastectomy also will develop distant metastases that radiation therapy does not prevent. Many studies have been conducted to test whether postoperative radiation will improve survival, and none of them has conclusively proved that it will.

Since it is no longer believed that combining radiation therapy with mastectomy will improve the chances of cure, it is given only to those women whose chance of a local recurrence is high. These women have very large breast tumors (5 cm, or 2 inches, or more), enlarged lymph nodes under the arm, or tumors that have invaded into the skin of the breast or into the pectoralis muscle underlying the breast. For these patients, keeping the risk of local recurrence minimal by adding radiation therapy is of definite benefit because a local recurrence is difficult to treat successfully and can cause unpleasant symptoms such as pain or bleeding. Fortunately, the majority of patients who have a mastectomy today do not have a high risk of local recurrence, and postoperative radiation therapy is not usually needed.

FOLLOW-UP SURVEILLANCE AFTER PRIMARY TREATMENT AND RECONSTRUCTION
WILLIAM C. WOOD, M.D.

After completion of primary treatment of breast cancer, patients are routinely placed under follow-up surveillance to detect and treat any recurrence of the first cancer or to discover any new breast cancer in the opposite breast at the earliest possible stage. As mentioned previously, women who develop breast cancer have an increased risk of cancer in the other breast (see p. 46). For women over 50, this risk is about 4% for their remaining years; for those under 50, it is about 14%. Although the risk is not as great as many women imagine, careful evaluation is mandatory. It is essential that a cancer in the opposite breast be detected as early as possible to increase the likelihood of cure, as is the case with a primary tumor.

Detecting a new breast tumor in the opposite breast is accomplished by a familiar triad: monthly breast self-examination of the opposite breast, clinical examination by a physician or nurse practitioner every 6 to 12 months, and annual mammography. This combination provides the greatest assurance of early diagnosis. More frequent examinations have not been shown to be beneficial.

Surveillance for evidence of recurrence of the initial breast cancer is also a collaborative effort on the part of the patient and her surgeon, oncologist, and physician. The goal of self-examination of the chest wall or reconstructed breast (or the irradiated breast if breast conservation was performed), like examination of the normal breast, is to detect an area that feels different to the examining fingers or looks different in the mirror. Lumps, thickenings, or areas of different color can all be normal, but they should be checked by a woman's surgeon as soon as they are detected. Any new lump or swollen lymph gland that is discovered may arouse anxiety. If it persists for several weeks, the surgeon should check it to make a diagnosis and confirm whether there is reason for concern.

Initially, follow-up consists of a brief history and physical examination performed every 4 to 6 months. Physical examination focuses on parts of the body that are common sites of breast cancer spread. In time, this interval can be increased and a woman can return to her normal "whole person care" examination by her internal medicine physician or gynecologist or family doctor.

The follow-up pattern of testing and its frequency are determined by a woman's physicians. Some physicians routinely order a number of additional studies such as chest x-ray films, blood counts, chemistry studies, blood tumor markers, and even bone scans. Others do not. Blood tests serve as screening tests for liver, bone, or bone marrow involvement. Chest x-ray films similarly can screen for asymptomatic lung metastases, and mammograms can detect recurrences and screen for second (new) cancers of the breast. The great majority of recurrent cancers and second breast cancers, however, are either detected by self-examination, by physical examination, or by mammography. Unless specific symptoms are present, there is little evidence to support additional studies that are inconvenient for the patient, cost substantial amounts of money, and do not appear to improve survival. Some would argue, however, that the reason for these routine studies is the periodic reassurance they provide to both patient and physician when they are normal. If a woman's physician recommends such studies, she should ask about the basis for ordering them so that she is convinced that they are necessary. On the other hand, any new symptom (e.g., ache or pain) or new finding (e.g., mass or lump) discovered on physical examination is a clear indication for specific studies. Because tumors that are faster growing recur sooner and more slowly growing tumors recur later, the interval between follow-up examinations can be increased over a period of years, but at no time should these examinations be discontinued.

Routine mammography of the reconstructed breast is not needed. Monthly self-examination of the rebuilt breast has proved the best method for detecting a recurrence. There is no evidence that reconstruction causes any significant delay in detecting the rare cases of recurrent disease behind or beneath the reconstructed breast.

IF BREAST CANCER SPREADS . . .
GARY A. RATKIN, M.D.

If the primary and adjunctive therapies are not totally effective in eradicating all disease, breast cancer can return and spread to other parts of the body. The unpredicted regrowth may occur within the first few years of the original breast cancer diagnosis or years later.

Once a metastasis has been found, an assessment of the patient's overall health and the degree of breast cancer spread is critical. Some metastases can be controlled simply with oral medications, others require local radiation therapy or surgery, and the most advanced might necessitate intensive chemotherapy. The goal of treatment is to control the cancer so that the patient is able to live comfortably. Although a cure is not usually possible, once a recurrence is found, treatment can permit good-quality life for many years. Breast cancer, unlike many other forms of metastatic cancer, can be well controlled for long periods of time with the use of medications or surgical techniques. Recently, much progress has been made in the treatment of such widespread breast cancer.

Hormonal Therapy

By altering the patient's hormonal balance the physician can often control her breast cancer even if there has been a relapse or spread. The detection of estrogen and progesterone receptors in the cancer tissue indicates whether the tumor is likely to be responsive to hormonal treatment (also see "Adjuvant Hormonal Therapy"). The chance of a response to hormonal therapy for patients with advanced breast cancer and positive estrogen receptors is 40% to 60%, whereas negative estrogen receptor tests indicate a less than 10% chance of response.

Hormonal therapy can take several forms. Today, tamoxifen (Nolvadex), an anti-estrogen, is the most widely used form of therapy in patients who have positive estrogen or progesterone receptors. This drug has few side effects and can be taken over a long period of time. (See p. 66 in this chapter for a discussion of these side effects.)

A woman who is still having menstrual periods might benefit from an oophorectomy, an operation to remove her ovaries, the primary source of estrogen in her body. In the past the adrenal glands or pituitary gland was removed to eradicate other sources of estrogen; however, there are medications available today to accomplish this goal. Aminoglutethimide (Cytadren) blocks the production of adrenal hormones, including estrogens, and is used in selected cases. This antiadrenal drug is difficult to use because of its side effects, including a severe skin rash, initial drowsiness, chemical imbalance, and nausea. A new group of drugs (LH-RH agonists) that blocks some pituitary gland function is under study for breast cancer.

Estrogen in medication form can be used in selected postmenopausal patients with metastatic breast cancer. Such conjugated estrogen preparations as Premarin and diethylstilbestrol are given in relatively high doses with a similar benefit to tamoxifen. Unfortunately, estrogen therapy produces more frequent side effects, including nausea, swollen ankles, breast engorgement, and phlebitis (blood clots in the legs).

Another "female" hormone that can be effective in controlling widespread breast cancer is progestational hormone such as megestrol acetate (Megace) or medroxyprogesterone acetate (Provera) in large doses. Progesterone has fewer side effects than estrogen, but an increase in appetite with subsequent weight gain is not uncommon. The use of male hormones such as androgens has been largely abandoned in breast cancer treatment since they are less effective and have many side effects.

Chemotherapy for Widespread Disease

Chemotherapy can be effectively used in the woman whose breast cancer has recurred locally or spread widely throughout her body. It is frequently used when there is lung, liver, or bone marrow involvement. These drugs may be used when there is a low chance of response to hormonal therapy or when a patient is so ill that hormonal therapy will not work fast enough or be potent enough to deal with the illness. Combinations of chemotherapy with hormonal therapy or radiation are often used.

When chemotherapy is indicated to treat a patient, a combination of drugs that are known to work in breast cancer are employed. These combinations have been tested to destroy the greatest amount of cancer cells and give the best response. Modern chemotherapy programs are usually given periodically such as every 3 or 4 weeks.

Normal tissues may be temporarily affected by the chemotherapy drugs, which produce side effects. Oncologists have learned a lot about the safe and comfortable use of chemotherapy in patients with metastatic cancer. By giving the medications less frequently the normal bone marrow and other areas of the body have a chance to recover.

Most chemotherapy combinations are given intravenously. Some of the most frequently used drugs in metastatic breast cancer are methotrexate, 5-fluorouracil, cyclophosphamide, vincristine, vinblastine, doxorubicin, mitoxantrone, and thiotepa. Typically, three or four drug combinations are given to obtain the best outcome. Side effects of chemotherapy for metastatic disease are similar to those described on p. 65 of this chapter.

The purpose of giving chemotherapy to control the spread of cancer and to improve symptoms should be clear to the patient. It is a good idea to also have a plan of evaluation after several courses of chemotherapy so that the success rate can be determined and long-term treatment plans can be made.

Taxol

Studies conducted at major U.S. cancer centers indicate that taxol (Paclitaxel), a drug made from the bark of the slow-growing Pacific yew tree, is highly effective in treating women with advanced breast cancer. Because of the scarcity of these trees, however, supplies of the bark are in limited supply. A synthetic form of taxol (Taxotere) has been introduced on the market and may have a particular advantage as it is well tolerated and can be combined with other drugs to treat breast cancer.

Intensive Chemotherapy and Bone Marrow Transplantation
ROGER S. FOSTER, Jr., M.D.

Many of the anticancer drugs used in chemotherapy can cause partial or complete disappearance of metastatic breast cancer if given in high enough doses. Two approaches are used to treat metastatic breast cancer. With one approach, chemotherapy is given soon after diagnosis, when there are fewer cancer cells to be eliminated. Standard doses of chemotherapy may be curative if there are not too many cancer cells to eradicate. Most current adjuvant chemotherapy programs given at the time of lumpectomy or mastectomy are based on this theory.

The second approach seeks to improve the tolerance of the patient to higher doses of chemotherapy. The theory is that if the chemotherapy can be given in high enough doses, then the last cancer cell might be eliminated. Unfortunately, these high doses of chemotherapy are not only toxic to the cancer cells but are also toxic to normal cells, particularly the bone marrow cells, so much so that the patient cannot survive without special procedures to aid recovery of the bone marrow and the blood cells it produces.

Bone marrow transplantation permits patients to tolerate high doses of chemotherapy. With this technique, the patient's own bone marrow is removed and stored and then the chemotherapy is given. Following administration of chemotherapy the bone marrow cells are transfused by vein and the bone marrow cells then "home" their way back to bone marrow space. Bone marrow progenitor (mother) cells can also be extracted from the patient's blood after various procedures have been performed to increase the number of these cells in the blood. These cells are then stored and transfused back after the chemotherapy; this process is sometimes called *peripheral stem cell support.* Another approach to supplementing bone marrow for the patient receiving high-dose chemotherapy is administering bone marrow growth factors to speed recovery of the few remaining bone marrow cells. Centers doing bone marrow transplantations commonly give bone marrow growth factors in addition to the bone marrow transplants.

All of these bone marrow procedures permit the administration of high-dose chemotherapy and are currently being tested on patients at high risk of cancer recurrence after surgery and on patients with recurrent or metastatic breast cancer. Most physicians regard these procedures as investigational. The role and appropriateness of high-dose chemotherapy with special manipulations to permit recovery of the bone marrow have not yet been clearly identified, and the number of cures produced by these procedures has not been fully established. There is some risk of early death with these procedures due to infections that occur before the bone marrow recovers. The Blue Cross and Blue Shield Association has begun financing studies for bone marrow transplants in breast cancer patients. However, these treatments are not currently covered by many health insurance policies.

Monoclonal Antibodies

Another area of research is focusing on attacking tumors by using monoclonal antibodies. Some scientists are injecting advanced cancer patients with monoclonal antibodies (immune system protein molecules) that have been found to shrink tumors in animal studies.

CLINICAL TRIALS: THEIR ROLE IN ASSESSING BREAST CANCER TREATMENT OPTIONS
ROGER S. FOSTER, Jr., M.D.

In the past, and sometimes even now, new treatments for breast cancer were introduced without first receiving the scientific scrutiny necessary to establish their value. Before these treatments are accepted by the medical community for use on patients, they need to be compared to alternative treatments in carefully conducted scientific studies.

The clinical trial represents an excellent method for comparing and assessing different treatment approaches to breast cancer management. In these clinical trials, groups of doctors and their women patients agree to participate in studies in which the cancer treatment alternatives that these patients will ultimately receive may be decided by randomization. Randomization means that neither the patient nor her doctor chooses between the alternative treatments; instead, the treatments are chosen arbitrarily, or totally by chance, to avoid any bias creeping into the study. Randomized studies are particularly important when the differences between treatments being compared are likely to be either small or nonexistent.

Clinical trials in breast cancer have now involved many thousands of women whose medical data have been carefully collected to answer a variety of questions about breast cancer. Out of these trials has come an understanding that breast cancer is not one disease but many different diseases, or perhaps a disease with many variations. Increasingly, appropriate treatment requires understanding these many variations of breast cancer.

Primary Treatment: Breast-Conserving Surgery vs. Total Mastectomy

The treatment of breast cancer by less than complete mastectomy has been studied in randomized clinical trials. Two large important trials in this area have contributed significantly to resolving questions that were unsatisfactorily answered previously. It has been shown that when carefully selected patients are treated by experienced surgeons and radiotherapists with breast-conserving operations, their survival at 10 to 15 years is comparable to the survival for women treated with operations that remove the entire breast. Some patients treated with breast-conserving surgery do, however, have a cancer recurrence in the remaining portion of their breast and require a total mastectomy at a later time. As further data develop from these studies, women and their physicians will have additional scientific information on which to base a decision regarding the alternatives of total mastectomy followed by reconstruction vs. breast-conserving surgery.

Adjuvant Treatment

Adjuvant treatments are those treatments given in addition to surgical removal of the cancer. Alternative adjuvant management approaches for breast cancer have also been the subject of investigation. For many years, the chest was irradiated after radical or modified radical mastectomy in the hope of improving the cure rate. Now, scientifically valid studies on radiation treatment have been conducted and demonstrate that the addition of radiation only decreases recurrence in the treated area and has no benefit on survival. We have learned that radiation treatment is best reserved for those mastectomy patients in whom cancer recurs or for patients with more advanced cancers at the time of diagnosis.

Randomized studies have shown that irradiation after breast-conserving surgery greatly reduces the chance of recurrence of cancer in the breast and therefore most of these patients are currently treated with radiotherapy. Other randomized clinical trials have investigated the question of alternative treatments for the axillary lymph nodes. These studies have shown that the axillary nodes can be treated by either surgery or radiation therapy with similar results. If the axillary nodes are not enlarged, they may simply be watched and treated only if they enlarge. These studies, which were conducted more than 10 years ago, proved that treating the axillary lymph nodes does not harm any immune response the patient's body may have triggered to fight cancer. Today, for most patients diagnosed with breast cancer under the age of 70, the axillary lymph nodes are routinely removed because up to 4 out of 10 patients will have microscopic spread of cancer into the lymph nodes, and that information is important in making decisions on additional treatments such as chemotherapy or hormonal therapy.

Randomized clinical trials have been important in studying the effectiveness of combining systemic treatments (those affecting the entire body) with local and regional treatments of radiation and surgery. Over the past 15 years these randomized trials have been conducted to assess the effectiveness of systemic treatment with chemotherapy and/or hormonal therapy. The studies have clearly shown that it is possible to decrease the recurrence rates and improve survival for patients with some types of breast cancer by using these adjuvant treatments. Despite these advances there is still a need for better adjuvant treatments.

Breast Cancer Chemo Prevention Trials

Observation of the beneficial effects that adjuvant (preventive) tamoxifen therapy has had in reducing the incidence of second primary breast cancer and cardiovascular deaths in breast cancer patients has led to the development of new clinical trials. These trials are designed to assess the value of tamoxifen in preventing breast cancer in women at high risk for breast cancer. The U.S. trial that is being conducted by the National Surgical Adjuvant Breast Project will involve 16,000 women: 8000 treated with tamoxifen and 8000 treated with a placebo. Since age is the most important risk factor for breast cancer, women over the age of 60 are eligible. Women under the age of 60, down to the age of 35, may be eligible if they have additional risk factors, including lobular carcinoma in situ, atypical hyperplasia, a family history of breast cancer, and are nulliparous (not having borne children). A computer-generated assessment of breast cancer risk is utilized to determine a woman's eligibility. The younger the patient, the greater the degree of risk that is necessary for acceptance into the trial. While the data on the benefits of tamoxifen in patients with breast cancer are compelling, the benefits must be proved in healthy women, with evidence that the benefits outweigh the side effects (see p. 66 for information on side effects).

Most breast cancer clinical trials require cooperation from physicians in many different medical centers. Numerous experts contribute to the design of each trial, thus providing "multiple second opinions." The National Cancer Institute reviews each trial design and commonly covers the expenses incurred in collecting the scientific data. In addition, each participating medical center has its own human investigation review committee that must approve the trial before it can begin at a medical center.

By participating in clinical trials, physicians are able to keep current with the most recent developments in cancer treatment, and patients can expect to receive either the best recognized treatment or a new treatment that a consensus of experts believes may represent an advance. In addition, information gained from the treatment will influence the future care of others.

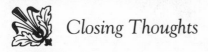 *Closing Thoughts*

The feelings of attachment a woman has about her breasts are profound and should not be overlooked by the physician treating her. These feelings will influence a woman's decision to seek help initially and eventually will help determine the type of therapy that she selects. Once the surprise of being stricken by a dreaded disease has passed, a woman desires and deserves honest information about her disease, her prognosis, and her options for treatment. In addition, she wants a physician who is sensitive to her psychological and aesthetic concerns. The physician who treats a woman afflicted with breast cancer must consider the relationship of therapy to ultimate survival, rehabilitation, and enhanced quality of life. To consider only management of her cancer is no longer sufficient.

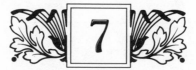

WHAT YOUR DOCTORS AND NURSES CAN DO FOR YOU

*It was frustrating. Each doctor wanted to do his part but
no one was coordinating the effort. I kept wondering where was
this team approach I've heard so much about?*

Today we live in an age of specialization. No where is this phenomenon more obvious than in the field of medicine, where a single individual is no longer capable of being current with all there is to know. Thus, when a woman has a breast problem, she may consult with several experts before she can decide on the appropriate course of action. Most likely she will begin by visiting with her primary care doctor, who is familiar with her medical history and whom she has grown to trust for advice about her health care. This doctor may be her gynecologist, family practitioner, or internist, and he is the person she will see for diagnosis of her problem and treatment advice. This doctor also will refer her to other specialists if he feels that they can contribute to the diagnosis or treatment of her suspected problem. When her doctor sends her to another specialist, he is not losing interest in her case, rather he is playing an important coordinating role by using his knowledge and taking advantage of recent developments in medicine to help her get the best care possible.

A woman's needs, of course, will vary with her individual situation. Sometimes her breast problem will be diagnosed as fibrocystic change by her primary care physician, and he will monitor her breasts with regular checkups and mammograms. These mammograms will be interpreted by the diagnostic radiologist. If a lump or another suspicious area is discovered on physical examination or on a mammogram and warrants investigation, she may be referred to a general surgeon for further examination.

If a biopsy is indicated, the story becomes even more complicated because a pathologist now becomes involved in the woman's health care. He analyzes the biopsy specimen and reports whether a cancer has been found, what kind it is, and whether it has spread to her lymph nodes. Even though the pathologist has no direct contact with the woman diagnosed with breast cancer or even with the woman whose biopsied lump proves benign, his report has a great influence on what happens to each of these women in the future. If the pathologist's report indicates cancer, then the general surgeon provides the woman with an explanation of her problem and some understanding of her treatment options (see Chapter 6). These options may include a mastectomy with possible breast reconstruction or breast-conserving surgery and irradiation. If cancer has spread to her lymph nodes, adjunctive therapy also may be required, and she may learn of chemotherapy, radiation therapy, and hormonal therapy. Depending on her individual situation and the therapy she ultimately selects, she may interact with a number of specialists associated with the breast management team; these experts include the radiation oncologist (radiotherapist), medical oncologist (chemotherapist), general surgeon, and plastic surgeon.

The thought of facing more than one doctor is often a frightening one. We don't adequately understand what each of these specialists does and who will coordinate care. It seems like an impersonal and expensive approach to health care. Women express confusion as to who is in charge. Furthermore, they don't always know what questions to ask these doctors or even how they can really help us. To clear up some of the confusion and impersonality surrounding these medical specialists, we have asked experts we know and respect in each of the previously mentioned fields to write descriptions of what they do and how they can help you. The descriptions are organized according to the role these physicians play in a woman's health care and the stage at which she might consult with each expert. Therefore the gynecologist and internist are included under a heading entitled "Primary Care: Diagnosis, Management, and Referral," and the diagnostic radiologist, general surgeon, pathologist, radiation oncologist, medical oncologist, and plastic surgeon are listed under "The Breast Management Team: Diagnosis, Treatment, and Rehabilitation."

The nurse's role is also included in the discussion of "The Breast Management Team." When a woman has a breast problem, she is usually referred directly to a physician. Nurses, however, are active in all phases of the woman's breast care and play a valuable part in patient education, therapy, and rehabilitation. Therefore we have asked two nursing experts we know and admire, an oncology nurse and a plastic surgery nurse, to describe what they do and how they can assist you during this difficult time.

The final member of the team is the woman herself. As one of our readers reminded us, "A woman has an important role to play in this team effort. She needs to maintain a positive attitude, keep herself informed, and take responsibility for maintaining good basic health habits with attention to nutrition and exercise. In other words, the woman does not passively submit to treatments imposed by her doctors and other team members; rather, she is an active participant in her own treatment and recovery." We couldn't agree more. It is in a woman's best interest to play an active role in her own health care and to become an integral part of this team effort that contributes so significantly to her ultimate health and survival. (See Chapter 8 for more information on the woman's role.) The first step in this effort is learning what these health professionals do and how they can help you.

All of the physicians listed are board-certified members of their specialties. We feel that it is important for a woman to choose a physician who has met this standard. All physicians can practice medicine after medical school or residency, but having board certification indicates that after training and an initial period of practice, they have passed an examination that tests their competence and shows that they meet the criteria for practice in the specialty.

PRIMARY CARE: DIAGNOSIS, MANAGEMENT, AND REFERRAL

A yearly visit to the obstetrician-gynecologist or internist is routine for many women. If they develop a breast problem, they look to one of these doctors for advice and help.

The Obstetrician-Gynecologist's Role in a Woman's Breast Care
JACOB KLEIN, M.D.

Specializing in the care of women and their reproductive organs, the obstetrician-gynecologist is in reality the primary care physician for most women and frequently is the only doctor that they see on a regular, ongoing basis. During a woman's annual or semiannual visits to her gynecologist he performs physical examinations that include a breast examination, pelvic examination, and Pap smear, which is a screening test for cervical cancer.

In the absence of breast disease the gynecologist is usually the physician who orders breast screening tests. It is his responsibility to be knowledgeable about the types of tests available, their advantages and disadvantages, and the frequency with which these examinations should be given. The newest developments in the area of breast screening must be part of every gynecologist's fund of knowledge.

The gynecologist is frequently the person most responsible for educating his patients about their bodies. This education includes information about the normal structure and function of their reproductive organs and what happens when these organs malfunction. In addition, it is the role of the gynecologist to stress the value of regular gynecologic examinations and the importance of breast self-examination for early detection of breast cancer.

It is vital for the gynecologist to educate patients about the need for regular, monthly breast self-examination as well as the best timing for these inspections. Because a woman's hormonal cycle has a profound influence on her breast tissue, she needs to understand these cyclic changes in order to know when to examine her breasts. Women have numerous reasons for not performing this test, including fear of discovering a mass, ignorance of inspection techniques or the importance of early diagnosis, and lack of awareness of the prevalence of breast cancer. The gynecologist needs to be sensitive to a woman's concerns and aware of her reasons for procrastinating about performing this health routine. With these reasons in mind, he should take responsibility for actually teaching his patients the appropriate techniques for breast self-inspection, and then he should monitor a woman's performance to make sure that her inspections are adequate and to help her gain confidence in her ability to successfully practice self-examination. He also can assure her that she will gain proficiency with this inspection if she makes it a monthly routine.

When a woman discovers a questionable breast mass, the gynecologist is usually the first physician she contacts. The relationship that exists between a woman and her gynecologist is a unique and particularly trusting one. It allows the physician to deal with the physical and psychological aspects of a woman's breast disease. Therefore a gynecologist must sensitively respond to the patient's breast problem, from a total perspective, realizing that the discovery of a breast mass provokes unparalleled fear and anxiety in most women. The stress caused by the discovery of a breast lump must be dealt with as well as the treatment for the actual breast problem.

The process leading to definitive treatment of a suspected breast problem is initiated by the gynecologist after a routine breast examination. His findings will either reassure him that a disease state does not exist or cause him to further evaluate the breast mass. The gynecologist will direct this evaluation by arranging for breast cyst aspiration, mammograms, or referral to a surgeon who is familiar with and sensitive to the issues involved with treating breast diseases. The patient will rely on her gynecologist for direction in her health care and will expect him to provide her with an explanation of the course of events that will probably follow. Once evaluation of her breast problem is complete and definitive treatment planned, a woman will frequently need to be reassured by her gynecologist that the other specialist's approach is medically sound. At this time the gynecologist plays an important role as a reliable source of information. He will continue the relationship with the patient concomitant with the care being provided to her by the surgeon, oncologist, radiotherapist, or plastic surgeon.

Prevention of breast disease and treatment of pathologic breast conditions when they do occur are an integral part of routine gynecologic care and should be expected and demanded by every patient.

The Internist's Role in a Woman's Breast Care

BENJAMIN A. BOROWSKY, M.D.

In current medical practice the internist is the specialist responsible for the comprehensive medical care of his patients and the monitoring of their ongoing health care needs. His involvement in the treatment of a woman with a breast problem or breast cancer is continuous, beginning before the disease is detected and continuing after treatment is complete.

As part of health maintenance counseling, the internist will advise women on the need for self-examination and physician examination, appropriate use of mammograms, and effects of various drugs and hormones on her breasts. As more data become available on the influence of diet and environment on the incidence of breast cancer, he will discuss this information with her as well. In short, the internist's first duty is to educate the patient about practices that will prevent cancer when possible and lead to prompt detection if it does occur.

Once a breast mass has been discovered, the internist's first effort is to confirm its presence by examination. He must then choose from several options. If he feels certain that there is no indication of malignancy, he may decide not to proceed further. Repeat examination at a more suitable time in the menstrual cycle may be needed. In some cases the use of mammography is helpful. If he is uncertain about the diagnosis, he may wish to refer the patient to a surgeon for another opinion or for a biopsy and/or definitive surgery.

In selecting a general surgeon for patient referral the internist is guided by more than the surgeon's technical knowledge and skills. He must also consider how the individual woman will relate to a particular surgeon. Each person differs in the extent she desires to be informed about the many surgical options now available. Some women (and their families) wish to play an active role in planning treatment, whereas others prefer not to have to make a choice. It is important for the internist, who usually knows the patient best, to consider her preferences in recommending a surgeon for her. It is also his responsibility to advise the surgeon as to the woman's feelings. The surgeon usually will be the source of technical information regarding the woman's surgical options, but the internist can help her and her family understand these options and can offer his advice when a treatment choice is to be made.

During and immediately after surgery the internist manages any other coexisting conditions a patient may have. He also will participate in decisions regarding postoperative x-ray treatment or chemotherapy.

After the initial therapy is complete, follow-up is a coordinated effort between the surgeon, internist, and oncologist and/or radiotherapist, when the latter are needed. It is usually the internist who carries out long-term follow-up and performs appropriate examinations to screen for signs of recurrent cancer. He also tailors his management of subsequent complaints to consider the effect treatment may have on the woman's breast cancer.

The internist functions initially in the areas of prevention and detection. After cancer has been discovered, his relationship as principal medical advisor becomes most important. In this role he guides the patient to the proper specialists and advises her when treatment choices are necessary. Finally, he continues follow-up care of the patient indefinitely to ensure, if possible, the long-term success of treatment.

THE BREAST MANAGEMENT TEAM: DIAGNOSIS, TREATMENT, AND REHABILITATION

Although the diagnostic radiologist is included here as a part of the breast management team, this specialist actually bridges the gap between the patient's primary care physicians and those members of the breast management team who will treat her breast problem. Screening or diagnostic mammograms may be ordered by any of these physicians, and the radiologist will confer with these specialists and with the woman herself to help screen for or diagnose any breast problems.

The Diagnostic Radiologist's Role in the Detection and Diagnosis of Breast Disease

BARBARA S. MONSEES, M.D.

The diagnostic radiologist is a physician with special training in interpreting imaging studies such as mammograms, chest x-ray films, computed tomographic scans, ultrasonograms, and magnetic resonance imaging scans. The diagnostic radiologist who specializes in breast imaging is a mammographer.

Under most circumstances, the diagnostic radiologist functions as a consultant to physicians who order imaging studies to diagnose and evaluate their patient's problems. In the case of mammography, however, unlike other imaging tests, the mammographer assumes a more direct role, consulting with the patient herself and helping her to understand the findings on her mammograms.

Although the radiologist does not position the patient for the mammogram and obtain the actual images (this is done by the radiation technologist), he or she determines the number and quality of images obtained, maintains a standard of quality control, and interprets the examination itself.

When a woman has no signs or symptoms of breast problems, she is usually referred for a *screening mammogram*. Her breast images are then taken by the technologist and later interpreted by the radiologist. In this situation the patient has no contact with the mammographer.

If an abnormality is detected on a screening mammogram, however, the radiologist takes the lead in evaluating the problem because, lacking any signs or symptoms, it isn't observable on physical examination. Other mammographic views or ultrasound studies may then be ordered by the radiologist to fully evaluate the problem so that the radiologist can advise the referring physician as to whether an abnormality is present and whether it is likely to be benign or malignant.

Often this information is also communicated directly to the woman herself by the radiologist so that she may seek consultation with a general surgeon who deals with breast problems. It is important for the radiologist to be sensitive to the patient's fears and to take the necessary time to explain what has been found on the mammogram and what that means for the patient.

When a woman or her physician finds a suspicious lump or thickening in the breast or a bloody nipple discharge, the woman should not be referred for a screening examination but for a *diagnostic mammogram*, which is performed under the direct supervision of the diagnostic radiologist. At that time the standard mammographic views will be taken, followed by a complete breast examination by the radiologist, who can then correlate the mammograms and physical findings and determine if any extra views are necessary to better evaluate the suspicious area. If an abnormality is suspected to be a cyst, ultrasonography (which is effective in distinguishing between a solid lump and a fluid-filled cyst) can be performed. If warranted, the cyst can be aspirated using ultrasound guidance. After all of the necessary images have been taken, the radiologist offers an opinion as to the type of follow-up needed, whether careful surveillance by the referring physician or surgical consultation. Frequently the radiologist will confer directly with the woman's primary care physician to expedite surgical consultation.

When a suspicious abnormality can be seen on the mammogram but cannot be felt, a biopsy is usually warranted, and the radiologist can assist in this procedure. The radiologist places a small hookwire into the breast (breast needle localization) using mammography to ensure its accurate placement. This wire is then used to guide the surgeon to the suspicious area so that a specimen can be removed for biopsy. With the recent advent of accurate equipment capable of placing a needle within even the tiniest lesion that can be seen on a mammogram, radiologists have also begun to perform closed biopsy of suspicious areas seen only on mammography. This technique, however, is still evolving and its indications are still being determined. (See Chapter 5 for more information on these techniques.)

The mammographer plays a key role in diagnosing breast problems. This specialist not only interprets the breast x-ray films, but also consults with the woman and her referring physicians, offering solace when necessary, answering questions, and helping to screen women for early signs of breast cancer and to diagnose preexisting problems.

The General Surgeon's Role in a Woman's Breast Care
KENNETH J. ARNOLD, M.D.

General surgeons are experienced in diseases of the breast, and this aspect of patient care represents a significant portion of their practice. A woman is usually referred to a general surgeon when a breast lump or abnormality is suspected, breast examination proves difficult, or the mammography results are questionable.

The surgeon ultimately decides whether to perform a breast biopsy. In arriving at that decision the surgeon reviews the patient's history, her risk factors, and her mammograms, if indicated. In general, one of three conditions will result in a recommendation for a breast biopsy: (1) a dominant lump, (2) a suspicious or indeterminate mammogram, or (3) bloody nipple discharge.

The surgeon can and should be more than just an arbiter of treatment options. He should be a resource to the patient, knowledgeable about diseases of the breast and their significance and able to answer the many questions that women have about their breasts.

For the woman who does not require a biopsy, the general surgeon uses his expertise to reassure and inform the patient about benign breast conditions and breast cancer, the need for breast self-examination and physician breast examination, and the necessity for cancer screening. The surgeon must be available to respond to the many questions today's informed women have about their breasts.

For the woman who requires a biopsy, the surgeon not only performs the biopsy, but provides the woman with the information and the emotional support that she requires. This means explaining the reason for the biopsy, the specifics involved in the procedure, the anesthetic to be used, the expected recovery, and the anticipated result. It is important for the woman to know when she will receive a definitive report on the result of this procedure.

For the woman diagnosed with breast cancer, the general surgeon plays a key role in her care. He must be able to sensitively and sensibly discuss with the woman the many controversies surrounding the issue of breast cancer and the various choices available to her. Because the woman is faced with so much information and misinformation, it is important for the surgeon to help her sort through the plethora of fact and fantasy that confronts her. In general, the surgeon will explain to the patient that there are two problems to be dealt with to increase the likelihood of cure: local control of the disease within the breast itself and control of the disease within the rest of the body. Dealing with these issues is time consuming, but it is important for the patient to feel that she has been given sufficient information so that she can make the choices that are available to her.

For the breast cancer patient, the surgeon must present all of the available treatment options with the benefits and risks of each and allow the patient an opportunity to ask questions and express feelings and preferences. Finally, the surgeon must be able to make appropriate recommendations for treatment and then skillfully carry out the agreed upon therapy, referring to other specialists as indicated. The surgeon will often act as the coordinator of a team approach to the woman's breast cancer treatment, coordinating her care and referring her to various other specialists such as radiation oncologists, medical oncologists, plastic surgeons, and support group personnel as they are needed.

When a woman decides to have a lumpectomy or a mastectomy to treat her breast cancer, the general surgeon will perform this surgery. For the mastectomy patient, he will also inform the woman of the option of breast reconstruction. Then, if the woman is interested in this option, she and her surgeon can discuss the timing for reconstruction. If she desires immediate breast restoration during the same operation as her mastectomy, the general surgeon often will refer her to a plastic surgeon, either the one on his breast management team or one with whom he has worked before.

A woman must feel comfortable with her surgeon and freely discuss any and all issues concerning her breast biopsy or cancer treatment. If she is unable to establish this relationship, she should consider seeking another surgeon with whom she can develop this rapport. Among the many questions a woman might consider asking her surgeon are the following:

- How should I examine myself? What time of the month is best and what am I looking for?
- When and how often should I see a physician?
- What are my risks of breast cancer and what can I do to lessen them?
- Is mammography necessary and will it increase my risk of developing cancer?

When a biopsy is necessary, she might ask:

- Should this procedure be done on an inpatient or outpatient basis and under local or general anesthesia?
- Can I have a fine-needle aspiration biopsy instead of an open surgical biopsy?

- If I have a surgical biopsy, what type of scar will be left?
- What are the aftereffects?
- Why is this biopsy necessary? Will the whole lump be gone or just part of it? When will the result be known with certainty?
- After biopsy, how long do I have to make up my mind on treatment if it reveals cancer?
- What do we do if it is cancer?
- What is removed in a mastectomy?
- Do I have to have an axillary dissection if I have a mastectomy?
- If I have a mastectomy, where will the scar be and will I be able to have breast reconstruction?
- Can I have breast reconstruction at the same time as the mastectomy?
- Do I have to have a mastectomy if I have breast cancer? Is any other treatment possible?
- What is removed in a lumpectomy?
- Do I have to have radiation therapy if I have a lumpectomy?
- Do I have to have an axillary dissection if I have a lumpectomy?
- What is the difference between a modified radical mastectomy and a lumpectomy?
- Is a lumpectomy as safe as a mastectomy?
- Will I need chemotherapy if I have a mastectomy?
- Will I need chemotherapy if I have a lumpectomy?

For the woman who ultimately develops breast cancer or for any woman conferring with a general surgeon, no question should be considered too silly or trivial and she deserves a thoughtful answer to every question.

The Pathologist's Role in the Diagnosis and Treatment of Breast Problems
JOHN S. MEYER, M.D.

A pathologist is a medical doctor specializing in the analysis and diagnosis of disease in the laboratory. He analyzes tissues obtained from biopsies or removal of organs and analyzes blood and other body fluids. He is an expert in cytology, which is the analysis of cells from tissues and fluids. In this role he will analyze Pap smears, smears of secretions from the nipple to detect malignant cells, and fine-needle aspirates of breast masses. To effectively diagnose breast cancer the pathologist must also have a thorough familiarity with the micro-. scopic anatomy of the breast and various disease states that affect it.

Although the woman with a breast lump will talk to and be

examined by her personal physician and surgeon, she is not likely to meet the pathologist who is responsible for diagnosing her condition if a biopsy is done. Ordinarily the specimen that the surgeon removes is sent to the laboratory, where the pathologist examines it in the light of the surgeon's findings, which are written on a form accompanying the specimen.

This examination involves two steps. First is the gross examination in which the pathologist uses his naked eye to scrutinize the specimen and select portions for microscopic study. After hardening and preserving these portions in formaldehyde or some other fluid, histotechnologists prepare microscopic slides on which very thin, transparent sections of the tissues are sliced and stained to make them visible under the microscope. Next, during microscopic examination of these slides, the pathologist analyzes the types of cells present and their relationship to each other.

When analyzing a biopsy specimen a pathologist does more than simply diagnose or rule out the presence of cancer. Breast cancer is actually not a single disease, but a classification containing many subtypes that have different implications for the patient and the doctors treating her. First, the pathologist decides whether the cancer is invasive (infiltrating) or intraductal (in situ). In situ cancer, either within the breast duct or lobule, does not metastasize and is virtually 100% curable by removal of the breast. If the cancer is invasive, it is classified as to the exact type. Certain invasive cancers are slow growing and usually do not metastasize. The great majority of women with these special types of breast cancer are cured by a mastectomy and axillary lymph node dissection without any further treatment.

Most invasive breast cancers are not the slow-growing types mentioned above. The pathologist can classify these cancers further by noting the characteristics of their cells (whether well differentiated or poorly differentiated) and their patterns of growth in the breast tissues and axillary lymph nodes. If an axillary dissection has been done, he examines the lymph nodes microscopically to determine the presence or absence of carcinoma. The chances of having a recurrence of cancer or a metastasis depend strongly on the number of lymph nodes that contain cancer.

The pathologist may perform a battery of tests or assays to identify specific oncogenes (genes that play a role in producing cancers) and growth factors that predict breast carcinoma prognosis. One oncogene that he looks for is the oncogene *erb B-2/neu* (also called *HER 2/neu*), a protein present on the surface of breast cancer cells that is associated with a high probability of distant cancer spread (metastasis) when a patient has positive axillary lymph nodes. This gene is thought to be present in up to 20% of women with breast cancer (particularly in women with a family history of breast cancer) and is capable of making tumors more aggressive and lethal. Tests are also conducted to measure the presence of epidermal growth factor receptors. Breast cancers with increased numbers of receptors for epidermal growth factor (a protein with growth-stimulating properties) have a relatively high likelihood of metastasis. The future role of these and similar tests is not yet clear.

The pathologist may also conduct tests to measure the enzymes that breast cancers secrete. These enzymes may attack surrounding tissues and help the carcinomas become invasive. One such enzyme that is related to breast cancer prognosis is *cathepsin-D*. Several studies have associated high levels of cathepsin-D with an unfavorable prognosis, but some questions remain about the utility of this test.

Much of the pathologist's attention focuses on growth rate measurements. Cancers with high rates of growth are more likely to produce recurrences within a few years of treatment than those with slow growth rates. Growth rates (S-phase fraction) may be measured by *flow cytometry*, which is an automated method for determining the *ploidy* (the amount of DNA in the cells). Tumors with abnormally high amounts of DNA are termed *DNA-aneuploid* and usually have a less favorable prognosis because they are faster growing than tumors with near-normal DNA content, which are called *DNA-diploid*. *Labeling indexes* and *Ki-67 assays* also are used to measure cell growth rate in tumors. Low labeling indexes are associated with a good prognosis and a smaller chance of tumor recurrence. Labeling index tests are technically difficult to perform, however, and are not available at all laboratories. Recent developments promise to increase the ease of performing these growth rate measurements.

Tests to measure the estrogen and progesterone receptors in cancer cells are an important means of determining the risk of cancer recurring, the subsequent need for further therapy (adjuvant chemotherapy, radiation therapy, or hormonal therapy), and which tumors are likely to respond to treatment with tamoxifen (an anti-estrogen) or other methods of hormonal therapy. Carcinomas that contain large amounts of estrogen and progesterone receptors, in general, are less likely to recur or metastasize within a few years of breast removal than are carcinomas with small amounts of these receptors or no detectable receptors. Thus information about the presence or absence of estrogen and progesterone receptors should be included in the pathologist's report.

The final report issued by the pathologist diagnoses the cancer and classifies it based on the various findings previously mentioned. This report is used by the general surgeon and other members of the breast management team in assessing the woman's risk of spread or possible recurrence of her cancer and in determining the appropriate treatment for her and the need for any adjuvant therapies designed to prevent recurrence.

The identification of a breast cancer might require a woman to consult with still other members of the breast management team who will help with her treatment and rehabilitation.

The Radiation Oncologist's Role in Treating a Woman With Breast Cancer

JOHN M. BEDWINEK, M.D.

A radiation oncologist (also called a radiotherapist) is a physician who specializes in the study of cancer and its treatment with ionizing radiation—a potent killer of malignant cells. The radiation oncologist determines if and when radiation should be used and is a part of the cancer team (surgeon, radiation oncologist, and medical oncologist) that decides what is the optimum combination of the three cancer treatment modalities: surgery, irradiation, and chemotherapy. The radiation oncologist also decides how much and what type of radiation therapy should be used and is directly responsible for delivering the radiation dose effectively and safely.

The radiation oncologist must have a broad range of training. He must have a thorough understanding of all types of cancer and a familiarity with the capabilities, limitations, and side effects of the other two cancer treatment modalities: chemotherapy and surgery. He should be well versed in nuclear physics and the physics of ionizing radiation, understand the effects of radiation both on tumors and on normal human tissue, and know the latest techniques for precisely delivering the right amount of radiation to cancerous tissue while sparing normal tissue. In addition, he must be knowledgeable in general medicine so he can manage his patient's problems and know when to refer to other physicians if problems arise outside his area of expertise.

The radiation oncologist's role can be separated into a number of different responsibilities beginning with the initial consultation, when he first sees the patient and studies all aspects of her condition. He reviews her current symptoms and past medical history, performs a physical examination, orders and evaluates all appropriate x-ray studies and blood tests, and reviews the biopsy specimen with the pathologist. Once the necessary data have been assessed, he confers with the surgeon and/or medical oncologist and they determine whether radiation is indicated or whether another form of treatment is more appropriate. Since he has conferred with the surgeon and/or medical oncologist, this decision carries the weight of a team approach. As mentioned in the section on "Breast-Conserving Surgery and Irradiation" in Chapter 6, it is the responsibility of the radiation oncologist and surgeon, acting in concert, to advise the woman whether mastectomy or breast conservation is the more appropriate treatment method for her.

Patient education is one of the radiation oncologist's most important functions. After deciding on the best mode of treatment he should be able to help the patient understand what that treatment is, why it is considered the best option, what are the anticipated side effects, and what is the expected outcome.

If radiation treatment is actually used, it is the radiation oncologist's duty to determine how much radiation to give and what specific areas of the body should be targeted. For example, he must decide whether to treat the breast only or whether to treat the breast and the adjacent lymph node areas. The radiation treatment must be planned so that a precise and uniform radiation dose is delivered to all tumor-bearing tissue while minimizing the dose to normal tissues as much as possible. He may use high-technology equipment such as a simulator with fluoroscopy, a three-dimensional treatment planning computer, or computed tomography to assist him in this planning process.

Care of the patient during the course of and after completion of radiation therapy is also the responsibility of the radiation oncologist. He must ensure that the daily radiation treatments are being given according to his plan and must monitor the effects of the radiation not only on the cancer, but also on the surrounding normal tissues. He must recognize which symptoms are side effects of the radiation dose and which symptoms are not and manage all side effects and problems that occur during the course of radiation therapy. Once radiation therapy has been completed, the radiation oncologist must assess the effectiveness of the treatment and monitor the patient at regular intervals to watch for radiation complications, regrowth of the cancer, and/or the development of new cancers.

Providing ongoing emotional support for the patient and her family pervades all stages of the patient's management. The patient needs to know that the radiation oncologist truly cares and will be there to answer all questions and to help with all problems.

A radiation oncologist must have compassion and sensitivity, qualities not easily taught in a formal training program. The patient who discovers that she has cancer has special psychological needs, and the radiation oncologist must be sensitive to these needs and be equipped to offer the necessary emotional support and understanding.

Equal in importance to compassion is the ability to communicate and teach effectively. It is crucial that the radiation oncologist provide clear and easily understandable answers to the following questions:

- What kind of cancer does the patient have, and how does it grow and spread?
- What are the treatment options for this particular kind of cancer? Will it be radiation therapy, surgery, chemotherapy, or a combination of these modalities?
- What is the specific purpose of each of the treatments to be used?
- What are the potential side effects and complications of the proposed treatment, and what are the chances of these occurring?
- What are the consequences of the complications if they occur, and what is the treatment for the complications?
- Will the patient be able to engage in normal daily activities during the treatment? If not, what are the restrictions, and how soon can normal activity be resumed?
- Are there any alternatives to the proposed treatment, and what are the chances of success and possible side effects of these alternatives?

These issues are the bare minimum that must be explained clearly and simply without the patient having to ask. There will always be more questions, and the patient should be given ample opportunity to ask additional questions after she has had time to reflect. The radiation oncologist must also make every effort to ensure that what is said is fully understood. Explanations and answers to questions should be given at least twice. It is the rare patient who can understand and fully grasp unfamiliar facts and concepts on the first explanation, particularly since she may still be in a state of shock and anxiety from recently being told that she has cancer. For this reason, the radiation oncologist should see the woman a second time a few days after the initial visit so that he can repeat earlier explanations and answer any questions that may have arisen since the first appointment. Also, it is helpful for the woman to have a close friend or family member present when explanations are given.

Being able to explain medical facts and concepts in an easily understandable fashion is, in part, a gift, but it is also a skill that can be acquired through patience, effort, and practice. The gift of explanation is not possessed by all physicians and not all physicians take the time and effort to develop such skills. This is unfortunate since being able to help the patient understand all aspects of her disease and treatment will greatly diminish her fear. Patient education is one of the most important responsibilities of the radiation oncologist. It is, in fact, one of the most important responsibilities of any doctor. Most doctors, unfortunately, do not know that the origin of the title "doctor" comes from the Latin word *doceo*, which means "to teach" or "to explain." A doctor should first and foremost be a good teacher. If he is not, then the patient should find another doctor who is.

The Medical Oncologist's Role in Treating a Woman With Breast Cancer

GARY A. RATKIN, M.D.

The medical oncologist's role in treating breast cancer has expanded with the development of therapies used after surgical treatment to lower the chances of breast cancer spread or recurrence. Improvements in the use of systemic treatment, both chemotherapy and hormonal therapy, have made consultation with an oncologist central to the management of most patients with breast cancer.

A medical oncologist is a specialist in internal medicine who is knowledgeable in the management of malignancies (including breast cancer) and in the use of medications to treat cancer. A woman who has had primary treatment for breast cancer consults a medical oncologist when adjunctive therapy is being considered. She usually is referred to the medical oncologist by her surgeon or primary physician (internist, gynecologist, or family physician). Close communication with each of these physicians is very important for the medical oncologist since he will be making important recommendations to the patient based on the information he receives. If metastatic cancer develops, the medical oncologist manages the overall treatment plan.

The oncologist reviews the original pathology report, hormone receptor and cell kinetic data (when available), and any clinical information such as x-ray films, laboratory tests, risk factors, symptoms, and physical findings. The medical oncologist can then advise the woman about the diagnosis, staging, and appropriate treatment.

Comprehensive knowledge of the latest drug therapies and experience in prescribing and administering chemotherapeutic drugs are required. When the patient requires chemotherapy or hormonal therapy, the medical oncologist is the one responsible for its administration. The common and unusual side effects of the drugs, how to prevent them, or how to treat them are addressed in the medical oncology consultation. In particular, the medical oncologist must have an in-depth knowledge of hematologic (blood) problems as well as broader experience in dealing with infectious diseases and lung, heart, or gastrointestinal problems. The oncologist must be aware of the many advances involving new chemotherapeutic drugs, new applications of hormones and chemotherapy, and current techniques that allow the most effective and safest administration of these agents.

The oncologist must also be aware of and understand the many physical and emotional problems that confront the cancer patient. He should be able to sensitively address the patient's concerns to help her cope with the various aspects of her cancer and its treatment.

To meet the patient's individual needs the oncologist should be aware of the resources available to that patient in her community and nationally and be able to make the appropriate referrals and suggestions. She may want to consult with experts in radiation oncology, pathology, surgery, or plastic surgery. Knowledge of local nursing resources is of critical importance as is information on pharmacies and medical supply businesses that cater to the needs of cancer patients. Appropriate community service organizations, dieticians, psychologists, physical and occupational therapists, and social workers may be of great value to patients. Most communities and many hospitals have cancer information services and support groups available that may be of service.

Finally, the medical oncologist must be a scientist as well as a humanist. This means he must be able to scrutinize and critically evaluate medical reports in order to arrive at the best treatment plan. Many oncologists in the United States and Canada participate in clinical research on new treatment programs through local medical school or national cooperative group efforts. Organized hospital cancer programs, tumor registries (organized by the American College of Surgeons), and the federally sponsored cooperative group efforts allow practicing physicians to contribute to the development of oncology as a science of cancer management.

A woman needs to understand the reason she is seeing an oncologist. Questions about the stage of her disease and the implications it has for her life or prognosis should be addressed to the medical oncologist. In addition, she should understand the goals of the suggested treatment. Further questions about the actual treatment program and how she can assess the effectiveness of treatment are very important. Some of the questions she might ask with anticipated answers include the following:

Why are drugs used to treat cancer?

Cancer cells can escape from the original tumor and spread throughout the body. Chemotherapy or hormonal drugs can travel through the bloodstream to reach the cancer cells wherever they may be.

How do you know which drugs to use?

Medical research has allowed physicians to compile experience with specific drugs to prove their effectiveness in controlling cancer. Once it is established which chemotherapy or hormonal agents work best, combinations are employed to increase their effect. By combining drugs we hope to see additional therapeutic benefit and less toxicity. In general, drugs that work by different mechanisms are additive and produce a synergistic combination $(1+1 = 3$ or $4)$.

Why are there side effects of chemotherapy?

Chemotherapy drugs work to kill or damage cancer cells throughout the body. The cancer cells are thought to be more susceptible to this type of damage while normal cells can heal themselves more easily. The side effects are the temporary effect of the chemotherapy on the normal tissue.

What can be done to prevent side effects of chemotherapy?

Many side effects can be minimized by using drug combinations in more moderate doses. Certain side effects such as nausea can be prevented by using anti-nausea medications before or after treatment. Simple measures such as holding ice in the mouth while certain drugs are administered intravenously can prevent mouth sores. Patients who receive a drug such as cyclophosphamide that can irritate the bladder can prevent these symptoms by drinking adequate amounts of fluids.

Why does my blood count have to be checked every time I go to receive chemotherapy?

Most chemotherapies can lower the red blood cell, white blood cell, or platelet count, which causes problems. If the white cell count is very low, the woman might be at high risk of serious infection. A low platelet count makes a person susceptible to bleeding or bruising. Anemia is the effect of a low red blood count and might require blood cell transfusions. The intensity of the chemotherapy regimen or the exact medications used determines how severely suppressed the count might be. Blood counts are usually allowed to recover before chemotherapy is safely administered again.

Are there other generalized effects of which the patient needs to be aware?

Many patients who are being treated with chemotherapy will notice fatigue, which may be worst when the white or red blood cell count is lowest. Depression and anxiety are common symptoms when patients are undergoing cancer treatments. Even the end of a preventive chemotherapy program might cause anxiety.

What are the most important side effects?

A suppressed blood count is usually the most serious aftermath of chemotherapy. If the white cell count is very low, the patient is at risk of bloodstream infection, which can be life threatening. A severely low platelet count may allow the patient to bleed internally, which could be critical or cause permanent damage to the body.

What should you expect from cancer treatments?

The goal of a cancer treatment should be clear to the patient. Many patients receive adjunctive or preventive treatment with chemotherapy or hormonal medications (usually tamoxifen). The goal of treatment, therefore, is to prevent any findings of breast cancer. The intention is to improve the cure rate if possible. There is nothing specific to check except to look for the absence of symptoms or physical findings.

Women with metastatic cancer may have a more specific goal of treatment since there are symptoms that might be alleviated, x-ray findings or laboratory tests that could be measured, or even physical findings. Physicians hope to improve symptoms and lengthen survival, but cure is unlikely.

• • •

The patient also needs to understand the benefits and the potential ill-effects of the treatment. Common side effects of chemotherapy must be clearly outlined along with means of preventing or minimizing toxicities. The woman then may have specific questions about the drug therapy as it applies to her, its timing, and even its cost. She may also have questions about her activities, job, or exercise. Possible drug interactions should also be explained before chemotherapy or hormonal therapy is started. The oncologist may want to make use of literature designed for patients by the National Cancer Institute about breast cancer, chemotherapy programs, and specific drugs.

Although a woman may have a primary physician and/or surgeon caring for her before referral to a medical oncologist, the pattern of patient follow-up may be very different after that referral. The oncologist will make suggestions about the frequency of routine examinations, laboratory tests, and x-ray films. During the course of adjunctive chemotherapy the patient will be examined frequently by the medical oncologist. After preventive treatment, follow-up visits will be coordinated with all of her physicians. For the patient with metastatic disease, this pattern may be different, with the medical oncologist serving as a primary physician instead of her family physician or surgeon. The exact pattern of care is established by close communication between the woman and her doctors.

The Oncology Nurse's Role in Caring for Breast Cancer Patients and Their Families
MARY ELLEN HAWF, R.N., O.C.N.

An oncology nurse is a professional registered nurse who is committed to providing optimal care to women diagnosed with breast cancer and their families. She is licensed in the state in which she practices and has completed educational training ranging from a diploma nursing program to a doctorate nursing program. He or she may also be certified in oncology nursing (O.C.N.), demonstrating a level of knowledge sufficient to perform the tasks necessary for competent practice. However, the level of education or degree should never be confused with one's level of competence. Frequently the oncology nurse has provided general nursing care prior to specializing in oncology. Much like physicians, nurses choose a particular area of expertise within the oncology field—surgery, gynecology, medicine, radiation, bone marrow transplantation, pediatrics, research, and hospice. The woman with breast cancer may encounter oncology nurses from several of these specialty areas throughout the course of her care.

Regardless of the nurse's specialty area, she must have extensive knowledge of the disease process, possible treatment modalities, and side effects of treatment and their management. She must also have a thorough understanding of the overall plan of care for each patient.

The nurse may be the woman's first contact when she arrives at the surgeon's office for consultation for a breast lump or for a breast biopsy. The woman is understandably anxious at this time, and the surgical oncology nurse can help alleviate this anxiety by explaining any planned procedures. After the consultation or biopsy, the nurse instructs the patient in care of the biopsy site or assists in coordinating additional tests such as mammography, ultrasonography, or surgery. Once pathology reports, surgical summaries, and x-ray/scan/laboratory reports are complete, more precise planning for definitive treatment will be recommended by the physician. Further discussion with the nurse regarding surgical options, expected recovery period, and post-surgical care is helpful for the woman and her family and permits them to freely express anxieties, fears, and concerns they may be experiencing during this difficult decision-making process. The surgical oncology nurse will focus on methods to minimize the impact of any subsequent surgery to facilitate a quick return to normal daily activity.

If radiation is recommended, the oncology nurse in the radiology department will explain the plan of treatment (radiation therapy alone or in combination with other therapy), type of radiation therapy to be used, dates of treatment delivery, overall length of treatment, location of the planned radiation "field" on the body, types of markings used, possible side effects to expect, and testing to be done to monitor tolerance to the treatment (skin reaction, laboratory results, weight, etc.). The nurse will monitor the patient's skin daily for signs and symptoms of infection or skin breakdown, inquiring about the patient's level of comfort and her ability to manage the symptoms. Suggestions to help the patient maintain healthy skin and to promote comfort will be given as needed.

Referral to a medical oncologist might indicate the need for chemotherapy as a form of treatment. Once again, the oncology nurse will play a vital role. In-depth explanations of recommended chemotherapy will be provided with ample opportunity before beginning therapy for the patient to ask questions and express concerns regarding expected side effects, scheduling of treatment, and anticipated life-style changes. Chemotherapy will be administered by a nurse who has been specifically trained to give chemotherapy drugs safely. This treatment will be given in an ambulatory care facility, hospital, or more frequently in the physician's office. The decision to administer the chemotherapy in one location or another is often determined by the intensity of the chemotherapy regimen prescribed, but it may also be determined by the physical surroundings and capabilities of the facility or patient preference. The nurse, along with the physician, will monitor any toxicities and make recommendations or adjustments in the treatment regimen to safely administer the chemotherapy while still maintaining therapeutic efficacy.

The woman may encounter other oncology nurses who work within the hospital. Some hospitals have a designated floor or "unit" for oncology patients. The nurses who choose to work in these areas are specifically trained to care for patients with cancer and have the knowledge and experience to minister to their needs. This is not to say that the lack of such an oncology unit indicates less knowledgeable or trained personnel. But frequently a designated floor or unit allows for easier coordination of multiple services and more focused attention on the needs of the oncology patient. Recently women with breast cancer are being offered peripheral stem cell/bone marrow transplantation as a treatment option. The oncology nurse working in this area must possess additional intensive care nursing skills to accommodate the potentially acute needs of the person undergoing transplantation. (See Chapter 6 for more information on bone marrow transplantation.)

Oncology nurses working at a home care agency or a hospice are often available to meet the needs of the woman whose cancer is in an advanced stage and those of her family. These nurses make sure that necessary care can be safely provided at home; they make referrals to community agencies and can make arrangements for the woman and her family in the face of imminent death.

Educating the woman and her family is a major responsibility of oncology nurses in all specialty areas. In addition to the details of a specific treatment modality, the oncology nurse will provide nutritional counseling with recommendations for follow-up care, including frequent physician examinations and breast exams, as well as early detection methods recommended for the woman, her family, and caring others. Referrals to community agencies, prosthetic suppliers, support groups, and home care services are also initiated and coordinated by the oncology nurse.

In addition to providing "hands-on" care to these women, the oncology nurse frequently acts as the liaison between the physician and the person with cancer. Although communication between physicians and patients is improving and certainly encouraged, women rely extensively on their nurses as a "sounding board" for their ideas, concerns, anger, grief, hopes, and fears. Given the predominance of females as nurses and males as physicians, a natural female bonding between patient and nurse frequently evolves. The nurse has the unique opportunity to become the patient's confidant.

Since multimodality therapy is commonplace in the treatment of breast cancer, coordination and timing of testing, surgery, treatment, and follow-up care can be quite a challenge for the woman. That challenge may be compounded by news that a newly diagnosed or recurrent breast cancer has been found, presenting a whole new set of decisions regarding treatment and care that needs to be made promptly. Though not intentional, it too frequently escapes the attention of medical professionals that this woman, regardless of her age, may also have a job that she enjoys (or financially needs), children that need car-pooling to and from school, an invalid spouse or relative dependent on her, or previously arranged engagements and commitments, to say nothing of the endless hopes and dreams she has for the rest of her life. The oncology nurse is uniquely aware of all of these pressures, and it is her responsibility to help coordinate a plan of treatment and care that is medically as well as emotionally therapeutic and accommodates a woman's needs and eases some of her tensions.

The role of the oncology nurse is a particularly rewarding one that enables her to establish lasting bonds with cancer patients that help these women cope with their disease and the problems it imposes. These women share with oncology nurses their joys and hopes, their idiosyncrasies, their family pictures and stories, their tears of sadness, as well as their tears of joy.

The Plastic Surgeon's Role in the Rehabilitation of a Woman With Breast Cancer
JOHN BOSTWICK III, M.D.

Plastic surgeons treat patients with a wide range of deformities. They perform aesthetic surgical procedures to counteract the effects of the aging process and reconstructive procedures to repair major body defects such as deformities resulting from birth defects, injuries and scars caused by accidents (including hand injuries and burns), and deformities resulting from cancer treatment.

Breast surgery is a major part of many plastic surgeons' practices.

Women consult plastic surgeons for aesthetic breast operations to enlarge, reduce, or elevate their breasts and for reconstructive breast surgery to replace their missing breasts and nipple-areolae after mastectomy. Recent developments in the field combined with the skills acquired from treating aesthetic breast problems enable plastic surgeons to create aesthetically successful breast reconstructions for patients with all types of mastectomy deformities.

A woman is referred to a plastic surgeon when she is interested in the option of breast restoration. Frequently this referral is made by the general surgeon before or after a planned mastectomy. It also may be made by her family physician or by another member of the breast management team, of which the plastic surgeon is a part. Many women come to the plastic surgeon after referral by other women who have been treated by him for similar problems.

When a woman consults with a plastic surgeon about breast reconstruction, he must consider her psychological state, the stage of her disease, and her need for additional therapy. Management of her tumor is a primary concern, and he will confer with the general surgeon and other members of the team to determine the best care for each woman and the best timing for reconstruction. When immediate reconstruction is planned, he works closely with the general surgeon to coordinate the mastectomy and reconstructive procedures.

The plastic surgeon is also aware of the ongoing concerns that a woman has about her cancer and must deal with her in a humane and sensitive fashion. A woman who is considering breast reconstruction has had to cope with the reality of breast cancer as well as with the loss of her breast. The emotional trauma that she has experienced should never be overlooked by the plastic surgeon in his dealings with her. He needs to provide support and understanding for the special problems and fears that she, as a cancer patient, is confronting.

The plastic surgeon also must be aware of some of the conflicts faced by the woman who inquires about reconstructive breast surgery. Although a woman may want to have her breast restored, she also may fear that reconstructive surgery will cause a recurrence of her cancer. The plastic surgeon needs to be sensitive to this fear and discuss it with his prospective patient. She also may worry that this elective surgery will be misconstrued as mere vanity on her part. The plastic surgeon's role is to reassure her that breast reconstruction is not merely a cosmetic procedure but a beneficial part of her total rehabilitation program.

The plastic surgeon's role in counseling patients is especially important. This interaction takes place before breast reconstruction and sometimes before mastectomy. Consultations should be conducted in a private, quiet atmosphere to enable a woman to feel comfortable and free to speak frankly.

As a counselor, one of the plastic surgeon's chief obligations is to be a good listener. If he does all of the talking, he will never really know what the woman's expectations are for treatment. He should ask open-ended questions that allow her to communicate her feelings and desires. He must understand what a woman expects so that he can design an operation that most nearly produces her desired result. If her expectations cannot be met, he needs to explain the limitations of what surgery can accomplish.

The patient's medical history and the status and treatment of her breast cancer provide the plastic surgeon with important information in formulating a plan for breast reconstruction. He also will perform a physical examination to assess the options for reconstruction. These options will then be discussed with the woman, covering such topics as the pros and cons, expected results, anticipated hospital stay and recovery period, and risks of each approach. If a woman chooses an implant or expander reconstruction, this explanation will also include a full description of these devices and any possible problems or complications associated with them. In addition, the patient will be given an informed consent document that comprehensively describes the pros and cons of these devices and operations. The patient must read this document and ask questions before she signs it and agrees to this operation. Breast reconstruction is a very personal procedure and the woman should understand that no one surgical technique is appropriate for all patients. She should be fully advised of all options. After these explanations, the plastic surgeon can formulate an operative plan that attempts to incorporate his patient's desires and expectations and is designed with her specific needs in mind. He should not assume, however, that a woman will naturally understand the details of her proposed surgery and should carefully review this plan with her.

The actual breast reconstruction is carried out by the plastic surgeon according to the preoperative plan that he and the patient have discussed and agreed on. After reconstruction, the woman returns to the plastic surgeon for periodic evaluations. On follow-up visits the plastic surgeon will continue to encourage his patient and to contribute to her rehabilitation from breast cancer.

The Plastic Surgery Nurse's Role in Counseling and Caring for the Breast Reconstruction Patient

LYNNE A. McCAIN, B.S.N., R.N.

Plastic surgery nurses provide a variety of services for the woman undergoing breast reconstruction. Educating patients about their reconstructive options is an important part of the nurse's role. Once a reconstructive approach has been selected by the patient and the plastic surgeon, the nurse provides specific information on the details of the procedure and her follow-up care.

During an educational session with the nurse the patient and her family may voice questions and concerns that the nurse can address. The nurse can show diagrams of the procedure followed by photographs depicting before and after views of women who have had similar reconstructive procedures. Many women request the opportunity to speak with other patients who have had breast reconstruction performed by the plastic surgeon. These names are provided so that she may contact these women who have already had the procedure that she is going to have. By talking to other reconstruction patients the woman will hear about the experiences of these other individuals and gain personal insights. Although pictures and diagrams are an important tool in educating patients about the different reconstructive techniques, nothing compares with the personal experience of speaking with another woman who has been there. It enables the woman contemplating breast reconstruction to realistically learn what to expect from this operation. It also gives her access to a networking system to share fears and worries and joys. Often women who have had reconstruction are willing to provide a "show-and-tell" session for a new patient so that she may visualize and touch a reconstructed breast.

During the reconstructive experience women encounter plastic surgery nurses from different specialties ranging from operating room and recovery room nurses to hospital and office-based nurses. All contribute to the care and recovery of these women. The operating room nurses are probably the least familiar to the patient since preoperative medications may have been administered before the patient's encounter with these nurses in the operating room. These nurses are attired in hospital scrubs, caps, and masks; they greet the patient, introduce her to the operating room staff, and try to comfort her, often by tucking the woman in with warm blankets, holding her hand until the anesthesia has taken its effect, and answering questions or calming fears. Once the patient is under general anesthesia these highly skilled nurses provide assistance to the plastic surgeon, ensuring that all the surgical instruments are available and that the operation proceeds smoothly.

When the surgery is completed, the patient is transferred to the recovery room where the next team of specialty nurses assumes care of the patient. These recovery room nurses monitor the patient's vital signs, provide pain relief, and reassure the patient that all is well. The recovery room stay may last 1 to 2 hours, depending on the patient's ability to recuperate from the effects of the anesthesia. The nursing staff releases the patient once she is alert, awake, and oriented. Both the operating room and the recovery room nurses are the silent caregivers who provide invaluable assistance to ensure that the operation proceeds smoothly.

The last specialty nurse that the patient encounters during her hospitalization is the bedside nurse. This skilled professional cares for the patient during her time in the hospital and prepares her for discharge by teaching her how to monitor the surgical site(s), how to change dressings, how to empty a surgical drain, how to take prescribed medications, and what restrictions on physical activity are necessary until recovery is complete. These nurses provide teaching sessions throughout the patient's hospital stay to help facilitate her recuperation. In addition to these verbal instructions, the nurse also provides the patient with written instructions that restate the "how to" of home care and recovery.

Nurses are readily available and attentive to the patient 24 hours a day during the patient's hospitalization and are often the first to detect problems that may arise. These nurses are trained to detect even the subtle changes in vital signs, in the surgical site, or in urine output and to respond to these changes before they become problems. The nurse will alert the plastic surgeon to changes and implement necessary alterations in the care plan that are needed to ensure optimal care of the patient to facilitate a speedy recovery.

All of these nurses and the office-based nurses respond to the patient's physical and emotional needs. They recognize that the reconstructive process is not necessarily complete when the incisions are healed. Breast reconstruction after a mastectomy begins a process of emotional healing. Losing a breast after mastectomy is an emotionally devastating experience. The patient finds herself overwhelmed by emotions ranging from anger, depression, isolation, sadness, and finally acceptance. Nurses are often the ones that women turn to for comfort as they try to cope. Many patients feel that they can open up to the nurse more readily because she has helped other women through the same experience and has worked closely with the woman through the reconstructive process.

Some plastic surgery nurses have become involved in organizing support groups for women undergoing breast reconstruction. These groups are often led by a nurse or social worker and they help women to educate themselves about reconstruction, to share feelings, and to know that they are not alone in this experience. During the meetings women discuss issues of self-image, the impact that mastectomy and reconstruction has on sexuality and body image, and other personal concerns that they are hesitant to share with others who have not gone through the same experience.

Plastic surgery nurses are a major source of support to the woman undergoing breast reconstruction. They serve as educators, counselors, and caregivers, ministering to the physical and emotional needs of these women.

 ## *The Team Effort*

Many specialists are involved in the care of the woman with breast cancer. Her primary care doctors she has known and visited for years. She feels comfortable with them and trusts their judgment. Others, however, are specialists she sees for the first time on referral for treatment of her life-threatening illness. The thought of seeing strange doctors is often intimidating to an already stressed woman. Knowledge of what these doctors do and the positive benefit they can provide for the woman with breast cancer might alleviate some of her fears of this experience and help her to feel more in control of her own destiny so that she can regard herself as a participating member of the team rather than a passive recipient of care. In addition, knowledge of the support that nurses can provide throughout this ordeal may help in this coping process. This chapter has been designed to provide this information for women and to demonstrate how the team functions at its best and how individual doctors and nurses, regardless of specialty, can deal with their patients with caring and sensitivity.

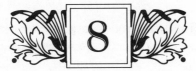

COMMUNICATING WITH YOUR DOCTORS

*I*n society we place so much emphasis on "communication" that it is surprising that the doctor-patient relationship is so often marked by frustration and inability to convey thoughts and feelings effectively. This setting may be the stage for acting out the most significant of life's dramas yet communication is often halting and bewildering. When a woman develops breast cancer, the difficulties in communicating become magnified by the seriousness of the disease itself. Breast cancer attacks a woman's life as well as her femininity; that makes it a powerful silencer. Silence, however, is no solution and women need to be able to relate to their doctors about their health care concerns so that they can make reasonable, educated decisions.

Obviously communication problems are more easily confronted on paper than they are in real life. They are sufficiently important, however, to merit attention and active problem solving. In the previous chapter we explained ways in which specific doctors can help you and listed some of the questions that you might want to ask them. That is only half of the equation. No matter how frightened or intimidated a woman may be by the specter of her disease, she must bring something to the communication process for it to succeed. With that in mind, this chapter attempts to provide women with concrete suggestions for evaluating and selecting their doctors and with skills to facilitate the communication process. The goal is to ensure that women get the information that will empower them to cope with the decisions they have to make and the therapy they must undergo. As most women have emphasized in our surveys and interviews, the worst part of breast cancer is the loss of control and helplessness that a woman feels. The goal of this chapter is to enable a woman to reclaim some of that control.

First let's examine what you as a patient need from the doctor-patient relationship. Those needs are as various as the women who will be reading this book. Some women want the facts presented honestly and in as much detail as possible. They want to know what they have to deal with and then get on with it. Others need a softer, gentler approach, the diagnosis and prognosis presented in a *Reader's Digest* format, softened and accompanied by the appropriate hand-holding and solicitude. Still others don't want to hear what they term the "gory details" and prefer to trust their doctors to do "what is best for them." Obviously these are stereotypes, and many of us will find ourselves somewhere in between. None of these approaches is to be condemned as inappropriate, but it is beneficial for each woman to understand what her expectations of her doctors are and how much information she really wants. Only then can she establish a satisfactory doctor-patient relationship.

Once you have addressed these needs, some basic questions and considerations will help you select a doctor who will meet your expectations.

QUALIFICATIONS AND COMPETENCE
What are your doctor's qualifications and training?

A woman has an obligation to herself to check her doctor out, to find out about his training and credentials, to ask for referrals, and to determine whether this is an area in which this physician has expertise. Information about a doctor's training is readily obtainable in the reference room of your local library in a book entitled *The Directory of Medical Specialists*, which lists only board-certified specialists (see Chapter 12). Board certification is an important credential. It means that after training and an initial period of practice, this doctor has passed a competence test showing that he meets the criteria for practice in the specialty. This book will list the doctor's year of birth, medical school, the year he was licensed to practice, the year of specialty certification, primary and secondary specialties, and type of practice. Other information on training and hospital and medical affiliations also is included. Doctors are listed geographically, making it easy to locate names of doctors in each community. The *American Medical Directory* is another helpful reference, but unlike *The Directory of Medical Specialists*, it does not indicate whether a physician is board certified.

Is your doctor on staff at a medical school–affiliated hospital? Does he have a teaching appointment with that hospital?

Association with a medical school suggests access to the latest techniques, technology, and developments in the field; knowledge of or participation in research efforts; and involvement in the education of residents. Breast cancer is a complex and life-threatening disease; you deserve the best care possible.

What professional associations and societies does this doctor belong to?

He should belong to one or more professional societies, indicating that he has a specific interest in his specialty area and that he has access to the latest developments in his specialty.

Does this physician specialize in breast cancer treatment?

It is not enough to just be a good doctor, the physician you choose, whatever his specialty, should have special expertise in treating breast cancer patients. You need to inquire what portion of his practice is devoted to treating breast cancer. How many breast cancer patients does he see in a year? How many has he treated this year? Last year? If you are consulting with a general surgeon, he should have experience with a variety of surgical techniques for treating breast cancer. You should ask if he performs lumpectomies and modified radical mastectomies and approximately how many of each in a typical year. You want a doctor who has the versatility to provide you with options for care. The same applies to a medical oncologist, radiation oncologist, or plastic surgeon. (More information on selecting a plastic surgeon is included in Chapter 12.)

You should also inquire whether the physician is a member of a breast management team. Comprehensive, coordinated treatment is provided by such a team effort. Members of a team are experienced in working with each other and pool their efforts to consult on your problems, to devise treatment plans that are individualized, and to ease some of the trauma involved in having to see various specialists. This team approach is common at major medical centers and will ensure that your doctors will have access to state-of-the-art technology and have the skills to use it. Ask what specialists are included on the team. At a minimum an effective team has a general surgeon, mammographer, pathologist, medical oncologist, radiation oncologist, and plastic surgeon.

REPUTATION

What is this doctor's reputation within the medical community?

Do you know any of his patients? Ask them about their level of satisfaction with this doctor's care. Patient referrals are an excellent way to find out about a doctor. Also, ask other physicians that you know and respect for their recommendations and their opinions of this particular physician. The local medical society will have a list of recommended physicians in your area, as will the specialty society for which he is board certified. Check all of these sources.

PERSONALITY AND PROFESSIONAL MANNER

A doctor's presence and style may not be the most important consideration for some patients, but certain characteristics are basic to a sound doctor-patient relationship.

Is he courteous?

Courteous treatment is a minimum standard of care that all patients have a right to expect.

Is he pleasant when he talks to you or examines you?

Has he taken the time and effort to learn something about you? Does he make an honest effort to relate to you? Not all doctors can be "Mr. Personality," but it is important for a patient to feel that her doctor is humane and caring; this makes it easier for her to cope with her disease. After all, as one of the women we interviewed explained, "When a woman develops breast cancer, she goes steady with her doctors. She doesn't have to love them, but it is important that she like them because she is going to be spending a lot of time with them." How well you relate to your doctor has a bearing on your treatment program and how you respond. Therefore it is important that he has your respect and regards you as a person, not just a patient.

Does he respect your sense of privacy and modesty?

Obviously there will be times when your privacy will be invaded; physical examinations and case photographs are two cases in point. At those times it is difficult not to feel uncomfortable. But your physician can avoid creating situations that lead to an invasion of privacy and put you at a disadvantage. One such situation is when a doctor tells his patient her prognosis or explains her proposed treatment plan when she is still undressed in his examining room. No woman can think clearly when she is struggling to keep herself covered with a flimsy sheet or gown.

Is he sensitive to your feelings? Does he allow you to express your emotions? Does he make light of your worries?

No matter how insignificant your concerns may seem to someone else, they are important to you and your doctor should never downplay your feelings as trivial. Your emotions warrant similar consideration. Breast cancer is an emotional disease; at times women need to cry, to vent the feelings that tend to surface suddenly and sometimes unex-pectedly. It is important to have a doctor who doesn't suppress or discourage these expressions of feelings. (It is also nice if he has a box of Kleenex conveniently located for those moments.)

ADDITIONAL QUESTIONS

Is he prompt or does he keep you waiting without an explanation? Is he tactful and diplomatic? Does he treat you like an adult? Does he address you by your first name, even though you have just been introduced? Does he seem brusque and hurried? Does he give you his undivided attention during your appointments? Does he refrain from taking phone calls during your examination and conference?

Unfortunately, far too many physicians lack good bedside manners and are woefully unaware of this deficiency. Many of the women in our surveys complained about their doctors keeping them waiting, some-times for hours, with no explanation and no apologies. Then when the doctor appeared, it was "business as usual" with no wasted time. Some even informed their patients that they were running behind "so let's get this over with." In response to just such a comment one women humorously wrote, "If he was in such a hurry, why couldn't he manage to get his butt in to see me 2 hours earlier when my appointment was scheduled?" Taking telephone calls from other patients during their consultations was another source of displeasure and frustration. Not only is this inconsiderate to the patient sitting in the doctor's office, but it is also a violation of privacy for the woman on the phone who thinks she is having a confidential conversation with her doctor.

Although the telephone provides an effective means of contact and communication between doctor and patient, it can be abused.

Our surveys provided ample examples of this abuse, but two cited by Mimi Greenberg in her book *Invisible Scars* merit repeating. One concerns the gynecologist who invited the patient into his office, informed her that she had breast cancer, and before she could respond asked her to step into the waiting room while he answered a call. The other, and one we have heard frequently repeated in various versions, concerns the surgeon who telephoned the patient regarding her breast biopsy results. He cheerfully began, "I have good news and bad news. The bad news is you have breast cancer. The good news is yours is the best kind to get."

• • •

There is a lesson to be learned from these vignettes. A diagnosis of breast cancer deserves and demands your doctor's full and undivided attention—in person, not over the telephone, and without interruption. No patient should ever have to settle for anything less.

COMMUNICATION SKILLS

Are his explanations understandable?

Does he confuse you with medical jargon that you cannot understand? Are his explanations filled with statistics? Does he explain how these numbers actually relate to your prognosis?

Does he take the time to inform you of all of your options?

A patient should demand to know her alternatives. It is unwise to make a decision based on partial information. That limits your alternatives right from the start. Learning all you can about your disease and the options means you can control the way your illness is handled.

Does he ask you if you have any questions? Does he answer your questions to your satisfaction or just gloss over them?

Frequently, particularly in an emotionally charged situation, a patient will not hear everything the doctor tells her during the first explanation. It is important to have a doctor who will take the time to repeat himself and to review his comments until the patient feels that she has a good grasp of what he is trying to tell her.

Is he offended if you inquire about a second opinion?

Second opinions are common in modern medical practice. Many insurance carriers insist on them before authorizing payment. A second opinion is an intelligent way to investigate options thoroughly. It is not meant as an insult. A doctor who implies that you are disloyal or says that he won't treat you if you get a second opinion is doing his patient a disservice.

Is he honest with you?

Your physician cannot always say what you want to hear, but you should expect honesty. He should tell you the truth and not circumvent the issue. A physician cannot promise a cure. What he can do, however, is bring honesty, integrity, and skill to bear on the problem. In all of our surveys with patients a perceived lack of honesty on the part of the doctor was judged to be the most damaging to the patient's well-being and was the main reason why many women said that they changed doctors. Fear of the unknown is far worse than fear of the worst known.

Does your doctor respect your confidentiality?

A patient has a right to expect confidentiality from her physician. It is her health problem, and no one else should be informed of it unless she agrees that this information can be divulged.

Does he listen to you?

Some of the most satisfied patients we have heard from are those who describe their doctors as good listeners. As one woman explained to us, "The best way a doctor can make you feel important is just to listen to you. Sometimes I just need to vent some of my frustrations or fears. I don't want someone to lecture to me; I just want someone to hear me. My doctor is very quiet, but he looks at me when I talk to him, he smiles and nods at the appropriate moments, and he makes me feel that he cares about me and about what I am saying. That makes all the difference to me; it also makes me more receptive to what he needs to tell me."

ACCESSIBILITY

How accessible is your doctor?

Is it difficult to get in to see him or can you arrange appointments with relative ease? Does he have regular and convenient office hours. Is he genuinely interested in having you as a patient or do you have the feeling that he is overbooked and too busy to see you? Is his office within reasonable travel distance?

Does he return your phone calls promptly? The same day?
Does he set aside enough time for you to ask questions at the
end of each visit?

Does he encourage you to ask questions? Does he seem rushed when
he is with you? Does he sit down to talk to you and establish eye contact or do you get the impression that he is in a hurry to get to his next
patient? It is important to feel that your doctor is willing to invest the
time that you need.

When you have problems, is your doctor willing to accommodate
you, to fit you into his schedule?

It isn't reasonable to expect your doctor to spend hours with you every
time you have an appointment, but if you need more time and you ask
for it, your physician should be able to schedule it.

A woman should check to see if her doctor has designated someone in his office to assist patients when he is not available and should
make an effort to meet this individual and talk with him or her.

• • •

The following list summarizes some of the fundamentals that you
should look for and expect in your doctors:
• He should be willing to answer your questions.
• He should explain what you do not understand.
• He should spend a reasonable amount of time with you when you
  need it.
• He should treat you as an adult.
• He should not suppress your expressions of emotion.
• He should not discourage a second opinion.
• He should respect your confidentiality.
• He should always be honest with you.
• He should be sensitive to your feelings.
• He should treat you as a person as well as a patient.

Basically you are looking for a doctor who is competent, caring,
and informative. In turn, you as a patient also must bring something to
this interaction. What can you do to facilitate communication? What
is your responsibility?

THE PATIENT'S RESPONSIBILITIES*

MIMI GREENBERG, Ph.D.

Let's take a look at the patient's responsibilities in the doctor-patient relationship. Following are some suggestions to help you improve the quality of this interaction:

Be prompt. If you want/expect your doctor to respect your time commitments, you must be willing to respect his.

Try not to cancel. Apart from the fact that cancellations, especially at the last minute, are usually annoying because they leave a big hole in the doctor's appointment schedule (and are not likely to increase your popularity with the nurses, technicians, and office staff), you may also wind up sabotaging your own treatment. Certain procedures are on timed schedules or doses (chemotherapy, radiation, and some surgical procedures), and you may be compromising your own prognosis and health. A good rule of thumb is this—don't cancel unless you are too sick to crawl out of bed. And frankly, if you are that sick, you need to be seen.

If you have several questions or wish extra time to speak with your doctor, tell the front desk when you set up the appointment. You will be given a time that is mutually convenient for both of you. Don't wait until the day of your appointment to request extra time. In all probability you won't get it because the schedule will be full. You will be disappointed and feel unnecessarily rejected.

Write down your questions ahead of time rather than trying to retrieve them from memory while you are talking with the doctor. If you don't, it's a cinch that you will forget them and then remember just as soon as you leave the doctor's office.

Take notes and write down the answers to your questions. This will save you many anxious hours and sleepless nights of wondering whether you are accurately remembering what was said.

Be direct in your communications. If you have a request, a problem, or a complaint, let your doctor know so that it can be resolved right away. Most physicians value your feedback and are genuinely interested in improving their services and meeting their patients' needs, but you have to let them know. Unfortunately, many of us insist on playing the role of the perfect patient who never complains and is

---

*Reprinted with permission from Greenberg M. Invisible Scars: A Guide to Coping With the Emotional Impact of Breast Cancer. New York: Walker & Co., 1988.

always nice. This is not to suggest that you become nasty, but if you are unhappy with your doctor, his staff, the treatment, and/or anything else that is breast cancer related, you owe it to yourself and your emotional well-being to make your concerns heard.

Follow the doctor's instructions. Don't improvise. If the instructions seem unreasonable, check to make sure you understood them correctly and discuss the possibility of modification or change. For example, if you are told not to drive for 2 weeks following breast surgery and axillary node dissection but you feel up to driving within a week, get the medical okay before you take matters into your own hands. Without it you may be compromising your treatment and cosmetic results as well as irritating the doctor, who may see you as a difficult patient.

A difficult patient is one who creates unnecessary problems that complicate treatment and/or recovery and are time consuming to the physician and staff. Please be reassured that one misunderstanding will not earn you the reputation of being a difficult patient. But certainly habitual and chronic disregard for instructions will. For instance, if your doctor tells you it will take 6 to 8 weeks before you can safely return to work, it is pointless to call his office every few days to report that you feel fine and wonder if he has changed his mind. Why not use the time constructively to give yourself a special treat—like going to museums, art galleries, concerts, or catching up on your reading or movies you have missed? Physicians call it "patient compliance" and patients call it "following doctor's orders." One reason some women find it a problem is that they tend to feel so controlled by their doctors and/or breast cancer that they grasp (sometimes mistakenly) for any little bit of power that will prove to them and their doctors that they are not helpless. Rushing back to work and driving prematurely are two cases in point.

Be businesslike with your bill payments and with your health insurance refunds. If your company mistakenly sends the reimbursement check to you instead of your physician, present the check immediately to your doctor's office. Also, unless you have been advised to the contrary, you are expected to pay for whatever your insurance does not cover.

Your doctor is only human. Avoid placing him on a pedestal. Once there, the only place to go is down . . . and with a thud! The main problem with idealizing your doctor is that he cannot possibly live up to your expectations and fantasies. Once the bubble bursts, you are apt to feel disappointed, angry, and anxious to switch physicians. And if you do switch, you are likely to repeat the same pattern all over again.

Even in the best doctor-patient relationships there are awkward, embarrassing, and comical situations. One such awkward situation is the fear/belief that your doctor has made a mistake or isn't giving you the right treatment. This is a universal fear that each of us experiences at some point. This is not the initial reaction of "Not me ... there must be some mistake." This is the wave of panic that washes over you at the moment you decide a serious and irreversible error has been made. When these panicky thoughts hit you, ask yourself two questions: (1) Why am I having these thoughts now? Usually you are upset at something or someone else, and without realizing it you seize the most convenient target. (2) What can I do to alleviate my panic? If you are certain you are not upset with someone else and are not transferring your feelings to your doctor or your treatment, then the healthiest and smartest course of action is to present your concerns to the doctor. This will give both of you a chance to examine the reality of the situation. There is no point in keeping your fears to yourself because it will only upset you and cause distance and mistrust in the doctor-patient relationship.

There is also no point in seeking a second opinion without first discussing the problem with the doctor who is treating you. Why? Because doctor No. 2 will need your records from doctor No. 1 to intelligently assess your diagnosis and treatment. In other words, doctor No. 1 is going to find out anyway, so why not give him the courtesy of finding out from you.

How does this affect the relationship? Most competent doctors will not try to talk you out of a second opinion. This is not to say that they love it, either. They don't. It's a big red flag that something is wrong in the relationship. Sometimes it isn't treatment competency at all, but rather the doctor's availability or bedside manner or a communication breakdown that is at the root of the problem.

In any case, you are not the first patient to feel that your doctor has made an error (or that you just feel more secure with another opinion), nor will you be the last. Doctors expect it. It comes with the territory. So take a deep breath, talk to doctor No. 1, and then for your own peace of mind talk to doctor No. 2 as well. You will sleep better for it. And if it turns out that it was all in your imagination, you needn't feel bad. . . .

BUILDING A RELATIONSHIP

Much of what you feel about your disease depends on the kind of relationship you have with your doctors and their attitudes toward treatment and toward you. It is important to approach this relationship with realistic expectations and with a commitment to be an active partner with your doctors in your own care. Just as you will experience bad days, doctors will also, and they are as individual and various in their personalities as the patients that they minister to. Therefore it is important to keep in mind that your doctors will have off days. Furthermore, not all are good communicators. Some are quieter than others; some tend to overwhelm you with information; others only offer it if they are prompted. The patient has to bring something to the communication process. You have to help your doctors understand what you need. If your doctor is one of the reticent ones and you feel he is the doctor for you, then it is your responsibility to ask the questions and probe for information. If you don't know what to say, if you are stunned or upset by his diagnosis or plans for treatment, it is your responsibility to say so. It is okay to ask to have someone accompany you to your appointments if you want someone else to listen to what the doctor has to say as a backup. You may also want to take a list of questions with you for your visit so you don't waste time trying to remember what you wanted to ask. Some people suggest taking a tape recorder to the doctor's appointment to record what is said. Personally, we feel this would tend to create an artificial barrier between the patient and her doctor. And, considering the litigious environment we live in, it may even make your doctor hesitate to speak openly with you. Let your doctor know if you need more help and information. Ask for information on support groups and names of other patients with similar problems that you can talk to. One woman we talked to felt her doctor didn't spend enough time with her. She described him as "a butterfly, flitting in and out of the room before I had time to ask him what I wanted." Her solution was a simple one. During one appointment she placed her arm on his as he was exiting the room and asked if he could please sit down, slow down, and give her some more time. Surprisingly, he hadn't realized how rushed he had seemed. His response was to smile, sit down, and talk to her. From then on their relationship improved. The point is this relationship is one worth working on.

In the years that we have been interviewing women on this topic we have seen attitudes change. Women have become more assertive about their own health care needs, less passive and accepting, and more consumer oriented. This new attitude puts them more in control and positively contributes to their ability to cope with their treatment. They are demanding that their doctors consider the psychological as well as the physical aspects of their disease. They are asking questions and expecting answers. When they don't get them and they don't feel comfortable with their doctors, they are making the necessary changes. Sometimes this means changing doctors; other times it means concentrating their efforts to salvage and improve the situation. Similar to a marriage, the doctor-patient relationship requires mutual participation; it is an active partnership in which both members contribute and ultimately benefit.

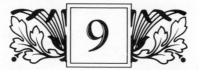

WHY WOMEN SEEK
BREAST RECONSTRUCTION

*I was planting seedlings one day and my prosthesis fell out
while I was bending over. Crying, I picked it up out of the muddy
water. I called a plastic surgeon that same day.*

*I ached to once again be able to put on a
beautiful nightgown and fill it all out. I wanted to shop for pretty
things and feel feminine and sexy again.*

*My breast was an essential part of my femaleness (not femininity)
and I wanted to be breasted.*

*I began to feel good about life again. I decided that I was going to live
and beat cancer. I wanted to look as good as I felt.*

*I was only 17, an oddity for breast cancer patients. I had a
long life to live, and I wanted to live it whole.*

This chapter opens with just five of the many different responses that we received when we surveyed and interviewed women who had undergone breast reconstruction. Their motives for seeking reconstructive surgery were diverse, but all were touching manifestations of the sense of personal loss that these women had experienced after their mastectomies. For some women, the mastectomy was an experience that left them feeling "ugly" and "lopsided." Reconstruction therefore represented a means of regaining beauty and wholeness—harmony of body. For these women, femininity was a core issue, and they felt that their "mastectomy appearance" deprived them of feeling fully female. They loathed the very sight of their bodies and found the simple act of bathing to be repugnant. The mirror had become a fearsome presence in their homes. Furthermore, they avoided any situation in which they might have to disrobe in front of others—dressing rooms, locker rooms, the beach. For a good number of these women, dressing and undressing had become a strictly private act, conducted in closed bedrooms, closets, or bathrooms, until they had their breasts rebuilt and no longer felt the need to hide their bodies.

As one woman explained, "I am again a woman in my own mind. I don't look down anymore and cringe. I just know that something is there, and it has changed my whole life." Clearly, an improved self-image was one of the chief reasons for desiring breast reconstruction expressed by all of the women we surveyed. This elective plastic surgery allowed them to feel more relaxed and more positive about the future.

Relatively few of the women in our survey sought breast reconstruction because it would improve the quality of their sex lives or help to save their marriages or relationships. Motivation for reconstructive surgery was usually self-inspired. Breast reconstruction, however, often had a positive impact on a woman's ability to contribute to and feel good in a relationship. By making her feel better about herself this operation allowed the woman to relate to others, especially loved ones, with increased confidence and self-assurance.

Many women did allude to their children as a powerful motivating factor. Young women, in particular, worried that their small children would be frightened by their scarred chests, would ask uncomfortable questions, or would fear for themselves. They did not want their children to see them "deformed." They also wanted to set an example for their daughters if they, too, must face breast cancer one day—to give them hope for restitution. Other older women said they had breast reconstruction to encourage their daughters to consider the same option. As one woman explained, "My daughter had breast cancer at the age of 28. She and I had our breasts removed the same year, and I thought that if I had reconstruction she would follow."

A family history of breast cancer also figured into a woman's decision for breast reconstruction. It was sobering to see how many of the women who answered our surveys had mothers, sisters, grandmothers, and aunts who had breast cancer. They had witnessed their loved ones' struggles firsthand. They sought to avoid some of the traumas that their relatives had experienced. As one woman related, "I grew up seeing my mother with a radical mastectomy on one side and a modified on the other; I saw her struggle getting clothes so that she would look 'normal.' I did not want to spend the rest of my life going through the same thing that she did." Other women referred to the positive reconstructive experiences of close relatives. One woman's identical twin had breast reconstruction, and she laughingly related that "she needed reconstruction also to maintain the symmetry. After all, if she remained breastless, they would no longer be identical." For these women, reconstruction represented a positive way to confront their heritage.

The search for restitution and return to wholeness was a strong motivating factor for all of the women we interviewed, and this reason also pervaded the answers to our questionnaire. Even when the results of reconstruction were not perfect, the woman's dissatisfaction seemed to be minimal because the breast was now a part of her body and could again be incorporated into her self-image. As one woman said, "The reconstruction is not like a normal breast; there are some problems. It is too hard and it shifts around, but I wouldn't go back to the way I was for anything. I love my new breast, hardness and all. I am not embarrassed to undress in front of someone now. I don't feel like a freak anymore. I feel like a sexual person again. I am whole again."

Elimination of the need for an external prosthesis was another important reason why many women elected to have reconstructive surgery. Women seemed to feel constantly aware of the presence of a false breast, worrying that it would become dislodged and the lopsided chest would be exposed. In their attempts to hide their deformity some women even resorted to using surgical tape to solidly fix their false breasts to their chests.

Other women who were large-breasted objected to the size and weight of the prosthesis necessary for symmetry with their remaining breast. For these women, the weight of the prosthesis created a physical imbalance and they felt as if they were being pulled to one side. Furthermore, the heavier the prosthesis, the greater its tendency to pull away from the woman's body, resulting in her effort to counterbalance this force by holding herself very straight. Some women actually said that they developed back problems and were unable to function without pain and disability. One woman, whose remaining breast was a bra size 41, had to be helped up from bed in the morning because the strain on her back had become so severe and debilitating.

The fit and coverage of the prosthesis was another area of concern and displeasure for women. Women with radical mastectomies consistently stated that the external prosthesis did not provide adequate coverage for their deformities. Their prostheses served primarily for filling out the form of their missing breasts; they did nothing to restore the anterior fold of the axilla or fill the upper chest area just under the collarbone.

Because a woman's prosthesis is fitted to provide breast symmetry when she is upright with her arms at her side, it does not move with her and is often unsuitable for the athletic woman who actively participates in sports. Accounts of prostheses that fell out on the tennis courts or slipped over to a woman's armpit during running or aerobic exercise were prevalent in our interviews and the source of much embarrassment to the women involved. With strenuous activity, this artificial breast was easily displaced or dislodged and could even float out of a bathing suit during swimming. It also could prevent the escape of heat from a woman's chest and cause skin irritation and skin rashes. Thus, for practical reasons of movement and comfort, many women felt that an external prosthesis was a nuisance and an inconvenience. "My prosthesis gets in my way. It interferes when I clean, exercise, or bend over." As one woman explained, "Prosthetic devices may be great in the beginning, but they are not totally comfortable. With breast reconstruction, one can feel whole again with no shifting of the prosthesis." The freedom afforded by reconstruction was emphasized by another woman who complained, "I enjoy being active; I am a swimmer and a golfer. My first prosthesis was large to match the existing breast, and it was cumbersome and floated when I dived."

For many women, one of the real bonuses of breast reconstruction was the increased variety of style and cut it allowed them in clothing. Reconstruction eliminated their need "to shop for clothes with higher necklines and specially designed swim wear." They now gained pleasure from the very act of shopping for clothing and once again felt excited about the possibility of purchasing lacy lingerie, pretty bras, and attractive blouses. Proud of their newfound ability to display a cleavage if they desired, they were also secure in the knowledge that when they were dressed there was absolutely no way that anyone could ever tell that their breasts had been reconstructed.

Before they had breast reconstruction none of these women regarded their prosthesis as a part of them or as a new breast. It seems never to have been incorporated into their body image, but instead was regarded as a necessity, a symbol of something missing and a constant reminder of the real breast. These women repeatedly emphasized their need to feel less obsessed with the cancer experience and a desire to rid themselves of their sense of deformity, which had resulted from having a mastectomy. Some felt that breast reconstruction relieved them of a cancer "stigma."

Interesting also was the reaction of older women we surveyed. Some of these individuals, in their late sixties and seventies, did not have reconstructive surgery because it was not a viable alternative when they had their mastectomies years earlier. They had lived so long without breasts they felt they were too old to bother with additional surgery. These women readily agreed, however, that if their daughters were to develop breast cancer and require mastectomies (and their daughters had an increased risk) they would urge them to have their breasts restored. Other women, in their seventies and eighties, had only recently developed breast cancer and their reaction was very different. They readily embraced the option of breast reconstruction, proclaiming that they had "lived this long with breasts and intended to live the rest of their lives with them as well." Age was not a deterrent, and these women expressed extreme satisfaction with their decision and were quick to recommend this option to their friends, who increasingly were being touched by this disease. For all of these women, breast reconstruction represented an exciting option and they felt that it would be "wonderful to have two breasts again."

In further examining motivations for seeking breast reconstruction, we noticed a definite correlation between age and marital status of a woman and her corresponding interest in reconstructive breast surgery.

Today, breast cancer is occurring with increasing frequency in young women. Moreover, breast cancer occurs with greater frequency in women who have never had children. Concomitantly, there are more childless women who are single than married. A mastectomy and the resultant deformity pose a number of especially uncomfortable and difficult questions for single women in the early stages of an intimate relationship.

How does one explain a missing breast to a potential lover? Some of the questions raised by women facing this situation follow:
• Do I tell my date I had a mastectomy?
• What is the right timing for this disclosure? Before or after discovery?
• Do I keep my body covered while we are having sex?
• Will I continue to be seen as desirable after I admit to a deformity?
• Can I feel sexy and good about myself with a deformity? Or is it easier to avoid sexual situations?

Many women take up the last option, preferring to steer clear of relationships that might lead to sexual intimacy. As one woman expressed it, "I could not face my life with just one breast. I was 42 years old and single when I had my mastectomy. I buried my sexuality for 13 months until I had the reconstruction."

Just as single and divorced women interested in meeting men and beginning new relationships often cite reconstruction as an attractive option, some widows reported feeling that breast surgery might be one step in a personal program of "starting over." Although many women who have had mastectomies after age 65 decide not to have additional elective surgery, age alone has no relationship to how women feel about themselves. Women at any age feel the sense of loss when they have a mastectomy. They still desire to return to wholeness. Many of the breast reconstruction patients we interviewed were over 50, and they felt that this surgery had renewed and invigorated them. In fact, some of the happiest and most satisfied women who have had breast reconstruction have been in these older age groups.

For many women, reconstruction is a symbol that they are completing the treatment and rehabilitation phase of their lives and are ready to get back to living. When the surgeon recommends reconstruction, he is saying that he feels good about the woman's chances for survival. In these cases, reconstruction represents a positive and reassuring statement from the general surgeon.

Reasons women seek reconstruction are as varied and individual as are the women themselves. Some women focus on the practical considerations of comfort and convenience, whereas others have psychological and aesthetic concerns; reconstruction bolsters their sense of femininity, self-confidence, and sexual attractiveness. Still other women seek peace of mind about the cancer experience, a realignment of their body image, and a return to wholeness. No one answer is better or more important than any other. The fact remains that after a woman's breast has been removed, a deformity exists and many women feel a deep sense of loss. The desire for restitution is a healthy reaction to this problem. It helps a woman to reconfirm her body image and bring her self-awareness back into harmony. For those women who feel the need to rebuild their bodies and replace their missing breast or breasts, reconstruction offers a positive source of hope for the future.

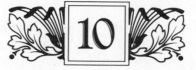

QUESTIONS FREQUENTLY ASKED ABOUT BREAST RECONSTRUCTION

B reast reconstruction is a frequently misunderstood surgical procedure. Although many women desire the operation, some hesitate to request it, fearing that it is not appropriate for them. Some worry that reconstruction can cause cancer or mask a recurrence; they may be concerned over the use of implants, which are foreign materials, and may be unaware of newer reconstructive techniques that allow women to have breast reconstruction using their own natural tissue. Others have anxieties about the appearance of the new breast, the prominence of scars, or the development of further complications. Still others are concerned about the costs and the correct timing of surgery.

Some queries are so frequently posed to the doctor half of our writing team that we have prepared the following list of questions and answers to serve as a primer.

Who is a candidate for breast restoration?

Today most mastectomy patients can have their breasts rebuilt; age is not a factor in determining a woman's suitability nor is her type of mastectomy or the placement of her mastectomy scar. Women who have had radical mastectomies (removal of the breast and chest wall muscles) or modified radical mastectomies (removal of the breast but chest wall muscles left intact) can now have satisfactory breast reconstructions. It does not matter how much time has elapsed since a woman's original cancer surgery. There is no statute of limitations for reconstruction and no disadvantage to waiting. Women have had successful reconstructive breast surgery 15 to 20 years after mastectomy.

How does a person's age affect the success of reconstructive surgery? Are you ever too old?

A woman's age is not as important a factor in determining the ultimate success of her breast reconstruction as is her motivation for the operation and her general health. Many women in their seventies have had successful reconstructive breast surgery and are very pleased with the results of this operation. A woman is never too old if she is in good health, is motivated to have breast reconstruction, and selects a type of reconstruction compatible with her general physical condition.

Does the size and extent of a woman's cancer have any influence on whether she should have her breast reconstructed?

Women with small tumors have the best prognosis for survival, and breast reconstruction is most frequently performed for these women. Immediate breast reconstruction is a viable and appealing option for women whose tumors have been discovered in the earliest stages. Women with large tumors that have spread to the lymph nodes also may have their breasts restored, but the timing of their operation is influenced by the type and sequencing of the adjunctive treatment they require.

Are women with advanced disease eligible for this operation?

Occasionally a woman whose breast cancer has spread beyond her breast region requests this surgery. When this happens, the surgeon must reconcile the woman's present health status with her desire for "wholeness." Should he operate on a woman whose prognosis is poor and who may not live to enjoy her restored breast? Is this surgery worth the time, pain, and money it will cost when the potential time for enjoyment may be limited? For this woman, reconstruction must be discussed and performed in the context of improving the quality of her remaining life. Many women desire this procedure despite the presence of systemic disease. As one woman explained, "Even if I die tomorrow, it was worth it. I want to go out just like I came in." If the woman's motivation is strong and if she is fully informed about this surgery, then her psychological and emotional needs are an important consideration. Some surgeons feel that these women with advanced disease are among their most satisfied patients. The decision for breast reconstruction cannot be made in isolation and requires consultation and follow-up with the breast management team. The final decision must be made by a well-informed patient.

Are there some women who are not suitable for breast reconstruction?

Yes, some women should not have breast reconstruction. Their emotional state, motivations, or personal circumstances may indicate that they cannot effectively cope with a major operation and recuperation.

Women also may not be suitable candidates for this operation if their general health status is poor. For example, if a woman has advanced diabetes mellitus, a recent stroke or heart attack, or severe chronic lung disease, she should not be considered for this procedure.

What are the timing options for breast reconstruction?

Reconstruction can be performed immediately, that is, right after the mastectomy or during the same hospital stay, or it can be performed on a delayed basis, that is, a few days, several months, or many years after the initial mastectomy. Today many women who are considering mastectomy learn about breast reconstruction and the possibilities for immediate reconstruction from their general surgeons *before* they have their cancer surgery. Frequently their surgeons will refer them to a plastic surgeon so that they can investigate the option of breast reconstruction and the best timing for this operation. Although most women have delayed reconstruction, immediate reconstruction is being requested and performed with much greater frequency because it offers women a reprieve from the deforming effects of mastectomy and a reduction in the number of procedures she has to undergo. Most medical centers now have breast management teams experienced in performing immediate breast reconstruction and are able to offer this option to many of the women considering mastectomy. Furthermore, with the development of tissue expansion, the use of autologous tissue (a woman's own natural tissue), and other new reconstructive techniques, the results of immediate reconstruction have improved considerably and the patient can reasonably anticipate respectable aesthetic results. Most women are pleased with the psychological and aesthetic results of immediate breast reconstruction. The ultimate decision about the timing of reconstruction must be made by a fully informed patient in consultation and agreement with her cancer surgeon and her plastic surgeon to ensure the best treatment for her cancer. (See Chapter 13 for more detailed information on the advantages and disadvantages of immediate and delayed breast reconstruction.)

Who are suitable candidates for immediate reconstruction?

Although immediate breast reconstruction is not appropriate for every patient, it is becoming a more frequently chosen approach for breast reconstruction. Today many breast cancers are being discovered at an early, more curable stage. Women with early breast cancer are the natural and obvious choices for immediate breast reconstruction should breast-conserving surgery not be selected; this would include women in general good health with small tumors (about 1 inch in diameter or less) and no involved axillary lymph nodes (indicating less likelihood that the cancer has spread beyond their breast tissue). Of these early cancer patients, young women, women with a strong desire for breast preservation, women with small breasts, and women who require bilateral (both breasts) reconstruction are particularly appropriate for an immediate procedure.

Who are suitable candidates for delayed reconstruction?

A woman who had a mastectomy before reconstructive procedures were offered or readily available is a natural candidate for delayed reconstruction. The woman with positive lymph nodes, indicating the disease has spread and additional therapy is necessary to treat her cancer, also is an appropriate candidate for a delayed procedure. Another candidate is the woman who needs time to evaluate whether she wants breast reconstruction. The delay between the mastectomy and the reconstruction gives her the opportunity to get acquainted with her plastic surgeon and decide on the best approach for her.

Are the aesthetic results of immediate breast reconstruction as good as those that can be obtained with delayed reconstruction?

Experience with immediate reconstruction over the past 10 years indicates that results are as good as and often better than those achieved with delayed reconstruction. With the newer mastectomy approaches aimed at skin conservation, the mastectomy scars usually can actually be reduced with immediate reconstruction. To achieve the best possible aesthetic result some plastic surgeons prefer to perform immediate surgery for women with small breasts because it is easier to match the remaining breast. Symmetry also is facilitated in women who are having both breasts removed. Women choosing immediate reconstruction need to understand, however, that the immediate operation is not the final operation. Similar to delayed reconstruction, additional procedures will be necessary to produce a symmetric, aesthetic breast appearance. (See the following questions for more information.)

A woman who desires an immediate breast reconstruction should inquire about how many immediate operations her reconstructive surgeon ordinarily performs (as compared to delayed procedures) and how the results he can obtain with an immediate breast reconstruction compare to those he can produce with a delayed procedure.

What are the psychological benefits from breast reconstruction?

Each woman benefits from breast reconstruction in her own personal and individual manner. Many women who have had their breasts rebuilt have said that this operation made them "feel better about themselves . . . normal or whole again." Some women indicated that it relieved them of a constant reminder of the cancer and the mastectomy. Other women were pleased at the freedom it afforded them compared to wearing an external prosthesis. (See Chapters 9, 11, and 18 for more information.)

How will a woman's breast reconstruction affect her relationship with her husband, family, friends, or loved ones?

Breast reconstruction usually does not change interpersonal relationships. It can, however, give the woman a boost in self-esteem, and as her feelings about herself improve, she can more thoroughly enjoy the normal relationships and activities of her life.

A woman will be disillusioned if she expects this surgery to remedy preexisting personal problems, repair a faltering relationship, or please another individual. To be worthwhile a woman's rebuilt chest must satisfy her personal, but reasonable expectations.

How many operations are needed for breast reconstruction?

Aesthetically acceptable reconstructions usually can be completed in two operations. The first operation includes the reconstruction of the chest wall and breast mound and adjustments of the remaining breast (if indicated). A possible operation on the other breast would include enlargement, reduction, or uplifting to eventually achieve breasts of comparable size and position (see Chapter 14). (For the immediate breast reconstruction patient, these adjustments are often accomplished during a second procedure.) The second procedure is less extensive and includes nipple-areola reconstruction (see Chapter 16) and any additional operations that improve breast symmetry. When a temporary tissue expander is used initially, the permanent implant is placed during the second operation and nipple-areola reconstruction is then delayed until a third operation, which can be performed on an outpatient basis. One-stage procedures (building both the breast and nipple-areola in one operation) have a higher incidence of malposition of the nipple-areola and breast asymmetries; these problems can be avoided with a two-stage procedure.

How many doctor visits are necessary for each different reconstructive approach?

Before the operation the patient usually sees the reconstructive surgeon once or twice to discuss the details of the surgery and address questions. A follow-up visit is ordinarily scheduled approximately 1 week after the operation, with another visit planned about 6 weeks later. When tissue expansion is done, a woman may need to return for up to three or four additional visits so the saline volume in the tissue expander can be adjusted. No matter which reconstructive procedure has been used, the surgeon will want to see a woman yearly for follow-up visits after her breast reconstruction.

Are blood transfusions necessary for breast reconstruction?

Blood transfusions are often necessary for flap procedures and microsurgical procedures and for some immediate breast reconstructions. Simple implant or expander placement usually does not require transfusion. To alleviate the fear and risk of blood-borne viruses, however, many surgeons request that patients donate 1 to 3 units of their own (autologous) blood for possible reinfusion in the operative and postoperative period. More blood will be needed for bilateral procedures and for mastectomies performed in conjunction with an immediate flap breast reconstruction. It is usually preferable to delay the operation for several weeks to allow enough time for the patient to donate her own blood. A few weeks' delay does not adversely affect the eventual treatment of the breast tumor, and it is best to prepare for the operation properly. Some patients prefer to obtain additional donor-directed blood (from relatives or friends) for transfusion when necessary. Currently, use of blood from the general donor pool is almost never necessary for breast reconstruction patients.

Will breast reconstruction cause cancer?

Breast reconstruction patients usually have already had a mastectomy in which the surgical oncologist removed as much breast tissue as possible. After mastectomy, sometimes a few cells from the breast tumor persist in the region of the mastectomy and later grow in this area (called a local recurrence). The likelihood of local recurrence is highest in women whose cancer has spread to the axillary lymph nodes. Radiation therapy and chemotherapy help to reduce that risk. The rate of local recurrence after a mastectomy for early breast cancer is generally low.

There is no evidence of any kind, however, that breast reconstruction causes cancer to grow or increases the chance of recurrence. Scientific studies have shown that the incidence of local recurrence after a mastectomy is not increased or affected by breast reconstruction, regardless of the technique used. Reconstruction with implant placement or the patient's own tissue does not increase the risk of local recurrence. It has also been noted that the type of tumors seen in local recurrence after breast reconstruction are the same as seen in patients who did not have breast reconstruction.

Will the reconstruction hide the recurrence of cancer or prevent the detection of a new cancer?

The site of local recurrence of breast cancer is usually in the mastectomy scar, in the skin flaps, or in the axillary (armpit) area. To monitor the woman's breast area for local recurrence after breast reconstruction with implants or expanders, the reconstructive surgeon places the breast implant behind the mastectomy area, usually under the underlying layer of muscle. When reconstructing the breast with a flap of the woman's own tissue, the tissue is placed behind the woman's chest skin. There is little difficulty in detecting an early local recurrence because the breast implant or the flap is beneath the skin and therefore does not obscure the frequent sites of local recurrence. Generally, if a small area of recurrence is discovered in the mastectomy skin, this area is surgically removed (often as an outpatient procedure). The implant, expander, or flap does not need to be disturbed or removed. Additional therapy (radiation or chemotherapy) may be required, however, to protect against another recurrence or possible spread of the cancer to other parts of the body. (Detailed information on breast implants is provided in Chapter 13.)

Will a woman be able to detect tumors as easily after reconstruction?

After reconstruction with an implant or expander beneath the muscle layer or with a flap* from the back (latissimus dorsi flap), the skin and scar are actually pushed forward and thus new tumors or local recurrences usually can be felt easily on breast self-examination (BSE). If the cancer recurs, it can be found by periodic checks of the skin to detect any new lumps. That is why it is equally as important for women to continue to perform BSE after a mastectomy whether they have had breast reconstruction or not.

Detection of tumors may be somewhat more difficult when a woman's breast has been reconstructed with the lower abdominal TRAM (transverse rectus abdominis musculocutaneous [muscle/skin]) flap or with the buttock (gluteus maximus) flap. Because this tissue is moved from a distant site and vascularity may be decreased, it sometimes develops firm, thickened areas of fat that may be confused with a local recurrence. These areas, however, are within the abdominal or buttock tissue and can be differentiated from a local recurrence. Sometimes mammography, ultrasonography, or a biopsy may be necessary for a definitive diagnosis. If a biopsy is needed, it can sometimes be done with a fine needle to avoid a surgical incision.

Does breast reconstruction compromise a woman's immune system?

There is no medical evidence that breast reconstruction or general anesthesia compromise a woman's immune system. Some believe, however, that a woman who has breast cancer may already have a compromised immune system.

What is the best placement of a mastectomy scar for the woman who desires breast reconstruction?

The best placement for this scar is in a low oblique position, extending from below the axilla to the inner lower breast area. This scar is easily covered by a brassiere, and frequently a portion of the scar can be reopened and the implant placed through it to avoid creating a new incision and thus a new scar. Sometimes, however, the primary cancer is located in an area of the breast that makes it impossible for the

---

*A flap is tissue that is moved from one area of the body and grafted to another site.

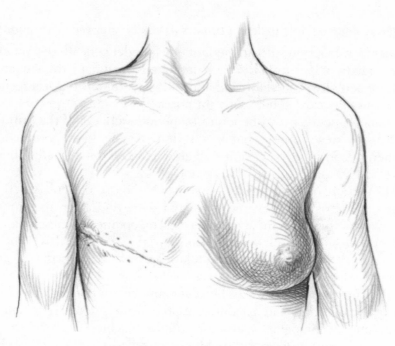

Mastectomy scar in oblique position

surgeon to leave an oblique scar, especially when it is high and medial in the breast area. When immediate breast reconstruction is done, the general surgeon and the reconstructive surgeon can plan the location of the incisions to ensure the best placement for the breast reconstruction. Sometimes a separate, shorter incision is also made to remove the tumor in the upper breast region.

What can be done if the mastectomy scar is in a bad location?

Breast reconstruction can be done with a mastectomy scar in any position. The scar position cannot be changed, but the reconstructive implant can be positioned through this scar and the scar revised to provide the best possible appearance.

Can the plastic surgeon totally remove the mastectomy scar when he restores the breast?

The scars from the mastectomy cannot be removed, although they sometimes can be reduced or made less obvious by a plastic surgery procedure called scar revision. A scar line will always be present where the original cancer surgery was performed. Initially the scars will be red and raised, a condition that will persist for several months after the operation. This redness (indicative of increased blood flow during the healing process) and thickness will subside over the next 1 or 2 years as the scars improve in appearance and become less obvious. Scars in fair-skinned women tend to remain red for a longer period of time. It takes less time for the scars of older women to fade. Some women heal with thick scars, and this tendency is obvious from the appearance of the mastectomy scar as well as any other scars that they may have.

What type of new scars are created by reconstruction?

Reconstruction using the existing tissues or by expanding the existing tissues is most frequently accomplished through the mastectomy scar. No new scar is created. Sometimes, if additional skin is needed to reconstruct the breast, other scars will be created when this skin is inset into the breast. New scars on the breast usually extend along the lower breast crease and either up to the old scar or up to the nipple level.

Whenever new tissue is added, scars will be left where the tissue is obtained.

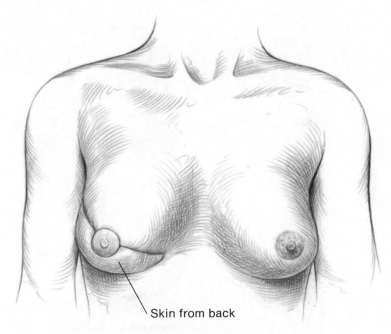

Skin from back

Breast reconstruction with a flap of tissue from the back (latissimus dorsi)

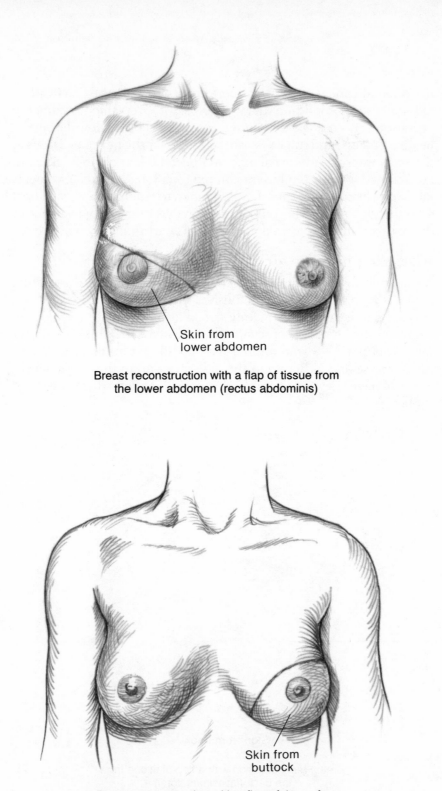

Skin from
lower abdomen

Breast reconstruction with a flap of tissue from
the lower abdomen (rectus abdominis)

Skin from
buttock

Breast reconstruction with a flap of tissue from
the buttock (gluteus maximus)

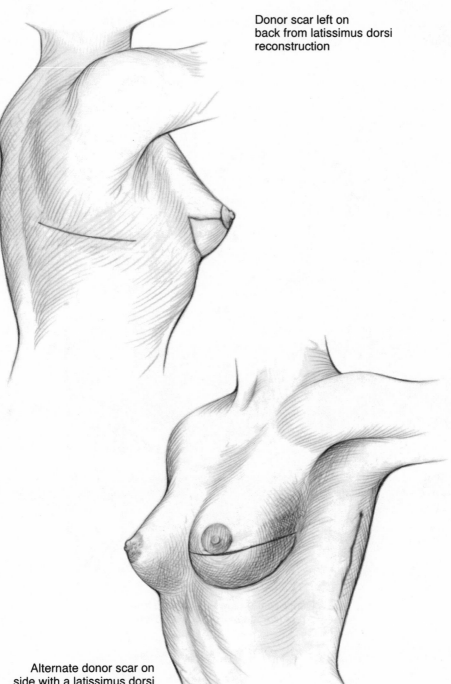

Donor scar left on
back from latissimus dorsi
reconstruction

Alternate donor scar on
side with a latissimus dorsi
reconstruction

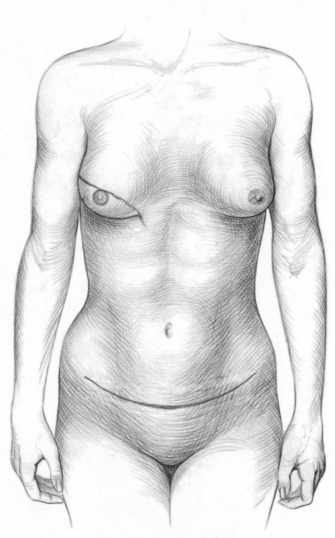

Donor scar on lower abdomen from
rectus abdominis reconstruction

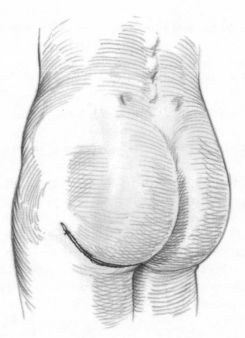

Donor scar left on buttock from
gluteus maximus reconstruction

Common donor sites are the back, side, abdomen, and buttocks. Scars on the back will either be left across the back or under the arm. The abdominal scar will usually extend across the lower abdomen just above the pubic hairline. The buttock scar will be in the crease or across the midportion of the buttock region.

How much skin is removed at mastectomy and can you be sure enough can be preserved for breast reconstruction?

When a woman has a mastectomy to treat her breast cancer, the oncologic surgeon usually removes some skin around the biopsy site as well as the nipple-areola. The incision extends to the axillary region to gain access to the lymph nodes. Studies have shown that it is not necessary to remove additional skin from the breast region as was done in the past. Therefore more skin can be spared and preserved for breast reconstruction. In some instances, particularly when a flap of the patient's own tissue is available for the reconstruction, the skin at the biopsy site and area of nipple-areola removal is replaced with the skin on the flap. Any additional skin that is needed is supplied from the remaining skin at the mastectomy site. With this approach, the skin of the restored breast has the same consistency and appearance as the skin of the opposite breast. Furthermore, when less skin is removed initially, the mastectomy scars are shorter and the extra skin that is left is filled out by the transferred breast tissue or the breast implant or expander that is inserted.

Actually, a woman's breast can be reconstructed regardless of the amount of tissue remaining after the mastectomy. When the pectoralis major muscle and sufficient breast skin are present, a simple reconstruction with an implant or expander can be done. When much of the skin or pectoralis major muscle is missing, a flap, either from the back, lower abdomen, or buttock area, is usually necessary.

If a woman knows that she would like to have breast reconstruction before her mastectomy, her general surgeon should be informed so that he can confer with her plastic surgeon (if she has already selected one) to ensure the best possible physical condition for the reconstruction.

Is it necessary for a woman's normal breast to be modified to match the new one?

Many times a good match can be achieved with tissue expansion and implant placement without touching a woman's normal breast. Sometimes, to avoid altering the opposite breast, it may be necessary to reconstruct the missing breast using a flap procedure. When the normal breast is very large and sags or is very flat and small, the surgeon may not be able to match it and some modification might be required. (See Chapters 13 and 14 for additional information on this subject.)

What areas can be reconstructed? Can large deformities and chest hollowness be filled in?

Predictably good restoration of the breast shape, contour, and size can now be achieved though breast reconstruction. It often improves the appearance of (but may not remove) scars, skin grafts, or radiation-damaged skin. The upper chest and axillary deformity after a radical mastectomy can be filled in and corrected. The infraclavicular area can be rebuilt, and the missing anterior axillary fold can be recreated. Restoration of these areas, however, requires the use of additional donor tissue from the back, lower abdomen, or buttocks and the subsequent creation of new scars in these areas.

Can the missing nipple be reconstructed?

Both the central projecting nipple and the darker surrounding areola can be reconstructed. This procedure is usually done as a second operation after the proper breast shape and size have been obtained. Although there are several different methods for reconstructing the nipple, some of the most effective techniques use tissue available at the site of the new nipple. The areola can be reconstructed from a circular graft of excess skin near the mastectomy scar or from the abdominal scar if an abdominal (TRAM) flap (see p. 302) has been used for the reconstruction. With increasing frequency, when extra skin is not available, a surgical tattoo can recreate the areola and the reconstructed nipple can be colored to the proper shade to match the opposite nipple. (See Chapter 16 for more detailed information on the different techniques for nipple-areola reconstruction.)

What types of implants and expanders are available for breast reconstruction?

The different categories of implants and expanders and a detailed discussion of these devices and associated benefits and risks are presented in Chapters 11 and 13.

How are breast implants and tissue expanders used for breast reconstruction?

A silicone implant or expander is often inserted under a woman's skin or muscle to create a breast mound during breast reconstruction. For breast reconstruction with implants to be successful, the implant must provide volume, projection, and size similar to that of the opposite breast. Just as the appearance of the normal female breast changes with age, breast implants may also need to be changed or adjusted over time to maintain ideal results. The use of tissue expanders makes obtaining the proper size for the breast reconstruction more likely. Changing the size of the expander is easier when the fill valve is left in place.

Can a woman's breast be built with her own natural tissue without the need for breast implants or expanders?

Reconstruction using flaps of the patient's own tissue (autologous breast reconstruction) is a viable and increasingly popular option for many women. The consistency and feel of the reconstructive breast closely approximate a normal breast. Sources of donor tissue are areas of excess tissue such as the lower abdomen, the back, or buttocks. The donor scar can also be hidden so that a significant deformity is not created. Many women who have gained some weight over the years find this an excellent opportunity to accomplish two goals at one time: rebuilding a full and natural breast while contouring an area of abundant fatty tissue. Many women have also noted some return of sensation to their breasts after they are rebuilt with their own tissue. The nerves of the breast are now being connected microsurgically to the flaps used for breast reconstruction to facilitate sensory return.

When breasts are reconstructed with the patient's own tissue, breast implants are usually not necessary. One of the prime reasons that many women choose this approach is to avoid the insertion of a foreign material in the body. If a woman is very slender and lacks the excess fatty tissue necessary to build a breast without the need for a supplementary implant, particularly if she needs to have both of her breasts reconstructed (bilateral breast reconstruction), she may want to consider selecting a simpler procedure involving implant or expander placement. (Autologous breast reconstruction techniques are discussed in great detail in Chapter 13.)

What is the TRAM flap? Is it the same as a "tummy tuck"?

The *t*ransverse *r*ectus *a*bdominis *m*usculocutaneous (TRAM) flap is a method of breast reconstruction in which a woman's lower abdominal tissue is transferred to the breast region and reshaped to form a breast that is symmetric with her opposite breast. Since this transverse ellipse of tissue is moved from the lower abdomen to the breast region, the blood supply is maintained because the tissue is left attached to strips or pedicles of the central abdominal muscle. The name "TRAM flap" is derived in part from the muscle it is attached to—the rectus abdominis muscle. This operation is often referred to as the "tummy tuck" procedure because the abdominal portion of the procedure in which the donor tissue is taken from the woman's abdomen is similar to the "tummy tuck" operation (abdominoplasty) to improve lower abdominal contour. In both procedures the abdominal area is closed and the scar extends across the lower abdomen.

How are microsurgical techniques used for breast reconstruction?

One of the major advances in plastic and reconstructive surgery over the past few years has been the development and refinement of microsurgical techniques for reconstructive surgery. These procedures are performed while visualizing the operative field through the magnification of an operating microscope, thereby permitting the repair and suture of tiny vessels and nerves. Microsurgical techniques are particularly helpful when tissue needs to be moved from a distant part of the body to an area to be reconstructed. Common donor sites for free flaps include the abdomen, buttocks, thigh (although the thigh flap donor scars are often objectionable), and back. The buttocks was one of the first distant areas used for breast reconstruction via microsurgery. Since the blood supply cannot be preserved when moving buttock tissue this long distance, a microvascular (involving the small blood vessels) technique is used to hook up the blood vessels of the buttocks to the blood vessels in the woman's breast region. Microsurgery can also be used to reconnect some of the sensory nerves in the breast area, thus providing the reconstructed breast with more sensation than might otherwise be possible with another type of breast reconstruction. The TRAM flap, described previously as a pedicle flap (one that is transferred while still attached to its blood supply), can also be transferred microsurgically as a free flap.

Is an implant or a woman's own tissues better for reconstruction?

This is difficult to answer because the specific method of reconstruction must be determined on an individual basis. Breasts reconstructed with implants or tissue expanders can look and feel quite natural. These operations can also be done without leaving additional scars. Sometimes, however, thick fibrous tissue develops around these implants (a condition called capsular contracture), causing them to feel firm and reducing the attractiveness of the breast. Placement of the implant under the muscle usually helps to minimize any potential hardening. More recently, implants with a rough or textured surface have also proved effective in reducing the incidence of capsular formation around these implants and in keeping the breasts soft and natural. These newer implants have thicker envelopes, which can sometimes be seen or felt through thin skin.

Reconstruction with a woman's own tissue avoids the use of a foreign implant material and produces a soft, natural reconstructed breast that will not become firm. She pays a price for these advantages, however. When the lower abdominal or buttock tissue is transported to a woman's breast area, the surgeon must create additional scars on the breast, lower abdomen, or buttocks. These are the most involved procedures for breast reconstruction and are associated with more pain, a longer recovery, and more postoperative complications. (This topic is discussed fully in Chapter 13.)

Does chest wall irradiation affect the success of breast reconstruction? Which techniques work best after radiation therapy?

Radiation therapy can reduce the blood supply to the chest wall skin and muscle. It can also damage the skin, reducing its elasticity and healing potential. After radiation therapy to the chest wall, breast reconstruction with tissue expansion is often not as successful because the skin may be damaged and less resilient; this means that the potential for complications is greater. Radiation can also affect the success of a breast implant or flap reconstruction by causing fibrosis (or thickening), capsular contracture, and breast firmness. Therefore, if radiation is anticipated, breast reconstruction may be delayed until after this treatment is completed. The best and least complicated breast reconstructions after radiation are done with autologous tissue—the TRAM flap, latissimus dorsi flap, or gluteus maximus free flap.

How will a woman's breasts look over the long term—5 or 10 years after reconstruction? Which type of breast reconstruction produces the most aesthetic long-term results?

Although it is impossible to predict with certainty how results will look in 5 to 10 years, generally some degree of capsular contracture will form after implant or expander reconstruction with each passing year. This usually results in some breast asymmetry as the reconstructed breast becomes elevated with time and the natural opposite breast droops subsequent to the aging process. With autologous reconstructions, the result is more lasting and less likely to change.

If a person gains or loses a considerable amount of weight, how will that affect the results of breast reconstruction?

General weight losses or gains are reflected in some women's breasts; in others they are not. After an implant reconstruction, a major weight change will probably produce a change in the normal breast that will result in breast asymmetry. This asymmetry may require an implant change (an outpatient procedure). Such a change is often not needed with the expander implant because of its internal valve. This implant has the flexibility to permit future implant size adjustments to accommodate weight changes that have altered the woman's breast size. This may be the best solution for a woman who wants a breast reconstruction but plans on losing weight in the future. Similarly, if the woman gains additional weight, the breast can be enlarged to match the other larger, fuller breast.

Reconstructions with a woman's own lower abdominal or buttock tissues usually remain symmetric under these circumstances because of the major fatty components of both the normal and reconstructed breasts.

What happens to breast symmetry as a woman's remaining unoperated breast ages?

Every woman's breasts age differently. Generally, however, there is gradual settling and lowering of the breast with time. Breast size also changes with aging; these changes are influenced by weight loss or gain, body fat content, and hormonal changes. When a woman's breast has been rebuilt with her own tissues, it tends to age more like her natural breast ages with better long-term symmetry.

What is the long-term appearance of a rebuilt nipple? Does it keep its projection?

If possible, the nipple built from the chest wall skin is usually made longer than the remaining nipple to counter the tendency of nipple reconstructions to become shorter and flatter over time. When built with a graft from the other nipple, symmetry is usually easier to maintain.

Can another person tell if a woman has had breast reconstruction?

A woman who has had breast reconstruction can expect to dress normally without anyone realizing that her breast has been rebuilt. Unless she is naked, her scars will not be noticeable to anyone, and her clothed breasts will appear the same as any other woman's.

If a woman has reconstruction, will she be able to wear V necklines and ordinary clothing without high necks?

A woman who has had a modified radical mastectomy with a scar that falls under her brassiere will be able to wear V necklines again. If she has had a radical mastectomy in which the pectoralis major muscle has been removed, reconstruction (which requires flap tissue) can still permit her to wear V-neck clothing unless the mastectomy scar extends into this central area of the chest and she is concerned about it showing.

Sports clothes also can be worn, but sometimes the style might have to accommodate any unusually positioned mastectomy scar or a donor flap scar on her back, underarm, lower abdomen, or buttocks.

How do the results of breast reconstruction compare with a woman's expectations? Do her breasts look and feel normal?

It is important for a woman to carefully define her expectations before she has this operation to make sure that the plastic surgeon knows what she wants and can tell her if it is possible. Breast reconstruction can fill in and rebuild the deformities resulting from mastectomy. A woman may be disappointed, however, if she expects her new breast to be the same as the one it is meant to replace. Her new breast with an implant will often be cooler, firmer, and more rounded than her remaining one. It will not move as naturally with changes in position or posture. Firmness is often associated with the use of implants. Also, the lower portion of the breast implant can sometimes be felt through the breast skin; this is not bothersome to most women and is considered a natural accompaniment of breast reconstruction with implants.

When the skin and overlying tissue cover is thin or irradiated, any irregularities or ripples in the breast implant or the actual textured-surface pattern of the implant can show through the skin. This rippling can give an unattractive contour to the upper part of the reconstructed breast and can be eliminated by placing the implant under autologous tissue or a layer of latissimus dorsi back muscle. A more normal breast "feel" and flow can sometimes be obtained by using the patient's own tissue from the lower abdomen or buttocks.

In what ways will a woman's rebuilt breast differ from her original breast?

It will be less mobile and have less sensation. It cannot produce milk. There are scars from the mastectomy and reconstruction. Furthermore, the nipple-areola does not totally match the other natural one and does not respond to stimuli.

What are the chances for breast symmetry?

The chances for breast symmetry are good. Each reconstruction must be individualized. Preoperatively the surgeon must determine if symmetry can be achieved with or without modification of the other breast. Bilateral reconstructions are often the most symmetric.

Will the reconstructed breast have projection?

Reconstructed breasts tend to be flatter and thus have less projection than natural breasts. Occasionally an implant is used to optimize projection after a flap reconstruction.

Is the reconstructed breast sensitive to touch and to sexual stimulation?

Because sensation or feeling in the chest wall area is lost during the mastectomy, the reconstructed breast is usually numb or at least has less sensation than the normal side. The underarm is also numb and feels strange to the touch. Some women say that shaving their under-arms becomes a rather uncomfortable experience. The underside of the upper arm is usually also numb. Sometimes, as some of these nerves grow back after the mastectomy, the woman may notice some radiating or "shooting" pains in the area of these nerves.

This lack of sensation is more common when an implant has been used for breast reconstruction. When a patient's breast is reconstructed with her own tissue (autologous tissue) from the lower abdomen, many of these women will develop some sensation to touch in the region of their reconstructed breast. Their chances for developing additional breast sensation are further enhanced when the reconstruction with autologous tissue is performed immediately at the time of the mastectomy. The best opportunity for preservation of breast sensation after mastectomy is probably offered by the newer microsurgical reconstructive techniques that surgically hook up or reconnect the nerves at the mastectomy site to the nerves in the autologous tissue flap that has been transferred from the woman's lower abdomen or her buttocks.

The special sensation associated with the nipple-areola area with its responsiveness to sexual stimulation is usually lost and does not return.

If a woman has breast reconstruction with implants, will her breasts be warm like normal breasts?

Usually the temperature of reconstructed breasts is determined by the thickness of the skin cover and adequacy of the blood supply. When the cover is thin, the cooler temperature of the implant will be noticeable and the breast will feel cold.

Will there be nerve loss?

No additional nerve loss is to be expected after breast reconstruction with implants. After autologous flap reconstruction, the area adjacent to the donor site is usually numb. With a TRAM flap, this numb area is above the abdominal scar; with a latissimus dorsi flap, below the back incision; and with a gluteus maximus flap, on the back of the leg.

What is the anticipated pain and recovery time?

After breast reconstruction a woman will experience pain in her chest area as well as in any donor sites where additional tissue was taken to build her new breast. The degree of pain and length of the recuperative period will vary with the individual patient, the extent of her defect, and the operative procedure chosen. The postoperative pain comes from the effects of the cut nerves in the breast region. As these nerves grow back, they can often be reeducated by massage of the skin a few weeks after the operation. (Specific information on these matters is provided in great detail in Chapter 13.)

A recent advance in pain control after an operation, the PCA (patient-controlled analgesia) unit, is now available to alleviate some of the patient's discomfort during her hospital stay. This device enables the patient to press a button when she needs pain relief. The machine then delivers a predetermined amount of pain medication. In the past it was necessary for a nurse to give an injection to relieve the pain every 2 to 4 hours. Current thinking indicates that better pain relief may be possible if pain medication is administered as the patient needs it. This approach allows the patient to be in control of her pain relief medication.

Some women do not handle any pain medication well, even the relatively small doses delivered by the PCA. A potentially distressing side effect for these women is nausea and vomiting from the effects of the anesthesia and the medication given immediately after surgery. This can be helped by reducing the dosage of the pain relief medication to the absolute minimum that the patient needs and can tolerate. A patient who does not tolerate medication well should alert the anesthesiologist and surgeon of this problem preoperatively so that some accommodation can be made to avoid nausea following the operation.

Is it painful to have the tissue expander inflated? How does it feel?

Most women describe a "full, tight feeling" during tissue expansion. For a minority of patients, expansion can be painful. To relieve the discomfort for these individuals the expansion process is paced more slowly, which means more frequent visits and lower volume expansion. In some cases some of the saline solution may even be removed temporarily until the patient feels more comfortable.

What aftereffects and adjustments should a woman expect after breast reconstruction?

Following breast reconstruction a woman's breast may be swollen and bruised. These are natural responses to healing and the patient should not be alarmed; the swelling will subside in a few days and the bruising will fade and disappear over a period of weeks, leaving her breast with a far more acceptable appearance. Her breast may also appear smaller or larger than expected and may not be completely symmetric with the opposite breast. Some asymmetries will lessen with time. If they persist, the breast usually can be adjusted a few months later during a second procedure and at the time of the nipple-areola reconstruction.

When an expander is used, the reconstructed breast will look smaller at first. It will be enlarged during several postoperative visits when additional saline solution is added to the expander.

If muscles are used for reconstruction, how will it affect movement and physical strength in the future?

The muscles and portions of muscles utilized for breast reconstruction are considered functionally expendable; other muscle groups usually take over when one of these muscles has been transferred. Therefore muscle flap reconstructions normally do not impose functional restrictions on a woman after the healing period is over. A postoperative exercise program can contribute to rebuilding strength.

What limitations or weaknesses does a woman experience after a musculocutaneous flap reconstruction?

Most of the activities of daily living, including sports activities, are not affected by breast reconstruction with a muscle or muscle and skin flap. However, a woman's ability to do sit-ups may be reduced after a TRAM flap. This problem is more noticeable if both rectus abdominis muscles (bipedicle) are used. Some activities that rely heavily on upper extremity strength, such as cross-country skiing, may also be more difficult after a latissimus dorsi flap procedure.

Will a woman have full use of her arm after breast reconstruction?

Breast reconstruction will not impose any permanent restrictions on arm mobility or strength. Because some free flap breast reconstructions and the latissimus dorsi flap require surgery in the arm area, a woman will be instructed to limit her arm activity for a few weeks after surgery to avoid complications.

When can a woman resume an exercise program after breast reconstruction? Will any activities be permanently restricted?

While each patient recovers at a different rate, most women who have implant reconstruction can resume normal upper extremity activity after 3 to 4 weeks. After a flap procedure, activity can be resumed in 6 to 8 weeks.

Is any depression experienced after this operation?

Some women go through a limited but normal period of depression after breast reconstruction. The operation, general anesthesia, postoperative pain, and medications may combine to produce these feelings. Because this operation represents a major step for a woman, there is an emotional buildup to prepare for it as well as heightened expectations for a lovely result. Therefore a woman may feel a let down once the operation is over because the postoperative appearance will not reflect the final result. Instead, her breast may look bruised and possibly flat, far removed from the result she expected. This depression usually subsides in a few days as the patient recovers and the appearance of her breast improves.

What are possible complications from breast reconstruction? When do they occur and why?

Complications of breast reconstruction appear either immediately after the operation or develop later. The type and degree of complications relate to the method of reconstruction used.

When an implant or expander is used to reconstruct the breast with existing tissues, a blood collection (hematoma) can develop around the implant; this problem usually requires drainage, often in the operating room. When the skin is thin or irradiated, actual exposure of the implant can occur because of the poor cover. Infection and delayed healing also may occur. Capsular contracture is the most frequent late problem associated with implant and expander reconstruction; this topic is addressed in Chapter 13.

Complications are more likely after flap reconstructions, particularly microsurgical procedures, the most complex of all. Hematoma may occur in both the site of the reconstruction or in the donor site. If the flap tissue that is moved does not have an adequate blood supply, a portion or occasionally the entire flap may be lost. With microsurgical reconstruction, sometimes the microanastomosis (where the blood vessels are connected) develops a blood clot and the patient may need to return to the operating room for a second procedure to remove the clot and resuture the blood vessels. (A more detailed discussion of the potential complications associated with the different breast reconstruction operations is included in Chapter 13.)

Is infection a serious problem after breast reconstruction?

Infection is an infrequent problem after breast reconstruction. It is more likely to occur after an immediate implant or expander reconstruction (a 2% to 10% chance). Infection after a flap procedure may result in partial flap loss, which would require revision of the flap during another procedure.

Do flaps used in breast reconstruction ever die or fail? If so, what can be done to complete the reconstruction?

Flaps are an essential component of some reconstructions. A flap is a portion of tissue that is moved from one area of the body to another. For the flap to be successful, transferred tissue must have a plentiful blood supply. If this blood supply is marginal or partially insufficient, a portion of the flap can die; this portion of the flap is therefore lost as a source of tissue for reconstruction.

Usually reconstruction can be completed after partial flap loss. Rarely is the entire blood supply to the flap impaired and the entire flap lost. Potential flap loss usually can be identified during the operation and appropriate measures taken by the surgeon to avoid this problem. Certain general health conditions of the woman can impair blood supply to flaps and result in flap loss; for instance, if a woman has diabetes, has received radiation to the flap vessels, or is a cigarette smoker, she may have reduced blood flow. (See p. 223 for more information on the risks of smoking.)

What is a worst case scenario for each of the different reconstructive procedures?

Implants and expanders can become exposed and infected, requiring removal. In this instance, reconstruction must begin again at a later date. Flaps can fail because of partial or total loss of the blood supply. When a flap fails, another reconstructive technique, either a different flap or an implant procedure, will have to be done to complete the reconstruction. More serious complications such as deep vein thrombosis and pulmonary embolus can develop, usually after longer operations; these are rare occurrences, but they are life threatening (see p. 242). Anesthetic complications, though rare, can cause serious consequences.

Can a woman die from breast reconstruction?

The risks to life from breast reconstruction are very low. One obvious risk is from anesthesia; today, however, administration of anesthetics is safe in the hands of well-trained anesthesiologists. Reconstruction with implants is also safe. Flap reconstructions, especially with the lower abdominal flap and buttock flap, carry somewhat more risk because of the length of these operations and the risk of blood loss and the development of venous blood clots in the woman's legs. It is possible for these clots to go from the legs to the blood vessels of the lungs (pulmonary embolus), a potentially life-threatening condition. The development of blood clots is linked to the length of the operative procedure; these clots are more likely to occur when the operation lasts more than 4 or 5 hours. The use of sequential compressive stockings (see p. 242) may enhance the blood flow and venous return from the legs during the procedure and in the postoperative period and thus decrease the possibility that this problem will develop. The surgeon may also decide to use an anticoagulant in a low dosage to reduce the possibility of a blood clot.

What are the costs of breast reconstruction?

The costs of breast reconstruction depend on the extent of surgical repair needed, the type of reconstructive operation a woman selects, whether this surgery is performed as an immediate or a delayed procedure, and the number of operations required. Simple insertion of an implant costs less than a procedure requiring a flap of additional tissue supplied from the back, buttocks, or abdomen. Creating a nipple-areola further increases the price. These decisions affect the length of hospitalization, the length of the operation, and the anesthesia that is required. Costs include the plastic surgeon's fees and the hospital charges. In addition, costs may vary depending on the region of the country. The cost of surgery, as with the cost of living, seems to be higher on the East or West Coast than in other areas of the country.

Immediate breast reconstruction usually costs less. The patient is already hospitalized for a mastectomy and is only anesthetized one time. She recovers from the mastectomy and reconstruction simultaneously. A surgeon's fee for immediate reconstruction without a flap and with the tissues remaining after the mastectomy usually begins at $2500 and goes up from there. The flap operations start at $5000; microsurgical flap procedures are even higher, starting at $8000. It is important to note, however, that some plastic surgeons prefer not to do a flap reconstruction as an immediate procedure because the complexity requires a longer operating time and a greater chance of complications.

If the breast reconstruction is delayed, costs are usually greater. Thus charges for reconstruction with available tissues and implants and expanders may start at $3000, reconstruction with the latissimus dorsi (back muscle) flap at $6000, reconstruction with the TRAM flap at $8000, and microsurgical reconstruction with the gluteus maximus (buttock muscle) flap at $10,000. A second procedure to restore a woman's nipple-areola usually costs upward from $1500 and can be done on an outpatient basis. Reconstruction with available tissues or tissue expansion, if performed as a delayed procedure, also can be done on an outpatient basis, thus lowering the costs. The cost for the implant is additional and now ranges from $1000 to $2000.

These costs are approximate and reflect a range seen in the country today. They are offered merely to give women an idea of the expenses to be anticipated when considering breast reconstruction. Your reconstructive surgeon will tell you the specific costs.

What is the expected hospitalization for the different reconstructive procedures?

The usual hospital stay for simple implant placement or tissue expansion is 1 to 2 days, although many women can have these operations as outpatient procedures. For the latissimus dorsi flap, hospitalization is 3 to 5 days; for the TRAM flap, 5 to 8 days, and for a microsurgical buttock or TRAM flap procedure, 6 to 8 days.

Will insurance cover the costs of breast reconstruction?

Most major medical carriers cover the costs of breast reconstruction after mastectomy based on the restrictions specified in their individual policies. This surgery is not considered cosmetic, but rather reconstructive, and many states have passed laws to ensure coverage by any company delivering health insurance within the state. Coverage varies, however, from state to state. It is wise to check with your insurance company before you have breast reconstruction to be sure that part or all of your expenses will be reimbursed. Persistence and assertiveness will sometimes be necessary to get the information that you need. If only a portion of the cost is covered, you need to inquire what percentage is covered and if this coverage is based on the actual cost of the surgery or on a preassigned payment schedule that identifies the "usual and customary fee" for a particular operation as determined by the insurance company. If there is a "usual and customary fee," you need to know what that fee is and how much of your anticipated bill will not be covered so that you can plan accordingly.

Dealing with the insurance company can be a frustrating experience. It may require additional letters and phone calls to the company, but you should not be turned off or discouraged. This is a legitimate reconstructive procedure that qualifies for coverage. It is your right to insist on information and specifically to know the extent of coverage before the operation. A letter from your doctor to the insurance company may be needed to explain your condition and the need for surgery. Although some insurance companies still do not cover rehabilitation of any kind, fortunately they are the exception, not the rule. The insurance company may, however, not be familiar with some of the more recently developed breast reconstruction techniques, and you may have to help educate them about the technique that you have selected. Your plastic surgeon can also assist you in this process with a telephone call to the insurance company and a follow-up letter.

Before a woman decides on reconstructive breast surgery, she should carefully read her insurance policy. Some policies stipulate that insurance will pay for either a prosthesis or breast reconstruction and not for both. If a woman receives reimbursement for the cost of her prosthesis, the cost of her reconstruction will thus not be covered later. It is necessary for her to be aware of these stipulations so that her eligibility for reimbursement for the costs of reconstruction, which are far greater than the cost for a prosthesis, will not be jeopardized.

In deciding whether she can afford breast reconstruction a woman needs to assess all aspects of her reconstructive surgery. What type of procedure does she plan to have done? Is it going to be done on an immediate or delayed basis? Is her other breast going to be modified? What is her insurance coverage? Does it cover both a prosthesis and reconstruction or does it cover one or the other? Does it cover modification of the other breast? Many policies will cover prophylactic mastectomies (the removal of breast tissue as a preventive therapy against the development of cancer in the future), but they will not cover what they consider to be aesthetic changes such as augmentation (enlargement), mastopexy (tightening and lifting of the breast), and reduction (reducing the size of the breast).

If a woman has implants from a former cosmetic breast procedure, she should check to ensure that this will not affect her insurance coverage. Unfortunately, because of the controversy surrounding implants, some insurance carriers have withdrawn coverage for women with implants.

For women with no insurance coverage and/or limited assets, breast reconstruction is often available through the plastic surgery divisions of university teaching hospitals.

If considering breast surgery, how should a woman become informed?

When a woman is considering an operation to restructure or reconstruct her breasts, she needs to obtain as much information as possible about the proposed procedure and to consult with a board-certified plastic surgeon with special expertise in breast surgery. (See Chapter 12 for more information on selecting a plastic surgeon.) During the consultation the plastic surgeon should review the patient's condition, discuss her options, and answer any questions she may have. If silicone breast implants and tissue expanders are being considered, the plastic surgeon should describe these devices, detail all potential benefits and risks, and answer questions concerning them or the implant surgery itself. He should also provide the patient with the manufacturer's informed consent documents (these are also approved by the FDA) and have the patient read these documents carefully and ask questions. The plastic surgeon can often provide reading materials to explain the different procedures. A woman should also discuss the operation with her other physicians, and if additional questions need addressing, a second opinion is in order. Only after all her questions are answered and she understands all of the possible risks and benefits should the woman make her decision.

How does breast reconstruction affect survival rates from breast cancer?

Many breast cancer experts believe that knowledge about breast reconstruction will save thousands of women's lives. Some women will come for treatment earlier on discovering a mass in their breast if they are aware of the chance for reconstruction after mastectomy. As one expert explains, "This procedure could conceivably have an immense impact upon the entire problem of early detection and treatment of breast cancer."

• • •

As breast reconstruction techniques become increasingly sophisticated and widely accepted, more women are seeking information about them. Before deciding for or against breast reconstruction, a woman needs to be apprised of the essential facts concerning this surgery. Her questions should be answered and her doubts should be addressed. This chapter has attempted to provide some of these answers.

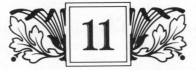

WHAT WOMEN WANT TO KNOW ABOUT BREAST IMPLANTS

S ilicone breast implants—problem or solution? This is the question that many women are pondering as they attempt to sort through conflicting reports about these devices that surfaced during the Food and Drug Administration (FDA) investigation. The enormous publicity surrounding this process with the unfolding drama of public hearings and media coverage was unduly frightening to many who were not privy to scientific information about these devices and had no means of evaluating their safety. In actuality, breast implants have been available for over 30 years now, and while they are not perfect, they have not proved an overriding cause for concern. Similar to all implantable devices, they have known benefits and risks and are subject to complications and potential problems. Even the FDA acknowledges that they do "not present a health hazard." The ongoing FDA investigation is not a cause for alarm; rather, it is an example of a government agency performing its designated duty to regulate the safety and efficacy of drugs and medical devices and to make sure that they meet certain standards. The real question is how safe are they and how safe is safe enough? This question has not yet been answered, but ongoing clinical studies are being conducted for this purpose and the FDA has mandated that use of these devices be monitored within these studies. Time will provide the answers to many of these questions. The concerns about implants will eventually be put in proper perspective, and undoubtedly, as with all technology, new improved devices will replace the ones that are currently being studied. New developments are already in evidence. In the meantime, questions linger. Many women are confused and concerned about potential dangers associated with breast implants. It is difficult to sort fact from fiction. The issues are complex and not all the answers are in. Furthermore, it is difficult to know whom to believe. The following discussion attempts to address women's questions and concerns, to present the facts, and to let women judge for themselves. To accomplish this goal this discussion has been divided into two parts. The first and largest is devoted to questions that women want answered about this topic. These queries are real ones posed by women in personal interviews and in surveys. The answers are based on published medical studies and reports, data supplied by experts, and documented scientific evidence as it is known today. The second and final section details our observations and those of other experts and attempts to assess the impact of the silicone breast implant debate and place it into perspective.

We begin by addressing women's frequently posed questions about silicone breast implants. . . .

What is the value of silicone breast implants?

Silicone gel–filled breast implants were originally developed in the early 1960s for women who desired breast enhancement. Some of these women's breasts had gotten smaller after pregnancy, and they wanted their breasts to be fuller once again; others felt their breasts were too small, poorly formed, or out of proportion to their total body shape. Implants offered a viable and effective solution for their problems. Building on patient satisfaction with implant surgery for breast enlargement, surgeons soon discovered that these devices were remarkably helpful for restoring breast shape and contour in women who had suffered breast loss after mastectomy for breast cancer. They also were effective for correcting breast and chest wall asymmetries and congenital chest wall deformities.

Since their introduction over 30 years ago over one million women in the United States have had breast implant surgery; most would choose to repeat the experience. Implants have made a difference to these women. They have offered a return to normalcy for women with breast cancer and an opportunity to put the cancer experience behind them and get on with their lives. Breast reconstruction has helped these women to feel whole again; they have reported feeling good about themselves once again, renewed self-confidence, and a new zest for life. Still others say that implants have provided them with a more normal body image, a more flattering breast form, or an improved self-image. The benefits of silicone breast implants have been both physical and psychological, and their value for women's health has become more obvious with time. Many cancer specialists believe and our experience would suggest that knowledge of breast reconstruction will save many women's lives because they will not procrastinate in seeking care for breast problems for fear of breast loss.

What are the psychological benefits of breast implants?

Since breast implants are used to enhance small breasts and reconstruct breasts after mastectomy, the benefit is mostly psychological. Women who have had breast implants report that their self-esteem is enhanced—that they feel more attractive, more feminine. Women who have had implants for breast reconstruction report that they no longer feel deformed as they did following mastectomy, that they feel more normal and less depressed over their appearance. Most relate a restored sense of well-being and relief at not having a "constant reminder of their cancer and mortality."

What are the physical benefits of implants?

Implants can be used to correct breast or chest wall asymmetries associated with developmental conditions or after trauma. They are also used for breast reconstruction after mastectomy. Many women who have had mastectomies report that the implant helps to restore a feeling of balance. For women with a large opposite breast, it may also alleviate back and shoulder pain and posture problems caused by the woman's attempts to disguise her uneven chest with a heavy external prosthesis. The implant can provide cover for the exposed chest wall, which may be sensitive after breast removal. It can also be used to replace an external prosthesis, thereby affording a woman greater freedom in selecting clothing styles and avoiding the discomfort and skin irritation that sometime accompany use of an external breast prosthesis.

What is the reported satisfaction rate of women who have had implant surgery?

A number of studies have been done to assess the satisfaction rate after breast implant operations. These studies have consistently shown that over 60% and sometimes as many as 80% to 90% of the women who have had implant surgery for augmentation are pleased with the results of the procedure. Even when women experience problems with breast implants, such as capsular contracture, they rarely choose to have their breast implants removed. There is an even higher satisfaction rate with implant surgery for breast reconstruction; however, because of the thin skin at the mastectomy site, the possibility of complications is greater with reconstructive procedures than with breast augmentation. Despite problems, these women report that they would choose to have implant surgery again.

What kind of breast implants are available? What type of fillings are used in them?

Basically there are two broad categories of implants to choose from: fixed-volume breast implants and implants in which the volume can be changed after they are implanted (tissue expanders). All of the currently available implants have an outer layer or envelope of silicone that is in contact with the body tissues. These implants are filled with either saline (saltwater) solution or silicone gel. Of the fixed-volume implants available, the ones most commonly used today are filled with saline solution. (Those with silicone gel can only be used if a woman is enrolled in clinical trials.) Alternate filling materials for the implant envelopes are under development; many of these materials would have the advantage of being radiolucent, as opposed to opaque, and easily eliminated or removed by the body if they leaked. Most likely these fillings will replace the silcone gel currently used; some of the fillings being investigated include water-based gels; gel-like solutions consisting of water, salts, and organic polymers; and synthetic peanut oil. These new products are not available yet and must face rigorous testing before premarket approval is granted by the FDA. This approval process could take as long as 3 to 5 years. Implants are also available with smooth and with textured silicone surfaces. Many surgeons feel that these textured surfaces have helped to reduce the incidence of breast hardness (capsular contracture) after implant surgery. (The different varieties of implants and expanders are described in greater detail in Chapter 13.)

Is one brand or type of breast implant safer than another?

The FDA monitors the quality of these devices through ongoing audits of the manufacturers' facilities to ensure the high quality of these products. Although some surgeons have expressed "less concern" about the safety of saline-filled implants and others prefer a particular type of implant because they have experienced more success with it, for example, in avoiding certain adverse effects such as capsular contracture, it will not be known for certain whether one brand or model is more effective than another until the FDA evaluates the safety and effectiveness of all breast implants. Ongoing clinical trials have been established to evaluate silicone gel–filled implants. The safety and effectiveness of saline-filled implants are also being scrutinized.*

Is silicone safe to use in humans?

Silicone, a commonly used substance for various implantable devices, is considered by many to be one of the least reactive biomaterials. Initially introduced for medical implantation in the 1950s, silicone was used for artificial joints, implantable pumps, shunts, drains, and other devices that required a material that was considered relatively nonreactive, nonallergenic, and easily tolerated by the body. Implantable silicone devices include pacemakers, breast implants, penile implants, and testicular implants. Anyone who has ever taken a capsule has ingested silicone, for it is used to coat capsules to make them more easily swallowed. Silicone is also present in processed foods, in cosmetics, in many drugs (especially antacids), and in our drinking water. Silicone is used to lubricate syringes, in intravenous tubing, and in shunts used for chemotherapy. Anyone who has had blood drawn or been given an injection has had some silicone introduced into his or her body. Infant pacifiers are usually made of silicone. As Dr. James Potchen, a radiologist at the University of Michigan explains, "Some systemic levels of silicone will be found in every patient with an implant. The fact is that a *very low* level of silicone is present in everyone. The relationship between use of insulin syringes by diabetics and systemic levels of silicone is just as impressive as that in patients with implants that bleed." If silicone presents any serious chemical hazards to the human body, they should already be apparent because of this chemical's widespread use; the fact is they aren't. Nevertheless, studies continue to rule out the possibility of currently unrecognized and rare problems. New silicone devices are routinely receiving FDA endorsement, such as the FDA-approved Norplant contraceptive device that is delivered from a silicone implant. Therefore, when the FDA was instructed by Congress in 1976 to begin evaluating medical devices, silicone devices, including silicone breast implants, were considered among the least worrisome. After reviewing implant safety, the FDA allowed them to remain on the market but instructed that they be monitored by the FDA.

---

*The formal review is scheduled for late 1993.

What problems are associated with implants and how often do they occur?

As with all devices, implants are not without problems. They are subject to rupture, possible leakage, displacement, and capsular contracture, the most common problem. They also may interfere with mammograms and cause calcium deposits and possible changes in breast and nipple sensation. These problems are not life threatening, however, and are usually easily corrected. Until the FDA studies and the registries provide definitive long-term results, we will not know for certain how frequently these problems occur.

What is capsular contracture? Does this pose a serious risk for women who have implant surgery?

A capsule is a firm, fibrous scar that forms around a breast implant. This is a characteristic response of the body to isolate any foreign substance; similar scar formation can be observed around hip implants, artificial joints, and pacemakers. In some cases, for unknown reasons, the scar tissue capsule may become thick and constrict the implant. This phenomenon is referred to as capsular contracture. This condition can make the breast harder and firmer than desirable, producing a rounded, spherical breast appearance; sometimes it can also cause pain. The severity of this problem varies with each individual. Ideally, the capsular layer surrounding the implant is thin and does not affect the shape of the breast. In some women it manifests itself as a small pulling or slight breast firmness, a minor nuisance. When the contracture is mild, no treatment is necessary. Most women find this minimal firmness acceptable and are not motivated to undergo further adjustments of their reconstructed breasts. In severe cases of capsular contracture a woman may experience significant discomfort and require an operation to release the scar tissue (capsulotomy) or remove it (capsulectomy). During this secondary operation the surgeon may reposition the implant under the pectoralis major muscle if previously placed over the muscle or he may replace it with a different implant with a textured surface after releasing or removing the capsule. These rough-surface implants seem to have a lower incidence of capsular contracture. It is usually necessary to remove the scar capsule around the smooth implant before replacing it with the textured-surface implant. Patients who continue to experience problems after surgical correction may decide to have their implants removed. After implant removal (explantation) the breast may require aesthetic correction for optimal appearance. A woman should be informed of this possibility.

Some women decide to have their firm breasts managed by removing the implant and scar tissue and replacing it with fatty flap tissue from the back, lower abdomen, or buttocks.

Although capsular contracture may be uncomfortable and produce breast distortion and asymmetry, it is not a health hazard. In severe cases this contracture may result in the implant being exposed through thin breast skin. It may also contribute to rupture, which is cause for concern. It does not, however, threaten a woman's life or health, and most women who experience this problem can have satisfactory correction by surgery. With the newer textured breast implants, capsular contracture is estimated to occur in approximately 2% to 4% of cases. Experience with these implants is relatively short term, however, and long-term follow-up may determine the incidence of contracture to be greater.

What can be done to avoid capsular contracture? Will exercises help?

Implants with a textured covering seem to reduce the likelihood of capsular contracture; it is thought that the rough surface prevents a smooth, uniform scar from forming and constricting the implant. When smooth-surface implants are used, some surgeons recommend breast massage of the implant throughout the breast pocket in an effort to prevent or reduce the incidence and severity of fibrous capsule formation around the implant. There is no scientific evidence, however, that breast massage is helpful in preventing contracture, and some surgeons have stopped recommending massage to patients with smooth implants. Massage is not necessary for implants with a textured surface.

What are calcium deposits? Can they endanger a woman's health?

Sometimes calcium forms in the capsule around the breast implant. These deposits may increase the hardening; however, they have a characteristic appearance and can be differentiated from calcifications associated with breast cancer.

What effects will implants have on breast sensation?

Women having implant surgery for augmentation may experience changes in breast and nipple-areola sensation. Most of these changes are temporary, but in some cases they prove permanent. Women having breast reconstruction with or without implants already have diminished sensation because of the nerves cut during the mastectomy.

Does a woman who has an implant reconstruction still need to have mammograms?

Mammograms are usually not necessary after a mastectomy and breast reconstruction. When an implant is placed in the other breast, this breast still needs to be monitored. Women who are having a mammogram must inform the mammographer that a breast implant or expander is present so that additional displacement views can be taken to help visualize the extent of the breast tissue. New evidence indicates that magnetic resonance imaging (MRI) may be an improved method for evaluating the breast implant integrity and the area behind the implant. This technology is quite expensive, and its application for breast imaging will require additional assessment.

Will breast implants interfere with mammograms?

Both silicone gel–filled and saline-filled implants can potentially pose some difficulty in breast imaging. These implants are opaque to x-rays; any breast tissue overlying the implant cannot be seen on breast films. Women who have implants in place should make sure that they inform the mammographer so that special *displacement* views can be taken (in addition to the "standard" or routine mammography *compression* views) to better visualize the breast tissue. Many physicians recommend that patients with implants who are having mammograms should have two additional displacement views. The displacement technique (also known as the Eklund or "pinch" technique) was introduced in the hope that it would allow more breast tissue to be visualized in women with breast implants. With these special views and in the absence of significant capsular contracture, satisfactory breast images can be obtained for most women and their breasts can be effectively monitored for possible breast problems. Both compression and displacement views provide better visualization if the implant has been placed *under* rather than *over* the chest wall muscle. (For more information on mammography and breast implants see Chapter 4.)

Should women with implants have mammograms more frequently?

According to Dr. Potchen, "The use of screening mammography in a patient with an implant should be no different than in any other patient. At Michigan State University we currently adhere to the American Cancer Society's recommendations that before age 40 women should have a baseline mammogram. Then, over the age of 40, they should have a screening mammogram every year or every other year, depending on the risk factors. Patients over the age of 50 should have screening mammography annually. We do not see a need for additional mammographic examinations in individuals who have an implant, and we would not advocate doing mammograms in younger patients."

Can implants slip, shift, or become displaced?

During the initial operation the plastic surgeon places the implant in the best position to provide the desired breast appearance. During the process of healing and over time the implants can shift or become displaced. This can occur because of the pull of gravity on a smooth implant or subsequent to a capsular contracture, which can elevate the implant. This problem rarely occurs when a textured breast implant has been used because the rough surface adheres to the surrounding tissue, thereby preventing displacement.

Can the implant be rejected by a woman's body?

"Rejection" means an allergic or immune response that causes the body to literally reject a foreign substance. In this sense, implants are not rejected. However, the overlying breast skin may become thinned, infection can develop, or healing may be incomplete, leading to exposure and necessitating removal of the implant. Although these are complications, they are not tantamount to rejection.

Can an implant be removed if it isn't satisfactory?

Yes, when an implant is not performing the function for which it was intended, or if the woman feels that she would be better off without the implant, it can be removed during a relatively minor operation, usually on an outpatient basis. She should discuss with her plastic surgeon if the capsule also should be removed. The procedure for capsule removal is called capsulectomy. (See p. 162 in this chapter and Chapter 13, p. 223, for more information on this procedure.)

If a woman needs to have her implants removed because of a problem or chooses to have them removed because she is fearful of the consequences, who will pay for this procedure?

Some insurance carriers will cover implant removal for certain types of problems; some manufacturers are also offering assistance with these expenses, as are some surgeons. Dow Corning is offering to pay $1200 for implant removal for women with their implants. The financial arrangements for implant removal should be discussed with your surgeon and your insurance company before any decision is made. You also may want to contact the American Society of Plastic and Reconstructive Surgeons (ASPRS), which can put you in touch with plastic surgeons who will remove the implants at reduced cost or sometimes at no cost.

How long do breast implants last?

The silicone breast implant has been used since 1964, and many of the original devices are still in place. Just as human and artificial organs can fail and require transplantation, breast implants also may have to be replaced.

No precise figures on the life span of silicone gel–filled or saline-filled implants are available at present. The ongoing clinical studies should help clarify this. What is known is that implants can last from a very short time to many years, depending on the patient and her implant. In any case, breast implants should not be considered "lifetime" devices. Women should be followed by their physicians for as long as they have their implants.

How strong are implants? Will they break upon impact? Can they be broken during mammography?

Breast implants are manufactured to specific standards requiring that they resist breast compression as well as multiple and long-term physical stresses. These devices, however, are not indestructible. Although the outer shell of the implant is quite sturdy, it can break as a result of physical trauma such as that experienced during a car accident. Compression views taken during mammography are calibrated to avoid undue pressure that could rupture a breast implant. According to Dr. Potchen, "There is no evidence that compression or displacement mammography has caused implant rupture."

What factors increase the chance that an implant will rupture?

The chance for rupture may increase with the length of time the implant has been in the body and with normal wear and tear. Trauma or injury to the breast also increases the chance of rupture, as may closed capsulotomy (a technique to correct capsular contracture in which strong pressure is applied to the breast to break up the scar tissue around the implant). This technique is less frequently used today and is not recommended by the manufacturers.

What percentage of implants rupture?

According to the FDA, the rupture rate for implants is "uncertain" but may be higher than they previously thought. Researchers at Washington University Medical School in St. Louis have detected a 5% to 6% rupture or leakage rate among the women with implants they studied. Earlier model implants, made with thinner walls and containing a more liquid silicone gel, are thought to have a higher rate of rupture and leakage. These implants, produced in the mid-1970s to the mid-1980s are no longer being made. The envelope failure rate seems to increase after 10 years of implantation.

How can a woman tell if she has a ruptured implant? Does implant leakage show up on a mammogram?

Any noticeable change in the shape, size, feel, or comfort of the breast could signal implant rupture. When such symptoms occur, a patient should see her plastic surgeon for evaluation. According to the FDA, "It is possible for a woman to experience rupture of the implant without symptoms, but women should not have routine mammograms (x-rays of the breasts) just to detect these 'silent' ruptures if they are not experiencing any symptoms."

Ultrasonography is an adjunct to mammography that can be useful in detecting implant rupture. Computed tomography (CT) scans have also been used but require a high dose of radiation as compared to mammography. Magnetic resonance imaging (MRI), which does not use radiation, is being studied but is not recommended for routine screening. Studies indicate that MRI is a useful adjunct to mammography for evaluation of the silicone implant for possible leakage as well as the actual breast for masses and cancer. Dr. Potchen reports that "MRI is currently the most accurate way of determining whether an implant has ruptured. It is an expensive and perhaps unnecessary approach depending on whether the rupture produces symptoms or is likely to create subsequent problems. It also depends on whether it is a *capsulated* [italics ours] rupture [in which the gel is contained in the capsule that surrounds the implant] or whether silicone has leaked into other tissues. Generally a crude estimate of rupture can be pretty well determined on a mammogram. Even at that, I would not recommend using mammography in patients younger than 30. One advantage of ultrasonography or MRI is that there is no radiation."

What happens if an implant leaks?

When the cover of a silicone gel–filled implant becomes thinned or ruptures, the gel usually remains within the fibrous capsule that develops naturally around the implant. Significant trauma can cause tears in the capsule, and the gel can extrude into the the breast and possibly migrate beyond the breast and form lumps (granulomas) nearby. Some of this silicone can cause enlarged lymph nodes in the armpit area (lymphadenopathy). When silicone escapes to other parts of the body, removal can be difficult. Gel migration outside the capsule rarely occurs, however, and, if it does, the viscosity (or thickness) of the gel seems to reduce its ability to migrate.

Gel migration is not a potential problem with implants containing only saline solution. However, there is the possibility of deflation if a leak develops in the implant covering. Currently available saline-filled inflatable implants have a very low deflation rate. If a leak occurs, however, the implant can be replaced. As with silicone gel–filled implants, saline-filled implants should not be considered lifetime devices.

What is silicone bleed?

Silicone bleed refers to microscopic amounts of silicone that "bleed" or seep through the implant's envelope. Although most of this is trapped within the implant pocket or the surrounding scar tissue, minute (microscopic) amounts of silicone could possibly migrate through the capsule. Implants made since 1981 have a thicker envelope (low bleed) design that reduces bleed and leakage.

Is there a test to detect silicone in the body or determine whether a woman is sensitive to silicone?

No. There is no widely available standard test to detect silicone in the body. Even if simple techniques for silicone detection were available, they might not be useful in detecting a rupture because small amounts of silicone ordinarily "bleed" even from intact implants. Furthermore, since silicone is ingested in food and many products, including commonly used medicines and cosmetics, individuals have quantities of silicone in their bodies regardless of whether they have breast implants; therefore it would be virtually impossible for these tests to determine whether the silicone came from the implant or another source.

As the FDA stated in its update, "Determining the presence of silicon or silicone in body fluids does not indicate whether a person is sensitive to these substances or at risk for any specific disease. There is presently no test to determine if a person is sensitive to silicone or silicon."

Do ruptured implants or leakage of silicone gel pose a major health hazard?

Drs. John E. Woods and Phillip G. Arnold, two plastic surgeons at the Mayo Clinic, wrote in *The Wall Street Journal* that "a significant number of patients will undergo implant rupture, or so-called sweating or leakage of implants. In the majority of these patients, there are no symptoms related to this. In fact, rupture is usually undetected, even by mammography. Because a membrane forms around implants (the capsule), when there is deterioration of the outside covering of the implant, the gel is usually contained within the capsule and simply lies free in this cavity and does not travel to other parts of the body.

"Over the years, we have removed many ruptured implants, not because the patient has complained of any symptoms but simply in the process of releasing capsules or exchanging the implants. We have not seen any serious consequences in patients with ruptured implants. Silicone gel is readily removed from the pocket and has only extremely rarely been associated with postoperative problems. We believe that when ruptures are known to exist, it is appropriate to remove the implants. In most patients, however, the presence of ruptured implants is not detectable, is asymptomatic, and is not likely to cause problems."

What should be done if an implant ruptures?

Most experts agree that a ruptured implant should be removed. Frequently the capsule surrounding the implant must also be removed at this time.

Can silicone gel–filled or saline-filled implants cause cancer?

There have been allegations that silicone gel–filled implants cause cancer. Silicone breast implants have been available for over 30 years and during that time have been studied extensively by plastic surgeons, implant manufacturers, scientists, and government regulatory agencies such as the FDA. In all of that time no scientifically documented cases of breast cancer have ever been attributed to breast implants nor is there any evidence that these devices have adversely affected the course of breast cancer when they are used for breast reconstruction. Two large population studies from Los Angeles County and Alberta, Canada, indicate that the incidence of breast cancer in women with silicone breast implants is the same or possibly lower than in women who have not had implants. As the FDA's current informed consent document states, "There is presently no scientific evidence that links either silicone gel–filled or saline-filled breast implants with cancer."

What do cancer specialists say about the dangers of breast implants? Is there a risk of cancer from breast implants?

Physicians at the Mayo Clinic in Rochester, Minnesota, Sloan-Kettering Memorial Hospital in New York, and M.D. Anderson Cancer Center in Houston have found that breast implants do not pose a health hazard. Large population studies seem to confirm this finding. Additional studies are under way to study implants and their long-term impact on a woman's health. The evidence presently available, however, indicates that breast implants pose no cancer risk.

What are connective tissue disorders? What symptoms are associated with these diseases?

These are rare disorders such as lupus erythematosus, dermatomyositis, scleroderma, and rheumatoid arthritis in which the body reacts to its own tissue as though it were a foreign material. A combination of symptoms may characterize these disorders, including the generalized symptoms of joint pain and swelling; tight, red, or swollen skin; swollen glands and lymph nodes; extreme fatigue; local symptoms of swelling of the hands and feet; skin rashes; and unusual hair loss.

The FDA advises a woman who experiences these symptoms to "see her regular doctor if the symptoms do not subside, because these complaints could be indicators of a variety of health problems, not just immune-related disorders."

Can implants cause connective tissue or autoimmune disease in healthy women?

There have been allegations that implants can cause or exacerbate immune-related or connective tissue disorders (also referred to as collagen vascular diseases or incorrectly as human adjuvant disease). This question has been carefully evaluated by respected immunologists and rheumatologists. They have found no conclusive scientific evidence to indicate that there is an increased incidence of such diseases in patients with breast implants. Although these conditions may exist concurrently, there is no evidence that a silicone implant has caused or contributed to autoimmune disease. The FDA's Advisory Panel on implants and the FDA's own update of May 1992 concur that "these disorders can occur in women with or without breast implants. Although some doctors have reported cases of these conditions among their breast implant patients, it is not known whether women with implants are more likely to develop these conditions than those without implants."

Further insight into this issue is again provided by Drs. John Woods and Phillip G. Arnold in their article in *The Wall Street Journal*. According to these experts, "There is no question that those with implants may develop rheumatoid arthritis, scleroderma, or breast cancer. There is no evidence, however, that they are more likely than the general population to have these problems. But because of the controversy surrounding implants, many of those with implants have been led to believe that every symptom they experience, from fatigue to joint pain to occasional fevers, are associated with implants. This is not grounded in fact."

A 1993 article from M.D. Anderson Cancer Center in Houston sheds further light on this issue. This article reports the results of a prospective study of 603 breast reconstruction patients and concludes that "the incidence of autoimmune disease in mastectomy patients receiving silicone gel implants is not different than in patients who had reconstruction with autogenous tissue." It also notes that "although case reports abound, no convincing evidence exists to indicate that the presence of these two events, autoimmune disease and silicone gel implants, is anything but coincidental. . . . Although many of the case reports used historical data as controls, much of the data concerning the incidence of these autoimmune diseases is inaccurate due to inadequate reporting." This study is the only prospective study to date comparing silicone gel breast implant patients with a matched control group with autologous tissue reconstruction. No difference was found in patients who were reconstructed with and without implants.

What advice should rheumatologists and immunologists give to patients contemplating implant surgery?

Dr. John Sergent, a respected rheumatologist, advises informing patients that "a few reports have indicated a relationship between implants and various rheumatic diseases. *The number of patients reported is small, and considering the total number of implants, it may not even be a valid observation.* If there is a causal relationship, it is clearly a rare event."

Should women diagnosed with connective tissue diseases or autoimmune diseases have reconstruction with breast implants?

These diseases are rare, and scientific studies are under way to define and better understand these conditions. As a precaution, however, if a woman has any of these conditions or has a family history of these conditions, she should probably not have silicone gel–filled or saline-filled implants until the results of current population studies and other information are available. As Dr. John Sergent explains, "My recommendation for patients with scleroderma is to minimize trauma of any kind. That would include all cosmetic surgery, not just implants. Many patients with scleroderma request cosmetic surgery to correct the perioral wrinkles they all have, and I strongly discourage them. Most of them do well with surgery; the skin heals quite well. However, there are some patients who have an exuberant fibrotic reaction. My across-the-board recommendation for patients with scleroderma is that all elective surgery should be avoided—implants or anything else."

Is it possible to be allergic to silicone implants or to the silicone gel within them?

As mentioned earlier, silicone has been used in medical devices and oral and parenteral medications for over 40 years, and there is no scientific evidence that individuals can develop allergies to these devices. It is, however, possible for antibodies to the silicone to develop. The mere presence of antibodies, however, does not indicate the presence of disease. The body's normal process of dealing with foreign bodies is an immune response with subsequent development of antibodies. Further studies will need to be conducted to determine if there are actually any allergic reactions.

What possible complications can occur with implant surgery?

As with any surgical procedure, there is the potential for complications, including infection, hematoma, bleeding, seroma, delayed wound healing, and reactions to anesthesia. (See Chapter 13 for a detailed discussion of potential complications for each of the different reconstructive operations.)

Are there any recorded deaths from breast implants?

There are no reports in the medical literature of breast implants being responsible for a single death. There is an inherent risk of serious complications and even death from any operation, but this is usually related to the risk of anesthesia for a period of time. This risk is somewhat higher for longer operations, particularly if the operation lasts for more than 4 hours. However, the risk is still considered very small.

How does the incidence of complications from implant surgery compare to the incidence of complications from other common surgical procedures such as appendectomies, mastectomies, and hysterectomies?

The rate of complications experienced after breast implantation is actually lower than the rate of complications from other commonly performed operations. Patients having breast implant surgery generally have a lower incidence of conditions such as infection, hematoma, pulmonary emboli, and deep vein thrombosis. However, reoperation because of capsular contracture or to achieve a better final breast appearance is necessary in a significant number of cases.

What should women with implants do to protect themselves against possible problems?

Women with implants should take the time to inform themselves about their implants. This means finding out specifically what type implants they have, the date of implantation, the manufacturer, and the model number. They can obtain a copy of the package insert (instructions accompanying the implant and providing information on possible risks and complications for that device model). Problems should be reported to their plastic surgeon and to the *U.S. Pharmacopeia* (see p. 183). It is also crucial for all breast cancer patients and for women with implants to practice monthly breast self-examination (BSE), to have regular physician examinations, and to report any problems, changes, or concerns to their doctors. They should keep in close contact with their doctors for adequate follow-up. Finally, joining a breast implant registry will help to ensure that women are kept informed about safety issues for these devices. (See p. 182 for more information about the types of registries.)

How do the risks associated with saline-filled implants compare to those associated with silicone gel–filled implants?

Hardening of the scar tissue (capsular contracture) and calcium deposit formation occur with both gel-filled and saline-filled implants. Rupture of the implant with subsequent implant deflation may be more likely with the saline-filled type. When a saline-filled implant ruptures, it is likely to deflate over a period of hours to days, requiring surgical replacement.

Although the safety of saline-filled implants is also being evaluated by the FDA, leakage or rupture of these implants results in release of saline solution (saltwater), which is not foreign to the body, thus avoiding some of the concerns associated with silicone gel. (The saltwater is absorbed within a few hours or days, resulting in deflation of the implant.) Because saline-filled implants do not contain silicone gel, fewer questions have been raised about an increased risk of autoimmune diseases or cancer. But since both types of implants have a silicone elastomer envelope, the long-term safety of which is being studied, the saline-filled implants may not be entirely without risk and are being reviewed by the FDA.

Is there a special risk for women with polyurethane-coated implants?

About 10% of women with silicone gel–filled breast implants have a certain type that is coated with polyurethane foam. The coating is intended to reduce the risk of capsular contracture. These implants are no longer available in the United States because the company manufacturing them has discontinued production.

The polyurethane coating can be chemically broken down under specific laboratory conditions to release very small amounts of a substance called toluene diamine (TDA), which has been found to cause cancer in laboratory mice. It is not known whether the foam breaks down to TDA in the body or if there is an increased risk of cancer from the TDA in women with this type of implant. Studies using the latest tests to detect minute levels of TDA are currently being conducted under the guidance of the FDA.

According to the FDA, the cancer risk, if any, is likely to be miniscule. If the polyurethane foam coating on these implants were to chemically break down in the body at the same rate as in laboratory experiments, the lifetime cancer risk for a woman with two implants would probably be less than one in a million, assuming she retained the implants for 35 years.

What about women who already have polyurethane-coated breast implants? Should they be removed?

According to the FDA, "Based on these risk estimates, there is insufficient evidence at present to support having polyurethane-coated breast implants surgically removed because of concerns about cancer.

The risks of the operation itself to remove or replace the implants are far higher than the risks of keeping the implants." Furthermore, removal of these textured-surface devices can be more involved than for smooth-surface implants and usually requires capsule removal, which can necessitate additional tissue excision.

Why don't women just have reconstruction with their own natural tissue from their abdomen, buttock, or back instead of facing the risks of a foreign material?

Many women want an operation that can be done either as an outpatient procedure or with minimal down time, expense, and inconvenience. For them, implant reconstruction is the best choice because it affords the convenience, short recovery period, and reduced cost they desire. This is also the procedure of choice for a woman who does not want any additional scars, a necessary part of most flap procedures. Implant surgery is a good choice for a slender woman who may not have enough fatty tissue for a flap procedure or for a woman with a medical condition that places her at increased risk if she has a more complex operation such as a TRAM (abdominal) flap, latissimus dorsi (back) flap, or a free flap. Furthermore, some surgeons experienced in breast reconstruction techniques with implants and expanders prefer these operations to flap procedures because they produce good results with a low rate of complications.

What are the risks involved with flap surgery? How do these risks compare to those encountered in implant surgery?

The decision to have a breast reconstruction with a flap or with a breast implant involves an analysis of the risks and benefits of the two approaches. Flap operations take longer, which means increased risks of major complications such as deep vein thrombosis, pulmonary complications, and fluid retention. The success of flap procedures depends on the blood supply of the flaps; if this is compromised, part or all of the flap can be lost. Fortunately, this is a rare occurrence. The shaping of the flap tissue into breast form also requires more skill and artistry on the part of the surgeon than that required for placement of a breast implant or expander. The obvious benefit of autologous flap reconstruction is that it creates a lasting, natural type of breast symmetry that is usually maintained for a lifetime and uses the woman's own tissues, usually without the need for an implant.

The perioperative risks of implant reconstruction are less serious and pose a lower chance of major complications. The benefits of breast reconstruction with breast implants are also significant for the patient who can have a successful procedure with minimal inconvenience and cost. The drawback of this approach is that a capsular contracture can develop around the breast implant and require additional procedures in the future. Additionally, implants are not considered lifetime devices and may have to be replaced at some point in the future.

How do the aesthetic results of operations with saline-filled implants compare to those achieved with silicone gel–filled implants?

Certain characteristics of the silicone gel–filled breast implants are preferable to those of saline-filled implants. The gel has a more natural consistency than saltwater and feels and flows more like a natural breast. These implants also offer flexibility in designing different breast shapes—some wider, some with additional projection to allow for individualization. Saline-filled implants are more limited in their shape; they are also heavier than silicone gel–filled implants and when overfilled are firm, spherical, and unnatural. When underfilled they can be soft, and their envelopes, which are thicker than those containing silicone gel, can develop noticeable and palpable folds, particularly through thin skin remaining at the mastectomy site.

What is the FDA's role in testing and evaluating implants and expanders?

The FDA has been charged with regulating all medical devices since 1976 and is involved in an ongoing evaluation of the safety and efficacy of breast implants. The FDA designates these devices as class III, which means that they must have premarket approval of their safety and efficacy. During the early 1990s the FDA conducted hearings on polyurethane-covered implants and silicone gel–filled implants. Saline-filled implants are currently the subject of scrutiny.

Why is the FDA evaluating breast implants if they are not dangerous?

The FDA investigation into the safety of silicone breast implants is merely an example of a government agency performing its legally mandated regulatory function. When the FDA was granted authority to regulate medical devices in 1976, 100,000 devices being distributed were permitted to remain on the market pending later review. Breast implants were included on the FDA's list for review, but devices such as heart valves and intrauterine devices (IUDs) were scrutinized first. In 1988, with the review process completed for some of these other devices, the FDA turned its attention to breast implants and officially placed them into a class III category, a designation assigned to most other permanently implantable medical devices. This classification requires manufacturers to submit comprehensive safety and effectiveness data in order to secure premarket approval. The FDA hearings and mandated clinical trials are a part of this ongoing review process as silicone gel–filled and saline-filled implants are being carefully scrutinized to ensure that they meet certain safety and effectiveness standards.

What is the FDA ruling concerning silicone gel–filled breast implants?

The FDA ruling requires all women desiring silicone gel–filled breast implants either for breast reconstruction or for breast augmentation to enter clinical trials. Any woman who needs an implant for breast reconstruction will be permitted to enter these trials or studies. That includes women who have had breast cancer surgery, women with traumatic breast injuries, and women with severe breast or chest wall deformities or asymmetries. Also eligible are women who have an existing breast implant that needs to be replaced for medical reasons. Only a very limited number of women will be able to receive silicone gel–filled breast implants for breast augmentation, and these women must be enrolled in strictly controlled clinical studies set up under an Investigational Device Exemption (IDE). Participants in all of these studies will be closely followed by their doctors after their operation and will be required to have periodic checkups for 5 years. Women in these studies must agree to read and sign a detailed informed consent form, have follow-up examinations after surgery and periodically for 5 years, and consider enrolling in a patient registry.

Now that the FDA has restricted access to silicone gel–filled implants, will women who want the implants for breast augmentation be allowed to get them outside of the clinical studies?

No. According to the FDA, "Any use of the gel-filled implants for breast augmentation outside the studies will be considered illegal. Women who are not in the studies can have their breasts augmented with saline-filled implants, if these implants are suitable. The saline implants continue to be available for reconstruction and augmentation." Saline implants are currently being evaluated by the FDA; their status and availability may change with the FDA's final ruling on their safety and effectiveness.

Why have women who want implants for augmentation been strictly restricted in their access while women who want implants for reconstruction are not subject to the same restrictions?

The decision made by the FDA panel seems to go beyond the scientific evidence available. The panel did not find information to link these devices with cancer or autoimmune conditions. Even so, they decided to restrict access to silicone gel–filled breast implants, making them available to all women who need them for breast reconstruction for "compassionate use" but only to a limited number of women desiring them for breast augmentation. All women receiving them must participate in carefully controlled clinical trials until more definitive safety data are available.

Some suggest that the FDA has applied a double standard in making this distinction, placing themselves in the role of judging the morality of a woman's reasons for choosing implants. Many physicians and breast cancer patients have questioned the logic of the FDA decision: why are implants not safe for healthy women but okay for women with breast cancer whose immune systems may already be compromised by their bout with cancer?

Why are women with older model implants being told by the FDA not to have them removed while access to the newer models is being restricted because of questions concerning safety and effectiveness?

The FDA wants more information on silicone gel–filled breast implants and therefore is requiring all women who get them to enter controlled clinical trials. Since there has been no information that the devices are harmful (i.e., cause cancer or autoimmune problems), and as long as they continue to give the patient some benefit, those patients who already have them in place have been instructed not to have them removed. The FDA and physicians believe that the risk of an operation, with the attendant anesthetic risk and that of operative complications, is far greater than leaving the devices in the patient.

How can the FDA justify allowing the sale of cigarettes, which have been scientifically linked to cancer, while restricting use of breast implants, which have never been linked to cancer?

Federal law does not place cigarettes and tobacco under the regulatory power of the FDA. These are regulated by the Federal Trade Commission, an example of the strength of the tobacco lobby, which has managed to keep tobacco, a known carcinogen and responsible for 400,000 deaths in the United States each year, beyond the scope of FDA review.

Has the FDA discovered any evidence to prove that silicone gel–filled implants pose potential dangers to a woman's health?

After studying the information about silicone gel–filled breast implants provided by its consultants, the FDA stated that more data are still needed about these devices, but there is no evidence that they cause breast cancer or autoimmune diseases.

If silicone implants are being so stringently regulated by the FDA, why aren't other silicone products subject to similar regulations?

The FDA is a governmental agency and thereby susceptible to the winds of politics, the press, and individual interest groups. The FDA determines its own agenda in response to these various interest groups. The individuals interested in this product made their positions known and lobbied the FDA to ban silicone gel–filled implants. The FDA responded accordingly. The FDA plans to review other silicone devices in the future, but lobbying efforts against other silicone products have not been as intense.

What should women who already have silicone gel–filled implants do about their implants?

It is important to bear in mind that most women do not experience serious problems with their implants. At this time the FDA is not recommending women have their implants removed if they are not experiencing any problems. Women with silicone breast implants should monitor their breasts just as if they did not have implants. This includes careful, monthly BSE, regular physician examination, and breast imaging as recommended. They should also schedule periodical follow-up visits to their plastic surgeon. (See Chapters 3 and 4 for specifics.)

What is the status of saline-filled breast implants?

Saline-filled breast implants, which contain saltwater rather than silicone gel, are still on the market. Manufacturers of saline-filled implants are submitting safety and effectiveness information for these products to the FDA.

Now that silicone gel–filled implants will be available only to women enrolling in clinical trials, will women who need them for reconstruction be reimbursed as before?

The FDA does not determine the reimbursement policies of health insurance companies. However, since the legal status of implants used for breast reconstruction has not changed because of the FDA's actions (and they are not considered "investigational"), there appears to be no reason why any reimbursement policies should be changed. To be certain about payment issues a woman should check with her insurance company before she schedules an operation.

How will the FDA's new regulations affect insurance coverage for women who have had implant surgery? Will women with breast implants be in danger of losing their insurance coverage?

This is, of course, a major concern for individuals with silicone breast implants. There is increasing evidence that individual insurance companies with individual policies are excluding coverage for future breast problems for women with silicone breast implants even when the problems are not related to their implants. Coverage varies with the different companies and group policies and with different health maintenance organizations and managed health care organizations.

If a woman wants to have breast implants for reconstruction, what should she do to make sure they are covered by insurance?

Most insurance companies do not cover "cosmetic" surgery; however, they do cover reconstructions related to the treatment of defined medical conditions such as breast cancer as a standard component of cancer rehabilitation. As a precaution, it is best to contact your insurance company before any anticipated operation. Your physician can often provide essential information to give to the insurance company related to the specific medical diagnosis, the specifics of the procedure, and the computer code numbers necessary for predetermination of coverage and an explanation of your benefits under the policy.

What is a clinical trial?

A clinical trial is basically a controlled study of patients who are receiving a prescribed treatment or combination of treatments. Clinical trials may be used to determine the usefulness of operations, drugs, devices, or treatments. Each study is designed to answer scientific questions and to find new and better ways to help patients. In breast cancer research, clinical trials have long been used for evaluating new treatments. Often one or more treatments are compared. Currently, clinical trials are being designed to study the safety and effectiveness of breast implants. (See p. 74 for a more detailed discussion of clinical trials.)

Specifically what are the silicone gel–filled breast implant clinical trials trying to evaluate?

The clinical studies are seeking answers to the following questions:
• What is the expected life of implants?
• How often do implants leak or rupture?
• What happens to gel that escapes into the body?
• How do you measure silicone in the body?
• How do you measure sensitivity to silicone?
• How often do women with implants suffer problems?
• Do implants cause or increase the risk of cancer?
• Do implants cause or exacerbate connective tissue disorders?

What is an IDE?

Investigational Device Exemption (IDE) is a permit for a physician to use a device that has not been approved for widespread distribution. Participation in an IDE study requires the investigator to supply additional information concerning the safety and effectiveness of the devices. Classification of the study under an IDE ensures that the clinical trials will be structured to gather this information under strictly controlled circumstances. Currently, silicone gel–filled implants used for reconstruction will not be included under an IDE, whereas those used for augmentation will be.

What does informed consent really mean?

"Informed consent" is a legal term that means that the individual contemplating a certain treatment be fully informed of all of the possible consequences of that treatment. To be truly "informed" this patient must be provided with this information in verbal and in written form and in terms that are clear and understandable. Risks and benefits of the procedure as well as possible complications and their consequences must be fully described and explained.

What type of informed consent does the FDA require for a woman getting silicone gel–filled breast implants?

The FDA has worked with the implant manufacturers to develop informed consent documents for silicone gel implants. (See Appendix C for an example of one of these documents.)

What is an implant registry? What is its purpose? Why should a woman participate?

An implant registry is a central computerized data bank that contains pertinent information on patients and their implants. The woman's name, address, and other personal data are kept on file. It also contains information concerning her silicone breast implant. For the registry to function optimally, this information should be updated periodically. The purpose of the registry is to provide ready access to women who are enrolled so that they can be contacted if there is new information concerning their implants. Information recorded in the registry can also be used to provide data to direct further study of the device.

Are there reasons why a woman would object to joining a registry? What are the potential problems?

Some individuals have pointed out that inclusion in a registry can pose a threat to a person's right to privacy. They also object to the fees that are sometimes required for participating in the registry.

Are there different types of registries? How can a woman find out how to join one? Is there a fee?

Presently there are two possible sources for registries: manufacturers and private organizations or foundations.

Each of the implant manufacturers still in the implant business is required to set up a registry for women using that company's implants. These are currently in place and are funded and organized by the manufacturers themselves. A patient can sign up for the prospective (for new patients) registry sponsored by the manufacturer through her doctor. There are no fees for participating in the manufacturer's registries. As a member of the registry a patient agrees to inform the registry via change-of-address cards or by calling a toll-free number if her name or address has changed and/or if her implant has been removed or replaced subsequent to implant surgery.

Medic Alert (a nonprofit foundation that provides bracelet identifiers for patients with medical conditions) has set up the International Breast Implant Registry. This registry is confidential and is not associated with the government or the manufacturers. The International Breast Implant Registry updates information on members twice a year, and the data are fed into their computerized data bank along with relevant information from researchers, manufacturers, and the FDA. Members and their physicians are contacted about any new findings or problems with specific implants and receive printed information. Members are also given the opportunity to participate in research studies. Women can find out more about the Medic Alert Registry by asking their doctors or by contacting Medic Alert directly (1-800-892-9211). A fee is charged for joining this registry during the first year, with a renewal fee every year thereafter.

If a woman already has implants, is she still eligible to join an implant registry?

The Medic Alert registry prospective study was designed to study the long-term effectiveness of implanted devices. The manufacturers also plan to offer a retrospective registry in addition to the prospective registry that is already in existence, but this has not yet been established. Once set up, it will be announced to the public at large.

How can a woman find out what type of implants she has?

Women who already have implants can find out what implant was used from their surgeons or from hospital records, if available. Those planning on having implants can ask their surgeons for a photocopy of the "sticker" that identifies the implant by brand name, type, product number, manufacturer, and date of implant. The manufacturers are also providing copies of a "Patient Card" that describes the specifics of the device that is being implanted.

How can a woman report problems with her implants?

She can report problems to the FDA by writing to the *United States Pharmacopeia* (USP) to obtain a problem reporting form, which she then fills out and returns. By using the form she can be sure that all important information pertaining to her problem will be included in the report, making her input as effective as possible. The form can be obtained by writing: USP, 12601 Twinbrook Parkway, Rockville, MD 20852. (The USP is under contract with the FDA to collect and organize the problem reports.) She may also report problems to the doctor who performed her implant surgery or to the company who manufactured them.

How can a woman sort through the media reports about implants to discover the truth about their safety and efficacy?

That is a difficult question. In our judgment the media is not the place to turn for objective scientific information. Rather, a woman seeking more information about implants should look to the scientific literature and to respected medical professionals for guidance. She may want to ask her physician to assist her by recommending articles, books, and videotapes that she can read or see on this topic. In addition, the information in this chapter and this book is culled from the scientific literature and from acknowledged experts. We have included an extensive bibliography to assist the reader in securing more information. The FDA has a toll-free telephone line for consumers (1-800-532-4440); by calling this number women can receive up-to-date, accurate information on silicone breast implants and their regulatory status.

What companies sell implants? How are these companies affected by the FDA ruling?

The bad publicity and subsequent litigation surrounding the breast implant controversy posed a tremendous threat to the existence of implant manufacturers. As a consequence, most manufacturers left the business in the early 1990s. Currently there are only three companies who continue to make breast implants: C.U.I., McGhan Medical Corporation (Inamed Corporation), and the Mentor Corporation. They are all carefully monitored by the FDA and must meet rigorous criteria for manufacture. These companies are participating in the clinical studies to provide additional information on the safety and effectiveness of these devices.

The companies remaining in the implant business are now subject to more stringent regulation; they are required to establish registries, participate in ongoing clinical trials, and conduct far-reaching product testing to ensure the continued safety and effectiveness of their products.

What steps have these companies taken to ensure the safety and effectiveness of breast implants?

These companies have completed or are in the process of completing numerous tests to evaluate the safety and effectiveness of these devices. They are also involved in research to develop and test new and improved devices. These studies have been ongoing for many years; in addition, new studies are now mandated by the FDA.

What part do these companies play in the clinical trials?

The companies play a pivotal role in the clinical trials. As a result, they will incur substantial expense in time and money to help implement the new studies. In the current studies the companies are required to work with specific doctors and centers around the country who agree to use their implants and to comply with the rules of the study. The companies are responsible for providing an FDA-approved protocol to these doctors so that they know how to proceed and for supplying these physicians with the necessary forms and paperwork to be completed on each patient. In addition, these companies must establish and support a patient registry and monitor each participating surgeon for compliance to the protocol. On request from the FDA these companies will also be required to collect and organize data on each patient for possible FDA evaluation.

Why have some companies gotten out of the implant business?

Many of the companies that left the implant business were large multinational companies, and for them the breast implant business represented an insignificant proportion of their overall business and a small contributor to their bottom line. In view of the bad publicity generated by scrutiny of implants in the national media, they decided that the best business decision was to withdraw from the market.

How will the FDA's regulations affect the price of implants?

Today, three companies remain in the business of manufacturing and selling breast implants and only two companies still manufacture and sell silicone gel–filled breast implants. These manufacturers are left with a smaller market, less demand for their product, and higher costs associated with implementing FDA regulations. They must fund the clinical trials and studies, deal with plaintiff's lawyers, and organize and finance registries. These additional financial and work-load burdens have understandably increased their cost of doing business. If they are to remain in business, this cost has to be passed on to the consumer. Consequently, the cost of silicone gel–filled breast implants has risen approximately 400% to 600% and most likely will continue to rise to enable these companies to continue to supply breast implants.

Is there any possibility that implant manufacturers will discontinue manufacturing silicone gel? If so, what alternate fillings will be available other than saline?

The likelihood is that within the next 2 to 3 years silicone gel in its present form will no longer be available as a filling for breast implants. Even though this gel has not been proved a health hazard, the litigation and bad publicity that is associated with this filling is causing manufacturers to seek alternatives. Currently, various new substances that promise to be radiolucent and easily absorbed by the body are under development. It is hoped that these fillings can be evaluated under the current clinical trials so that they can receive FDA approval in time to be used as substitute fills if silicone gel is no longer being manufactured.

What role have the manufacturers played in the silicone implant debate?

The manufacturers have played a key role in the breast implant debate, and these companies have been the subject of intense scrutiny and publicity. They have been both praised and condemned. All parties acknowledge that over the years these companies have invested enormous resources in developing these devices. They have poured millions into sophisticated technology aimed at testing and improving their products. They have also worked with the plastic surgeons using implants to get feedback for future design modifications. They have been committed to conducting ongoing research in support of these products. Although the profit motive remains a strong factor in all businesses, and implant manufacturers are no exception, these companies have always maintained a scientific interest in the products that they produced and have expressed a commitment to providing a service to women desiring these products. Critics feel that more attention should have been paid to assessing the long-term durability of these devices. Some say the companies were lax in conducting the specific studies needed to assess the long-term efficacy and safety of these devices and to meet FDA standards for premarket approval. Many believe that they should have taken the lead in coordinating follow-up with the plastic surgeons implanting these devices so that they could accurately assess the rate and severity of complications and the impact these problems had on the patients involved. Some plastic surgeons feel that they relied too heavily on the companies for supportive data, and now they question the accuracy of some of the information that they received. Nevertheless, most would agree, including the independent investigators who have studied these problems, that there were no major cover-ups or signs of wrongdoing and none of the information that has been disclosed indicates that these mistakes resulted in increased risk to the health and safety of women with implants. Furthermore, these companies are fully cooperating with the FDA to provide full disclosure and to produce the safety and effectiveness information that the FDA has demanded. It is unfortunate that this information was not gathered years earlier so that it would have been available to answer the FDA's queries and to prevent the concerns and fears that resulted.

What role have lawyers played in the silicone implant debate?

Reports in the press and media have pointed out the close relationship of the plaintiff's bar and the consumer advocacy groups that have been vocal in pressing the FDA to ban breast implants. Prior to the escalation of the breast implant debate, lawyers' groups set up special committees and organizations to solicit women as potential plaintiffs in lawsuits against the implant companies. The plaintiff lawyers' trade group, the Association of Trial Lawyers of America, set up a special Breast Implant Litigation Group. Numerous ads were placed in newspapers and on television encouraging women to contact these attorneys to report problems with implants.

The plaintiff's bar requires continuous product liability activity in order to thrive. Contingency-fee lawyers get approximately one third or more of the money awarded in such cases. The banning of these implants would provide them with a virtual gold mine in potential lawsuits to be filed against the implant manufacturers. As *The Wall Street Journal* reports, "The business of the contingency-fee lawyers . . . is speculating in litigation, hoping to hit deep pockets with big awards, of which they pocket a third or more." Numerous suits have been filed against implant companies and individual physicians. And, as reported in the *Boston Globe* in a story headline that reads "Lawyers Fight Over Limits of Implant Trials," these lawyers are also locked in battle with each other over the perceived rewards.

With so many different consumer groups speaking for women's interests in the implant debate, how is a woman to know which groups truly represent her interests and which ones are special interest groups that seek to profit from this debate or to address grievances?

It is often difficult to distinguish among the many consumer and support groups that speak for women's interests. Many women have complained that these groups misrepresent themselves as impartial support groups for women seeking information, whereas in reality they represent a specific bias. Women have complained that these groups do not provide them the balanced information they desire.

Conflict-of-interest charges have been raised against the most vocal of these consumer groups, the Public Citizen Health Research Group, led by Dr. Sidney Wolf, and its relationship with the FDA and with plaintiff attorneys. Some have suggested that Public Citizen Health Research Group can profit substantially from the banning of these devices and that this organization is indebted to plaintiff attorneys for funding. In an article in *Forbes*, several plaintiff attorneys were quoted as openly admitting to supporting the organization "overtly, covertly, in every possible way." Additionally, *The Wall Street Journal* reports that "the Public Citizen Health Research Group has prepared how-to kits on suing implant manufacturers; plaintiff lawyers pay the group $750 per kit."

To determine if a group will provide the unbiased scientific information you seek we suggest that you start by asking your physician about the names of groups that may be helpful. Many hospitals have support groups set up to aid breast cancer patients and their families. You might also check with the local chapter of the American Cancer Society (ACS) for names of groups in your area. In addition, Y-ME, the largest national support organization for breast cancer patients, is an excellent, reliable source of balanced information. (Appendix A includes a list of reputable support groups throughout the country that can assist you in obtaining information.)

What is the American Cancer Society's position on silicone gel–filled breast implants?

The American Cancer Society requested that the FDA continue to allow women access to silicone gel–filled breast implants for breast reconstruction. According to their background information on silicone breast implants, "Breast implants are considered an important and effective rehabilitation option for women who have had mastectomies. The American Cancer Society is aware of the importance of breast implant devices for these patients and has provided information about the benefits and risks of this procedure to patients and health professionals through its ongoing public and professional education programs."

The Society's position statement resolves: "The American Cancer Society believes that breast implants should continue to be made available as an option in cancer rehabilitation. Any decision regarding breast reconstruction should be discussed by the woman and her physician to determine the individual's benefits and risks. The American Cancer Society supports further research into long-term safety issues related to breast implants."

What experts should a woman consult about the advisability of breast implants for breast reconstruction or cosmetic breast surgery?

The woman considering breast surgery that involves breast implants should obtain detailed information about these devices before deciding if they are for her. Information in this book has been obtained from a host of sources. Additionally, she should seek input from her individual physicians: her family doctor, gynecologist, internist, oncologist, and surgeon. Plastic surgeons are well informed about breast implants and can give detailed information. If questions remain after the consultation, she should consider seeking opinions from other board-certified plastic surgeons with expertise in breast surgery. (See Chapter 12 for more information on selecting a plastic surgeon.) The FDA documents on silicone breast implants are another source of information as well as materials supplied by the manufacturers and the American Society of Plastic and Reconstructive Surgeons.

PUTTING THE ISSUE INTO PERSPECTIVE

Now that the initial evaluation has ended, what does it all mean? What are the ramifications for women desiring implant surgery? Are the dangers real or have they been distorted? What is the impact on women, their choices, their health care, and ultimately their peace of mind?

Evaluating the Risks

We would all like to have simple answers to these questions, but that is not likely in the immediate future. Fortunately, there are also no clear-cut dangers that should unduly alarm us. The preponderance of available scientific evidence suggests, and many credible experts seem to agree, that most women are not in any serious danger from silicone gel–filled or saline-filled implants or expanders. The FDA has concluded that "these devices do *not* [italics ours] present a health hazard." As is true of all surgical procedures and all implantable devices, benefits must be weighed against associated problems, risks, and complications, and women need to be alert to these dangers and fully informed about them.

Most women, however, do not experience serious complications from breast implants and expanders. Ongoing surveys of women who have had breast implant surgery indicate a high satisfaction level. When queried, most women indicate that they would choose to have implant surgery again. These devices have been on the market for 30 years, and if they had been linked to serious, debilitating health problems, surely we would have heard about it by now, not only in association with implants but in connection with the numerous devices, medications, and products that contain silicone and are widely ingested, injected, or implanted. Silicone is a commonly used material; there are few people in our society who do not have minute quantities of silicone in their bodies as a result of normal activities of daily life.

Defining the Problems: The Scientific Process

What of the women who have experienced serious health problems after implant surgery? Their concerns and anguish are not to be minimized, but the source of their problems needs to be scrutinized more closely. Are these conditions a result of the operation itself, are they associated with the implants, or are they coincidental? This investigation should be conducted not by lawyers in a courtroom, not by expert witnesses receiving payment for their testimony, not by the media in the headlines and on the talk shows, not by self-proclaimed consumer groups receiving funding from malpractice attorneys, but by skilled scientists with expertise in this area who have no special interests beyond the quest for answers to these women's problems. We need to examine the source of these problems to determine why they occurred and how they can be prevented or alleviated. It would be a disservice to women to attribute particular symptoms to implants when in fact these problems may have another cause that could be effectively treated if correctly diagnosed.

Peer review and randomized studies are the raw materials that have long supported the scientific process. These well-respected scientific methods have been largely ignored as the FDA hearings became politicized and sensationalized. It is time to redirect our efforts in the interest of women and of scientific progress.

FDA Ruling: Positives and Negatives

Although some may disagree with the FDA evaluation process and the specifics of its ruling, most would concur that the goal of obtaining reliable scientific information to answer the question of whether implants are safe and effective is an admirable one and worth pursuing. The FDA wants more information about possible health problems related to the use of these devices. The ruling calls for detailed scientific studies while allowing the use of breast implants under certain provisions. Additional data will be collected to answer basic questions about the safety and effectiveness of silicone gel–filled breast implants.

These clinical trials should have positive benefits. They can ensure comprehensive informed consent and follow-up for all women having silicone gel–filled implants for breast surgery. They are designed to provide a means for discovering the true incidence of problems experienced by women who have had these devices implanted, such as the rate of rupture, infection, and contracture. Additionally, they can look for possible links between these devices and other health conditions.

Access to these clinical trials and to silicone gel–filled implants is available to all women seeking breast reconstruction after mastectomy or for other breast deformities but is strictly limited to a small number of women requesting breast augmentation. The distinction between breast reconstruction patients and augmentation patients seems to interject a moral judgment in what should be a scientific investigation. The trials should study the safety of these devices, not whether some women have a "better" or more "pressing" need for them.

Impact of Breast Implant Controversy on the Doctor-Patient Relationship

The implant controversy called into question the competence and motives of medical professionals. They became targets of much media criticism; malpractice attorneys sought to isolate them, along with the implant manufacturers, as villains in the implant debate, even though implants, the object of these attacks, have never been proved unsafe. As a result, women's confidence in their doctors (particularly in plastic surgeons since they perform implant surgery) was eroded. This was unfortunate. The ties that bind patients to their doctors are crucial to patient well-being. Women facing breast cancer need to have a positive attitude and faith that their doctors will recommend the best treatment and provide the best care possible. They need to know that their doctors are on their team and are committed to helping them.

Few will benefit from this erosion of confidence, certainly not women or the doctors who care for them. If plastic surgeons erred in this scenario, it was by acts of omission, not acts of commission. They could have taken the lead years earlier in establishing registries for better patient follow-up and designing and implementing clinical and research studies on the long-term safety and viability of these devices. They could have worked with the manufacturers to provide a comprehensive, understandable informed consent document to be used for all patients contemplating implant surgery. Most likely they were lulled into complacency by the high level of patient satisfaction and low incidence of complications that they saw after implant surgery. If these measures had been taken, the hysteria generated over the safety of breast implants may have been averted. The much-needed supporting studies and data would have been available to address questions raised.

The female half of this writing team has spent the past 18 years observing and working with doctors and has generally been impressed with their genuine desire to provide optimal health care. Some are indeed more skilled than others, some are better communicators than others, and some are more devoted to their patients than others, but this is true of all people, all professionals. The ongoing FDA scrutiny of breast implants should not reflect on the motives of all caregivers who used them, often in response to patient desires. This is not to excuse those individuals who may not have acted in the best interest of their patients, particularly those physicians who were not qualified to perform implant surgery. (See Chapter 12 for information on how to investigate a doctor's credentials.) But a few bad actors should not cast doubt on the total performance. It would be unfortunate if the implant debate served to permanently undermine the doctor-patient relationship. When a woman is diagnosed with breast cancer, she needs to have confidence that her doctors will help her survive and overcome this life-threatening disease.

Impact of Breast Implant Controversy on Women

For breast cancer patients who have had reconstruction with implants, the breast implant controversy was anxiety provoking. Some of these women were led to believe that their reconstructive implants posed as serious a threat as the cancer they survived. Some were made to feel that they had "time bombs" implanted in their breasts; others were hounded by guilt for having wanted to restore their missing breasts. An atmosphere of fear was generated in the name of women, but not in their interest.

The restriction of silicone gel–filled breast implants primarily to breast reconstruction patients has unfairly penalized and stigmatized women who seek to enhance their self-image. Furthermore, it served to negate some of the positive psychological benefits of reconstructive surgery, sending a message to breast cancer patients that implants are not safe for healthy women. For many breast cancer patients, the doctor's recommendation for breast reconstruction is a sign that their prognosis is good and he considers them candidates for the same type of breast surgery as normal, healthy women. Now this positive reinforcement has been blunted. This may not have been the message that the FDA intended to send, but it was the message that the process delivered.

Healthy women have also been affected by this decision. Many cancer experts believe that breast reconstruction is a lifesaving option for many women who would delay seeking care for breast problems for fear of breast loss. (Implant reconstruction represents the least expensive, least complicated, least time consuming, and therefore most frequently selected method of breast restoration.) If women are aware of this source of rehabilitation, the hope is that they will be encouraged to practice BSE, to get regular physical examinations, and to go for regular mammograms. Thus, if a cancer is found, it will be in an earlier, more curable stage. Unfortunately, many women will now continue to regard implants, all implants, as hazardous despite the results of subsequent studies. Our surveys and interviews with women over the past 10 years confirm that some will choose to avoid or delay seeking treatment for a breast lump because of their overwhelming fear of breast mutilation. According to some reports, only 50% of the women who discover a breast lump see a doctor within 1 month, and 20% wait a year or more before seeing a physician. Delay in seeking treatment could be a serious blow to the progress that has been made in the early detection of breast cancer.

A Woman's Right to Choose

Women's rights continue to be assailed from many quarters. The FDA in its ruling regarding silicone gel breast implants limited a woman's right to make an informed decision in consultation with her doctor about her own health care. This is a personal decision, but the FDA has inserted itself between a woman and her doctor. As Peter Huber (author of *Galileo's Revenge: Junk Science in the Courtroom*) aptly points out in his 1992 article in *Forbes*, "If the state can regulate whether or not a woman can put a bag of silicone into her chest, it obviously can also regulate whether she can put an aspirator into her uterus or a contraceptive pill into her mouth. . . . Given all the recent publicity, no one can even plausibly claim that a woman who now opts in favor of a silicone implant has not been fully informed of the risks. If anything, she has been overinformed. The choice should now be hers. . . . When you compromise on the principle of personal autonomy—of freedom of individual choice—you are soon left with all compromise and no principle. . . . A breast implant, safe or dangerous, intact or ruptured, is still just a bag of plastic. When a woman stands in her doctor's office discussing a breast implant, there's only one body and one life involved: her own."

•   •   •

The decision of the FDA and the sensational stories of the media that surfaced in 1992 portrayed women as pawns and second-class citizens. According to Peter Huber, "The entire debate has revolved around a vision of vain, foolish, helpless women—women at the mercy of manipulative doctors and conspiring chemical companies, women more like children than adults, women incapable of making intelligent, individual choices for themselves." Those of us who know and work with women with breast cancer know that this is not the case. Women can only gain control over this devastating disease if they have the necessary information and knowledge, and most women who investigate breast cancer treatment and breast reconstruction do so with great intelligence and diligence.

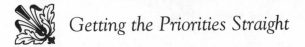

Getting the Priorities Straight

Breast cancer is an overriding threat for all women. It is the most common malignancy in American women, with approximately 180,000 new cases diagnosed each year. It is also the second most common cause of cancer death in women; this year alone over 40,000 women will die from this disease. It seems somehow frivolous for the media and the government to focus so much time and money on breast implants when the real culprit remains virtually ignored.

The breast implant debate has now subsided, and as time passes, many women reading this material will be unaware of the controversy that raged and will not be faced with the same issues and concerns. Breast implants are not perfect, but they are not the public enemy that they have been portrayed, and they probably did not warrant all of the attention that they received. The positive psychological, aesthetic, and physical benefits they confer have been all but overlooked in a media blitz of unparalleled proportions. If these devices had not been implanted in women's breasts but rather in some other area of the body, they probably would not have received such widespread attention.

This discussion has attempted to examine the issues and controversies surrounding silicone gel and saline implants based on logic and scientific evidence. Although women's choices have become more limited, we hope that this discussion will help alleviate some of the anxiety that has been generated and allow women to direct their attention to a far more ominous threat that confronts them. Breast cancer is the enemy, and women need to be fully empowered to face this serious challenge.

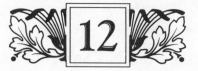

SELECTING AND COMMUNICATING WITH A PLASTIC SURGEON

Having made a decision to seek breast reconstruction, a woman needs to choose her plastic surgeon carefully. Today, one sees ads for plastic surgery in newspapers, the *Yellow Pages*, and even magazines on the newsstand. These ads, however, are not discriminating and therefore are not the best means for selecting a plastic surgeon to perform breast reconstruction or for choosing any doctor to provide medical care. Many highly trained physicians choose not to advertise at all. Rather than selecting a plastic surgeon based on ads, a prospective patient should consider the following guidelines for making this choice.

TRAINING

The physician a woman selects should be trained in plastic surgery and have met the qualifications of the American Board of Plastic Surgery, which grants board certification in this specialty. To be able to take the board examination a surgeon must have 3 to 5 years of training in general surgery or in a surgical subspecialty and an additional 2 to 3 years of specialized training in the broad aspects of plastic surgery. Furthermore, he must demonstrate competence by completing an approved residency training program; this means the doctor's peers have approved his moral and ethical qualifications as well as his knowledge in the field. Approximately 1 to 2 years after residency training is completed, he is eligible to take board examinations and once again subject himself to the scrutiny of peers in order to obtain board certification. Once certified, he may apply for membership in the American Society of Plastic and Reconstructive Surgeons (ASPRS).

EXPERIENCE

The plastic surgeon a woman chooses should have experience with the different techniques appropriate for breast reconstruction and have a record of successful operations. If he has a teaching appointment at a medical school–affiliated hospital, this association suggests access to the latest surgical techniques, involvement in the education of residents, and awareness of recent developments in the field. It is not enough to be just a well-trained plastic surgeon. A good doctor must know about the specific procedures that apply to the patient's problem if he is to render optimal care.

HOW DO YOU INVESTIGATE A DOCTOR'S CREDENTIALS?

Getting information about a doctor's training is easy to do and worth the effort. This information is available in the reference room at the local library. It can be found in a book entitled *The Directory of Medical Specialists*, which lists only board-certified specialists. It will list the doctor's year of birth, medical school, the year he was licensed to practice, the year of specialty certification, primary and secondary specialties, and type of practice. Other information on training and hospital and medical affiliations also is included. Doctors in this book are listed geographically, so it is easy to locate the names of doctors in each community. The *American Medical Directory* is another helpful reference, but, unlike *The Directory of Medical Specialists*, it does not indicate if a physician is board certified.

FINDING A PLASTIC SURGEON

How do you find out whose surgical competence is highly regarded? How do you know who is experienced in breast reconstruction? Most people do not know where to go for reliable information. This information, however, can be obtained from numerous sources. One of the best sources of referral is another physician in the community or another member of the breast management team. The general surgeon is a knowledgeable person to ask; frequently he works with a plastic surgeon as part of a team. He also may have patients who have had breast reconstruction and are willing to discuss this topic and recommend their doctors. Other women who have had breast reconstruction provide an excellent source of information and reliable recommendations about their plastic surgeons; they have firsthand knowledge of this surgery and can personally relate to the surgeon's skill and bedside manner. A woman's gynecologist or family physician also may know the names of plastic surgeons who have performed successful breast reconstructions.

The American Society of Plastic and Reconstructive Surgeons (444 E. Algonquin Rd., Arlington Heights, IL 60051; 708-228-9900) provides information on breast reconstruction; it also will supply a list of board-certified plastic surgeons performing reconstructive breast surgery in different communities throughout the United States. The American Cancer Society, through its Reach to Recovery Program, is now providing information on breast reconstruction. By contacting this organization through the local chapter of the American Cancer Society, the woman desiring information on breast reconstruction will be placed in contact with a woman who has had her breast reconstructed and will share her experiences. Breast cancer and breast reconstruction support groups also provide valuable information and access to other women of similar age and background who have had breast reconstruction. Many times these support groups are affiliated with local hospitals. The local medical society is another source of information; it often has lists of specialists in the community and their areas of interest. (See Appendix A for more information on this topic.)

FINDING THE RIGHT PLASTIC SURGEON

Locating a qualified plastic surgeon does not necessarily mean a woman has found the right surgeon for her. She needs to determine if this physician will meet both her physical and emotional needs. Breast reconstruction is a very emotional experience; a woman's breasts have far greater psychological implications than their anatomy and physiology would suggest. A woman needs a doctor who listens, who treats her as an individual, and who has time to deal with her concerns.

Remember, as with any anticipated surgery, a woman should consider a second opinion before finally selecting a surgeon. Some women, however, hesitate to request another opinion for fear it will offend their doctors. They are intimidated by their doctors and are reluctant to question their statements and seek more information. Time spent in finding the right plastic surgeon is well invested, however. Unfortunately, most people do not devote the necessary effort in making this important choice. As one woman in our survey so aptly explained, "Most women devote more attention to buying a vacuum cleaner than they do to selecting a doctor."

QUESTIONS TO ASK A PLASTIC SURGEON

Before selecting a plastic surgeon a woman needs to know that he is receptive to her questions and concerns. To assist in making a satisfactory choice of a plastic surgeon, we have included some questions a woman might ask during her consultation.*

- How many breast reconstructions have you done and what type of results have you achieved?
- May I talk with several of your patients who have had this surgery?
- What are the different options for breast reconstruction?
- What are the benefits and risks associated with the different reconstructive techniques?
- What are the benefits and risks associated with breast implants?
- Is it possible to have reconstruction with my own tissue and without an implant?
- Which reconstruction approach is appropriate for me and why?
- What is involved in this surgery?
- What type of anesthesia will be used: local or general?
- How many different procedures and hospitalizations will be needed? How long will I be in surgery for each operation?
- What type of scars will I have and exactly where will they be placed?
- What are the expected results of surgery? Can I expect good long-term results?
- Will my breasts be symmetric?
- How long will it take me to recuperate?
- What are the anticipated costs of surgery?
- Will you help me file for insurance coverage?
- What are possible complications from this surgery?

   Some plastic surgeons may have photographs of breast reconstructive patients. These might help the patient understand the results that can be achieved for a deformity such as hers.

*Chapters 9 through 13 are totally devoted to answering women's frequently asked questions about breast reconstruction.

QUESTIONS TO ASK YOURSELF BEFORE YOU SCHEDULE SURGERY

- Is this the plastic surgeon I want to do my breast reconstruction?
- Is he properly trained and qualified?
- Does this surgeon seem to understand how I feel and is he sensitive to my needs?
- Has he taken the time to understand what I want done?
- Has he provided me with enough information so that I can make an informed decision?
- Is he going to spend the necessary time with me to answer my questions and deal with my concerns?
- Does he have the necessary skill to perform this surgery?
- Has he explained what he plans to do in terms that I can understand?
- Does he treat me as a responsible adult?
- Does his plan for surgery agree with my expectations for what I would like done?
- If there is a problem, do I feel comfortable with this surgeon handling it?

COMMUNICATING WITH A PLASTIC SURGEON

Good communication not only helps the patient find the best plastic surgeon to perform her breast restoration, but also enables her to work with him to achieve the result she desires. Preoperative consultations provide the patient and surgeon with an ideal setting for discussing their thoughts and exploring their expectations for a final result.

A typical consultation with a plastic surgeon about breast reconstruction should begin with an explanation of the woman's concerns and expectations for this operation and a complete review of her medical and surgical history. It is in a woman's best interest to have a plastic surgeon who is well informed about all aspects of her health and tumor care so that he can consider these factors in discussing reconstructive options with her. It is helpful if he has copies of the general surgeon's operative report and the pathologist's report. He also needs to be aware of the radiation and chemotherapy that she has received, the status of her opposite breast, and her feelings about it.

After this initial discussion the plastic surgeon will need to physically examine the woman's chest, back, and abdomen to determine the extent of her deformity and the reconstructive approaches that are appropriate for her physical situation.

Preoperative photographs are taken during this initial examination by a plastic surgeon, and a woman should expect to be photographed during her visit. If she visits more than one doctor, she usually will have pictures taken by each doctor. Although these photographs do not show the patient's face, sometimes this picture-taking process is unsettling for the woman. These photographs are important, however, because the plastic surgeon will use them for evaluating her condition and planning her operation. They also provide a record of her treatment. He may eventually use them (with the woman's permission) for educational purposes to demonstrate the results of this surgery to other patients and physicians and for publication in the professional literature.

Once this examination has been concluded, the woman can again meet with the doctor to review the different options for breast reconstruction. Final determination of the operative plan must often wait until the plastic surgeon has consulted with the other members of the breast management team.

If a woman has a husband or if there is another important person in her life (many physicians call this person a "significant other"), this individual should accompany the patient on her preoperative visits with the plastic surgeon. Mutual expectations can then be aired and discussed and the influence of the man's feelings on the woman can be observed and evaluated. Even though the man and woman share in the learning process, the final decision about surgery must be made by the woman herself. At no time should a woman feel pressured into this surgery by a relative, friend, husband, or even the plastic surgeon with whom she is consulting.

If a woman has a consultation with her plastic surgeon before her mastectomy, they should discuss the correct timing of reconstructive surgery, whether immediate or delayed. If she desires an immediate reconstruction, the general surgeon and plastic surgeon need to confer and agree on the suitability of this approach for her. Before an immediate breast reconstruction is done, the details of timing, operative care, and team cooperation must be carefully planned.

The woman who consults with a plastic surgeon after her mastectomy should remember that reconstructive breast surgery is never an emergency procedure. In the interest of good communication she may require several visits to her plastic surgeon to answer all of her questions, to clearly explain her expectations for reconstruction, and to work with him to define a specific surgical plan appropriate for her. There are many methods for reconstructing breasts today, and a well-trained plastic surgeon will probably be knowledgeable in a number of different procedures. It is important, however, that the type of reconstruction a woman selects be the simplest and safest procedure yet still is the most likely to meet her expectations for a good result.

SURGICAL OPTIONS FOR BREAST RECONSTRUCTION

A s recently as 20 years ago a woman who had a mastectomy had few options if she desired breast restoration. Breast reconstruction techniques had not been perfected, and the most a woman could expect was the creation of a breast mound that bore little resemblance to her remaining breast. Without reconstructive surgery she faced the prospect of living with a lopsided chest or wearing a breast prosthesis to hide her deformity. A prosthesis, however, was not always the solution to her problem. Sometimes it made a woman feel increasingly self-conscious because she worried that her artificial breast would become dislodged and be obvious to others. Betty Rollins' humorous yet poignant account of her attempt to find a suitable external prosthesis after her mastectomy reveals the frustration felt by many women in trying to appear whole again.

Today, with the development and refinement of techniques to satisfy the requests of women seeking breast restoration, the results of reconstructive surgery have improved dramatically. Women who require or choose a mastectomy can now select from a number of reliable procedures that meet their psychological and aesthetic expectations for breast restoration. Breasts can be rebuilt using implants or expanders and the tissue remaining after the mastectomy or with flaps of muscle or muscle and skin (musculocutaneous) obtained from the abdomen, back, or buttocks and then transferred to the chest wall. The choice of reconstructive method depends on the amount and quality of the tissue remaining after the mastectomy, the surgeon's experience with each technique, and the patient's preferences and expectations. In addition to these basic operations, the patient may request additional procedures to enhance breast appearance.

In deciding which surgical option is appropriate for her a woman first must resolve her feelings about her remaining breast. Does she like the way it looks and want the rebuilt breast to match it? (Most women have strong feelings about preserving their remaining breast intact.) Is she willing to consider an operation on her normal breast if this will make both breasts appear symmetric? If her remaining breast is large and full and she does not want it modified, will she agree to a flap procedure that will provide sufficient tissue to match her large breast but will also result in an abdominal, back, side, or buttock scar? Her feelings about her remaining breast will affect the type of procedure chosen and the ultimate success of the reconstructive effort.

This chapter is designed to be a woman's guide to the different techniques available for breast restoration, their indications for use, and their advantages and disadvantages. Additionally, the various types of implants and expanders and their applications are described. The optimal timing of breast reconstruction is also considered, with a full discussion of the benefits and risks of immediate and delayed breast reconstruction. No one procedure is advocated above any other. The particular approach must be selected with the individual woman's needs and her deformity in mind.

IMMEDIATE VS. DELAYED BREAST RECONSTRUCTION

Once a woman has decided that she wants breast reconstruction, timing becomes an important consideration. When should this elective surgery be performed? Should she have breast reconstruction immediately at the time of the mastectomy or wait until some time after the mastectomy for a delayed breast reconstruction? For some women, the decision is made by circumstance because they are unaware that reconstruction is possible until long after the mastectomy has been performed. Today, however, with increased emphasis on informed consent, many women learn of the option of reconstruction from their general surgeons or other doctors before they have their cancer surgery and have the opportunity to contact a plastic surgeon (or more than one for second opinions) to discuss reconstructive surgery and the correct timing for this procedure.

The past 10 years have witnessed important changes in breast cancer detection and management. Today the diagnosis of breast cancer does not mean that a woman must experience permanent breast loss after breast cancer treatment. Increasing experience with conservative surgery and radiation therapy and mastectomy and immediate breast reconstruction have demonstrated the validity and efficacy of these approaches in providing women with optimal treatment of their cancer with minimal deformity. Furthermore, many breast cancers are being detected at an early, more curable stage, breast reconstruction techniques have improved, and cooperation between reconstructive surgeons and general surgeons or surgical oncologists (surgeons who specialize in cancer surgery) have increased. Immediate breast reconstruction is now being requested and performed with much greater frequency and with better results. General surgeons have come to accept immediate reconstructive surgery as a viable and appealing option for many breast cancer patients who desire breast preservation have an excellent prognosis, and are not candidates for conservative surgery and irradiation.

Before the decision for immediate breast reconstruction can be made, the general surgeon and the patient must address the proper management of her breast cancer as the foremost consideration. No aspect of treatment should be compromised. The possible need for adjunctive treatment, either radiation therapy or chemotherapy, is a key factor in the timing of breast reconstruction. Breast reconstruction should not delay the administration of chemotherapy. Often it is wise to delay the breast reconstruction until after radiation therapy has been completed. The potential for achieving the most aesthetic breast appearance is also an important consideration. To help the patient make the best decision the reconstructive surgeon should let her know which approach he thinks will produce the optimal result.

The choice between immediate and delayed reconstruction makes the decisions a woman must make before her breast cancer treatment even more complex. Not only must she decide on the appropriate tumor management, but she also has to select the best reconstructive technique, the correct timing for her breast reconstruction, and the plastic surgeon to perform it. A sense of urgency pervades her decision making if she is not to delay or compromise the treatment of her cancer. She has much additional information to process and more specialists to consult. All of this can be overwhelming for some women, and they understandably choose not to respond promptly but to face treatment one step at a time. Others opt for an immediate procedure to avoid breast loss and the trauma of yet another major surgical procedure. Fortunately, access to information and care is now more readily available to many women interested in immediate reconstruction. With increasing experience, many breast management teams have now fully incorporated immediate breast reconstruction into the choices for management presented to the patient during her initial discussions about tumor management. The plastic surgeon is often part of these initial discussions, and the scheduling of appointments and the actual operation can be streamlined through this type of teamwork. Ultimately, however, the decision to have immediate or delayed reconstruction is a personal one influenced by the patient's individual needs, the stage of her cancer, and the recommendations of her general surgeon and her plastic surgeon. She makes this decision after she has had full opportunity to weigh the advantages and disadvantages of each approach and choose the one that is best for her. (See p. 54 for more information on immediate breast reconstruction.)

What Are the Advantages of Immediate Reconstruction?

Immediate reconstruction, or reconstructive surgery performed at the same time as the mastectomy, has a definite psychological appeal for many women. Dealing with a life-threatening disease and simultaneously coping with the loss of a breast are devastating to most women. Some woman even delay medical help and refuse a mastectomy because they fear losing a breast. Some women will not consider a mastectomy unless they can have immediate breast reconstruction. Others decide to have a lumpectomy and radiation therapy even though this may not be the best treatment for them. In recent interviews with young women in their twenties and thirties who had chosen mastectomy and immediate breast reconstruction, many explained that they felt that immediate reconstruction was a compelling necessity for them in order to adjust to their diagnosis and to continue to conduct normal social lives. The desire to be seen as "normal" among their peers and to be able to interact with the opposite sex was crucially important to them.

Obvious psychological and aesthetic advantages are associated with an immediate procedure; the patient who requests it is usually pleased with her decision. The breast management team is sending her a message that her prognosis is positive enough to justify beginning her rehabilitation without delay. The patient feels that her doctors are addressing not only her tumor but her overall concerns as well.

Cooperation between the oncologic surgeon and plastic surgeon can often result in more attractive reconstructed breasts, sometimes with less scarring. Improvements in immediate breast reconstruction have led many plastic surgeons to believe that the results they achieve with immediate reconstruction are often as good or better than those they attain with delayed reconstruction. Often immediate reconstruction can permit the surgeon to remove less breast skin than would ordinarily be removed for a mastectomy alone, thus reducing or shortening the breast scar. The preserved skin used to cover the new breast reduces the need for skin expansion and requires less transferred skin from the abdomen, back, or buttocks if autologous breast reconstruction has been selected. The surgeon can also help preserve the landmarks of the breast such as the inframammary fold (where the breast meets the chest wall) and the medial (central) and lateral (side) limits of the breast; these boundaries can then be used to more accurately rebuild the woman's breast, resulting in a reconstructed breast that often exhibits optimal symmetry with the remaining breast.

Studies by Schain et al., Noone et al., and Dowden reveal that immediate reconstruction has positive psychological benefits for women who wish to rid themselves of their preoccupation with cancer and breast loss. Furthermore, these women are, for the most part, satisfied with the results of their immediate surgery. The study by Schain et al. indicates that women having immediate breast reconstruction experience less overall psychological trauma and recall the pain of their mastectomy less intensely. Their new breasts are incorporated more quickly into a redefined body image and they exhibit a lower level of distress, probably because they awaken from the mastectomy with a breast contour intact and thus do not experience the sense of mutilation that so often accompanies breast amputation. They also do not feel the anxiety associated with camouflaging the defect or having the external prosthesis become dislodged. These women are particularly grateful that they did not have to live without their breast or breasts for any period of time. These studies have also shown that the survival rate of immediate breast reconstruction patients is comparable to that of patients who have not had reconstructive surgery and that the local recurrence rate is no higher in this group.

Essentially the same techniques are used for immediate breast reconstruction as for delayed breast reconstruction, sometimes with specific modifications to accommodate the mastectomy. The primary procedures used include implant or tissue expander reconstruction

with the available tissues left at the mastectomy site or breast reconstruction with autologous tissue (the patient's natural tissue) from the
lower abdomen, back, or buttock. Immediate breast reconstruction also provides for a quicker resolution of the mastectomy deformity and
reduces the number of operations the woman has to undergo without
significantly lengthening her hospitalization. She benefits from the
reduced cost of having one operation under general anesthesia performed during one hospitalization. She can recover from the mastectomy and the breast reconstruction at the same time without the need
to schedule additional time for another operation for the reconstruction at a later date.

What Are the Disadvantages of an Immediate Procedure?

Symmetry is sometimes difficult to obtain in one operation, and the
patient should anticipate the need for another procedure to improve
the result. If the nipple-areola is placed at the time of mastectomy, its
final and ideal position is difficult to determine. Therefore immediate reconstruction usually does not include a nipple-areola; this is delayed until a later operation. Sometimes, when the cancer is preinvasive, the nipple-areola can be preserved. Furthermore, some surgeons
do not want to operate on the remaining breast at the time of the
mastectomy.

There is a higher complication rate from skin loss, hematoma, and
infection with immediate reconstruction, especially with implant
surgery. The mastectomy wound, fluid accumulation (seroma), and
low-grade infection add to the potential for fibrous formation around
an implant, possibly resulting in capsular contracture or hardening of
the reconstructed breast. Infection can pose a problem if a tissue
expander is in place; the expander may have to be removed to allow
time for the tissues to heal before once again attempting reconstruction, this time on a delayed basis. The reconstructive surgeon may suggest that some latissimus dorsi muscle be transferred from the back to
enhance implant cover and lower the chance of infection or implant
exposure.

Immediate breast reconstruction with an implant or expander
typically requires about the same amount of time as the mastectomy.
When a TRAM flap is done, it usually takes twice as long as the
mastectomy. Free flaps can take even longer. The woman who elects
immediate reconstruction must have realistic expectations about her
breast appearance after immediate reconstruction. It will not be a

replica of the breast that she lost. Sensation will also be decreased and lactation will no longer be possible. Furthermore, the breast reconstruction will not be complete with this one operation. A second and sometimes a third procedure are necessary to complete the process, depending on the type of breast reconstruction selected, the individual healing process, and the expectations and preferences of the surgeon and the patient.

Some plastic surgeons fear that a less than perfect reconstruction could cause further emotional distress for an already stressed patient. Since the patient has not seen the mastectomy deformity, she measures the reconstruction against her normal breast. Many plastic surgeons and women who have had a delayed reconstruction feel that the mastectomy experience is traumatic enough without adding reconstruction to it. Since reconstruction is for a lifetime, the woman should have the best possible result, which additional time may help the surgeon to achieve.

Close teamwork between the general surgeon and the plastic surgeon is required for this surgical approach. The general surgeon should be supportive of the decision for immediate breast reconstruction, and he must work with the plastic surgeon to plan and perform this operation.

There are obvious benefits and risks to be considered in immediate reconstruction. They are summarized as follows:

Benefits	Risks
Possible improved aesthetic result	Less time for physicians to assess
Avoidance of trauma attending the mastectomy experience	the needs for additional therapy that may be required
Reduced cost and hospitalization	Higher complication rate and
Potentially shorter mastectomy scar	longer operative time
	Additional anesthesia time

What Are the Advantages of Delayed Reconstruction?

Delayed reconstruction can be performed from a few days to years after the mastectomy. For patients with stage I disease who do not require chemotherapy or radiation therapy, many plastic surgeons prefer reconstruction 3 to 6 months after mastectomy.

Delayed surgery affords the woman time to cope with her initial cancer. In recent interviews, 14 women who had delayed reconstruction were asked if they would have preferred their reconstruction done immediately. Although four admitted that they could have had the procedure earlier than they did (after 11-, 9-, 6-, and 3-year delays), they all felt that a waiting period was necessary to allow them to "cope with their cancer, get their emotional lives in order, and separate the negative cancer experience from the very positive reconstruction." In addition, these patients also felt delaying their surgery gave them more time to investigate reconstructive surgery and thus they had more realistic expectations about what reconstructive surgery could provide.

By delaying her reconstructive surgery a woman has time to fully evaluate her decision to have her breast rebuilt; some women change their minds after a waiting period and decide not to pursue this option. This time also allows a woman to recover from any additional therapy that might be required and to fully explore the topic of reconstruction, find the right plastic surgeon, get to know him, and decide on the correct reconstructive approach.

For the plastic surgeon, delay offers the psychological benefit of a patient committed to this procedure. In addition, for health considerations, the plastic surgeon and general surgeon often prefer to know and to help the patient understand the full extent of her disease and the anticipated treatment before she embarks on further surgery.

Delayed reconstruction allows the breast tissues time to heal, soften, and settle. There is less chance of infection, seroma, and implant extrusion. For the woman having breast reconstruction with her own tissues, she can plan the timing, select the surgeon, and donate her own blood prior to a more involved procedure, which has a longer recovery. The surgeon can then plan his surgery more effectively to achieve breast symmetry and accurate placement of the nipple-areola (if it is to be reconstructed). The plastic surgeon may feel he has better control of the variables than when a new operation is initiated at the end of a mastectomy operation.

What Are the Disadvantages of a Delayed Procedure?

One of the primary disadvantages of a delayed procedure is the period of time that a woman must live without her breast and the associated psychological and emotional trauma she will experience. A second operation also involves another hospitalization, another general anesthesia, and additional pain, recuperation time, and cost. Some women who do not have this procedure at the time of their mastectomy may not ever have the opportunity for breast reconstruction again.

Again, there are risks and benefits of a delayed procedure:

Benefits	Risks
Time to recover from mastectomy	Time to dwell on cancer
Time to recover from adjunctive therapy	Patient may experience depression from mastectomy status
Time to get acquainted with plastic surgeon	Patient may never "get around" to having reconstruction
Time to make an informed decision	Additional cost of two surgeries (both financial and time)
	Additional potential for problems from two surgeries and two anesthetics

What Is the Correct Timing for Breast Reconstruction if the Patient Requires Chemotherapy or Radiation Therapy?

Most physicians recommend that patients with positive lymph nodes or disease that has spread beyond the breast area have chemotherapy, hormonal therapy, or radiation therapy before breast restoration. Most adjunctive chemotherapy now lasts for 6 months. Chemotherapy can impair the body's ability to resist infection by lowering the white blood cell count; therefore it is important to delay breast reconstruction for at least 1 month and preferably 2 to 3 months after the completion of chemotherapy to be sure that the patient's blood count has returned to normal. Because radiation therapy causes some changes in the skin, the reconstructive surgeon also will recommend that the patient wait at least 6 weeks after radiation therapy to reduce the possibility of healing problems after the operation. Some women do not want to wait until the adjunctive therapy has been completed and decide to have immediate reconstruction and then radiation and/or chemotherapy.

What Timing Is Suggested for Patients With Advanced Disease?

Once the woman with advanced disease and her surgeon decide to proceed with reconstructive breast surgery, they need to determine the correct timing for this procedure. On the one hand, these women have a less favorable prognosis than if they did not require chemotherapy; thus they often prefer to go ahead with reconstruction without delay. On the other hand, they also have a greater risk of developing local recurrences, and the systemic chemotherapy can affect their blood count and modify the wound-healing potential. Surgeons usually prefer to delay breast reconstruction until after chemotherapy or radiation therapy. Because some patients with advanced disease have earlier recurrences or relapses after cessation of chemotherapy, some oncologists suggest that reconstructive surgery be delayed 1 to 2 years after chemotherapy. However, the blood count and other variables that can affect wound healing usually return to normal by 1 month. Each case is individual and the reconstructive surgeon and medical oncologist should confer concerning the proper interval after chemotherapy. The surgeon half of our writing team usually advises patients with advanced disease to complete chemotherapy and wait 2 to 6 months before having reconstruction. (See p. 128 for more information on the timing of breast reconstruction.)

Results With Immediate Breast Reconstruction

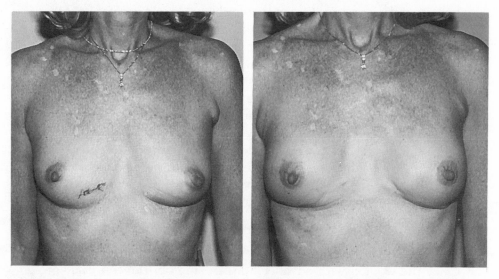

Lumpectomy and axillary lymph node dissection were used to treat this woman's left breast cancer. An extensive intraductal component and positive tumor margins were found on pathologic examination. Bilateral total mastectomies and immediate breast reconstruction were then performed with breast implants placed beneath the muscle. No new scars were created and her nipple-areolae were spared.

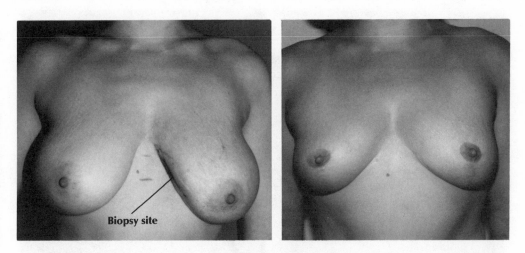

This 28-year-old woman desired a lumpectomy to treat her left breast cancer. Since she wanted smaller breasts, lumpectomy was combined with reduction of both breasts.

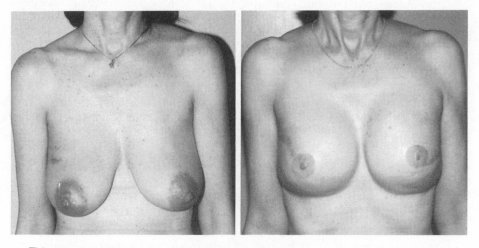

This 44-year-old woman had bilateral prophylactic mastectomies and immediate reconstruction with tissue expansion. The patient is shown 2 years after nipple-areola reconstruction.

Results With Immediate Breast Reconstruction—cont'd

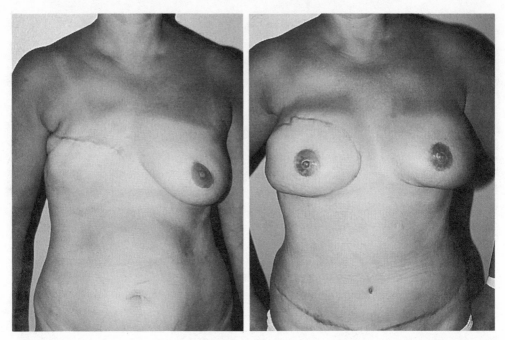

This woman, who previously had a modified radical mastectomy of her right breast, elected to have a left prophylactic mastectomy and immediate TRAM reconstruction and delayed TRAM reconstruction of her right breast. Skin-sparing incisions were used around the areola and in the inframammary fold. This patient illustrates how the length of incisions can be reduced when immediate breast reconstruction is performed.

RECONSTRUCTION WITH AVAILABLE TISSUE

Despite their desire for breast restoration after treatment for breast cancer, many women will forego reconstructive surgery if it means a lengthy or complicated operation, convalescence, and rehabilitation. Constraints of time and money or psychological needs often limit their choices to a simple procedure or to no procedure at all. Women who choose these simpler procedures do not object to the use of a foreign material in their bodies and do not express overriding concerns about breast implants. Their chief goal is breast restoration in the simplest and most convenient manner. For these women, implant or expander reconstruction provides the perfect solution. Unlike the more complex flap techniques, the operative variables are not increased, new scars are not created, and the potential for perioperative complications is minimized. Furthermore, these procedures do not rule out other procedures, especially flap operations, should they become necessary in the future. The patient who chooses implant reconstruction should be aware, however, that this reconstructive approach is not necessarily a one-stage procedure. A second operation will be required to reconstruct the nipple-areola and if necessary to make appropriate adjustments in implant size. Similarly, tissue expansion will require additional office visits to inflate the expander and for implant placement or adjustment and nipple-areola reconstruction. Under most circumstances these secondary procedures can be performed on an outpatient basis.

Before we discuss implant and expander reconstruction techniques and their expected postoperative care and recuperation, a brief review of the available implants and tissue expanders is appropriate.

Types of Implants and Expanders

Basically there are two broad categories of implants: fixed-volume breast implants and implants in which the volume can be changed after they are implanted (the latter are called *tissue expanders*). All current implants have a silicone layer or envelope that contains the filling; this covering is the outer material in contact with the body tissues.

Of the fixed-volume implants available, the ones most commonly used today are those that can be inflated with saline solution. (Those with silicone gel can only be used if a woman is enrolled in clinical trials.) Alternative implant fill materials that are radiolucent on mammography, compatible with the surrounding tissues, and absorbed by the body if a leak occurs are under development and should be available within the next 3 to 5 years.

Implants that contain only saline solution do not have the potential for silicone leakage. They may not, however, have the natural feel that implants containing some gel do. When saline-filled implants are soft and have good cover, they can feel natural. When there is thin tissue over these implants, a margin of the implant may be felt or the breast may have a rippled appearance. If leakage develops, they will deflate, whereby another procedure is needed to replace the implant. Although leakage and deflation were problems associated with earlier saline implants, today's saline inflatable implants have a much lower incidence of deflation.

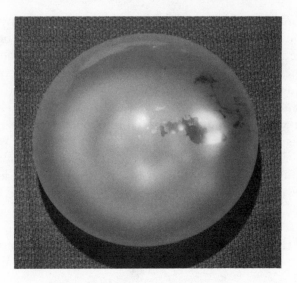

Saline-filled textured-surface implant

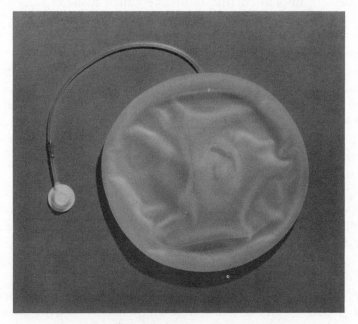

Textured-surface permanent expander implant

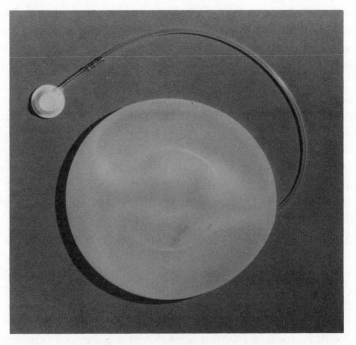

Postoperatively adjustable saline-filled
textured-surface implant

Tissue expanders are adjustable implants that can be inflated with saltwater (saline) to stretch the tissues at the mastectomy site. These tissue expanders have a silicone shell that can be filled with saline solution and adjusted after their placement. The saline solution is injected through the skin and into a valve leading to the implant. This fill valve is either a separate valve connected with tubing near the breast reconstruction site or it is attached to the front of the implant. After the breast has been expanded to the proper volume and shape, the expander is left in place as the definitive implant or is exchanged for a permanent fixed-volume implant.

There are two basic designs of tissue expander valves through which the saltwater is injected to inflate the expander and stretch the tissues. One type of valve is connected to the tissue expander through silicone tubing. (This is the kind found in the permanent expander implant and the postoperatively adjustable implant.) This valve may be removed or in the case of the smaller valves (less than ½ inch in diameter) it can be left in for an extended period of time to permit future adjustments in breast size. Another type of valve is an integral part of the tissue expander. A metal disk is incorporated in the back of this integral valve, and a magnetic finder is then used to locate the site for injection of the saline solution. This valve can sometimes be felt through thin skin cover.

The postoperatively adjustable implant and permanent expander implant are alternatives to the temporary expander and are being used with increasing frequency for many implant breast reconstructions. Both of these devices permit postoperative adjustments in breast size. The *postoperatively adjustable implant* contains only saline solution; it is basically a saline implant that has separate tubing connecting it to a small fill valve, usually located in the underarm area. The *permanent expander implant* has two envelopes as opposed to the single envelope used in the postoperatively adjustable implant. The outer envelope contains a thin layer of silicone gel. This silicone layer can produce a more natural feel without the rippling that is sometimes evident through thin skin when only saline is used; it also reduces the possibility of saline leakage from the inner compartment. The quantity of silicone gel in the outer envelope is minimal. (Most likely, within the next few years this gel will be replaced with one of the new substances currently under development.) Similar to the postoperatively adjustable implant, the permanent expander implant has separate tubing connecting the implant to a small valve placed under the skin, usually at the side of the breast, below the breast, or in the axilla. With these two models of expander implants the small separate fill valve can remain in place for months or even years so that breast size can be altered over a long period of time, or it can be removed when breast volume is judged ideal. Most women tolerate the small valve without a problem and appreciate the option of changing their breast size and volume should it be necessary or desirable. Once the valve has been removed, these expanders become permanent fixed-volume implants.

One of the more recent developments in implants and expanders has been in the surface texture of these devices. Initially all silicone implants and expanders had a smooth outer envelope. Today the surfaces of these devices often are textured to lessen the incidence of firmness produced from scar formation (capsular contracture). The textured tissue expander seems to produce softer breasts in a higher percentage of patients. Initial results would indicate that patients with these textured devices experience a lower incidence of capsular contracture— less than 5%.

Implant Reconstruction

Implant reconstruction using the available tissue remaining after the mastectomy is often the choice for the woman who has sufficient healthy tissue at the mastectomy site to adequately cover a breast implant, a permanent expander implant, or a postoperatively adjustable implant. This method is appropriate for the woman who has had a modified radical mastectomy in which her breast is removed but her chest muscles are preserved. The skin remaining at the mastectomy site should not be tightly stretched across the chest wall; the surgeon should be able to move the skin over the muscle, which indicates the presence of tissue beneath the skin that can be used to provide a smooth contour for a pleasing breast shape. Reconstruction with this technique is particularly suitable for obtaining a symmetric appearance in a woman whose remaining breast is of normal size and does not sag.

When immediate reconstruction is planned, the same general indications apply, but the preferred candidate's breasts should be somewhat smaller. There are limitations to the size of the silicone breast implant that can be placed at the time of the mastectomy to avoid complications and not compromise healing. These size limitations make tissue expansion, which permits more flexibility and accuracy in sizing the reconstructed breast, an appealing option for an immediate operation.

Surgical Procedure and Postoperative Appearance

Breast restoration using the tissue remaining after the mastectomy is the simplest technique available today. This operation normally takes 1 to 2 hours to perform. If the remaining breast is to be altered, this modification can be made during the same operation, and any further adjustments on the reconstructed breast can be made during a second operation to rebuild the nipple-areola. Either a general (the most common) or local anesthetic can be used with adequate sedation. This operation may be done on an outpatient or inpatient basis.

The plastic surgeon places a breast implant beneath the patient's skin and upper chest muscles to produce a breast shape. To avoid creating new breast scars the surgeon will frequently reopen a portion of the mastectomy scar and insert the implant through it. If an immediate reconstruction is being performed, the implant can be placed through the mastectomy incision. The plastic surgeon may even remove the entire mastectomy scar and resuture it to produce a better, thinner scar line. When the mastectomy scar is not in the best

Breast Reconstruction With Implants

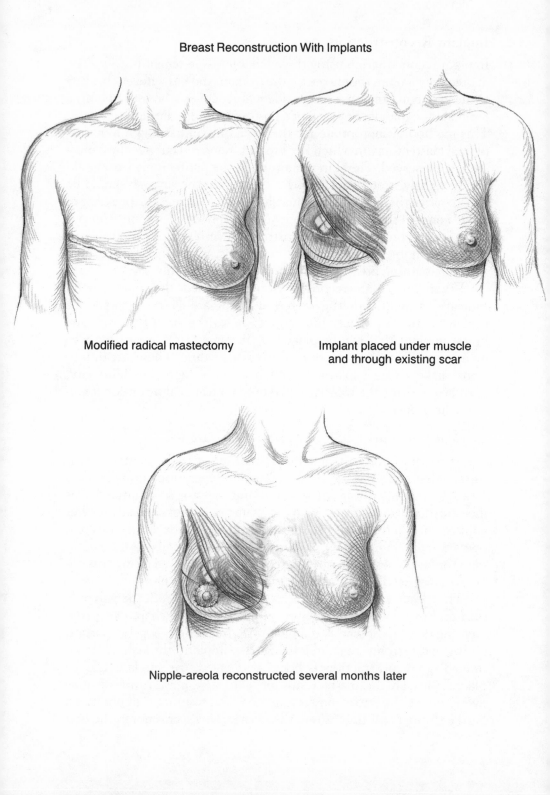

Modified radical mastectomy

Implant placed under muscle
and through existing scar

Nipple-areola reconstructed several months later

location, a small incision can be made near the new inframammary crease (where the lower part of the breast joins the chest wall). The implant is then placed through this new incision. Because this infra-mammary scar falls in a crease, it is barely noticeable.

The technique for immediate breast reconstruction is similar to that just described. After the general surgeon removes the breast and the pathologist examines it, the plastic surgeon begins the breast reconstruction. He elevates the layer of muscular tissue just under the breast, selects a breast implant or expander, and positions it for the best symmetry with the other breast. He then closes the muscle layer and sutures the skin incision. Sometimes a strip of latissimus dorsi muscle, obtained through the mastectomy incision, is used to give better cover, protect the lower portion of the implant, and reduce postoperative complications.

Although this approach is designed to produce a reconstructed breast of the correct volume and shape at the initial procedure, in practice, this goal is not always attainable in one operation, especially if the breast is to appear as natural and symmetric as possible. It is fre-quently necessary to adjust the implant during a second procedure. If the adjustments are minor, nipple-areola reconstruction is done dur-ing the same operation.

The newly restored breast often appears flattened immediately after reconstruction with available tissue (immediate or delayed). This flatness results from the implant being positioned behind tissues that are relatively tight. These tissues will stretch and soften over the next few weeks and months to provide better breast projection and shape. When a permanent expander implant or postoperatively adjustable im-plant is used, further adjustments can be made later to improve pro-jection and give the patient some control over final breast size.

Postoperative Care

After surgery a drain is often inserted into the reconstructed breast and left for 1 to 3 days to remove any excess fluid from the operative sites. The postoperative dressing selected should provide the best sup-port for the new breast. A brassiere is chosen if the implant needs to be guided upward; an elastic "tube top" or light dressing is selected if it is to be maintained in place or allowed to move downward. If non-absorbable stitches are used, they are removed approximately 1 week after surgery. This is usually not painful because the skin in that area is numb and reasonably insensitive. Today, however, most reconstruc-tive surgeons use absorbable sutures that do not require removal.

Because the breast has decreased sensitivity, the patient should not use a heating pad to relieve breast discomfort; she could accidently burn herself. After the stitches have dissolved or are removed, the surgeon may suggest that the patient massage and move her new breast around to keep it as soft and natural as possible. Massage is not needed, however, if textured implants have been used for reconstruction.

In a few weeks the scars will become red; this is a natural healing response and should not be alarming to the patient. This redness will fade with time. When the woman has fair, translucent skin, the increased blood flow into the healing scars will make them appear red for a longer period of time, sometimes for several years. Some patients naturally tend to heal with thick, raised scars. (A woman can get some idea of how she will heal by checking the appearance of any other scars she may have.) There are various recommendations for improving the appearance of these thickened scars, even though time is often the best solution; they will often fade and soften naturally over a period of months to years. Some surgeons will recommend that surgical tapes be placed over the scars for several weeks or months to support the scar and to reduce the likelihood that they will widen and thicken. These scars may also be treated by injecting a cortisone solution into them or temporarily taping silicone sheeting over them to provide gentle pressure to flatten and help fade them. In more severe cases the surgeon may re-excise, revise, and resuture the scars. When the scars are tight, they can be lengthened with a technique called a Z-plasty. With this technique, the skin is cut in the shape of a Z and then reshifted and sutured to relieve some of the skin tension and tightness.

After reconstruction the patient's breast skin may be dry because of contact with the dressings. A nonallergenic skin moisturizer can help relieve dryness. In addition, if there are no drainage problems, some surgeons may suggest the use of vitamin E oil or cocoa butter; the patient can lightly massage this oil into her scars to help them soften and fade. Vitamin E oil can cause a rash, and if so, it should be discontinued.

Complications

Implant reconstruction with available tissue has a low rate of complications. Complications are somewhat more common with immediate breast reconstruction. The most troublesome problem is excessive formation of hard fibrous tissue around the implant—the body's normal reaction to all foreign material. This reaction is called *capsular contracture*. There is some scar formation around all implants, and most reconstructed breasts feel firmer than the normal breast. To reduce breast firmness some surgeons use implants that have a textured surface. Surgeons recommend placement of smooth-surface implants under the chest wall muscle to help avoid this problem; in this location the implant is covered and protected by a thick layer of muscle. Although textured implants work equally well to reduce breast firmness in either location (above or below the muscle), many surgeons feel that they are best placed under thicker cover so that their texture is not visible under thin skin. When a smooth-surface implant is placed, many surgeons suggest that the woman massage her breasts on a regular basis to keep them soft and natural in appearance. Massage is not necessary for women with textured-surface implants; in fact, it may disturb the tissue adherence that the texturing promotes and that serves as a deterrent to fibrous scar formation.

Sometimes this fibrous formation around the implant becomes tight, the implants become hard, and the breast appears deformed. This problem is often managed by a capsulectomy, a procedure in which the hardened capsule and implant are surgically removed and the implant repositioned or replaced (for example, a smooth surface may be exchanged for an implant with a textured surface). Alternatively, a strip of latissimus muscle may be inserted between the breast skin and implant to cover and cushion the implant. For some patients, the implant is removed and a flap of autologous tissue from the abdomen or buttocks is substituted for the implant.

Problems with implant leakage and displacement may also occur and are usually treated by removing the implant and replacing it during an outpatient procedure. (See Chapter 11 for more information on implants and possible complications.)

Bleeding and infection are rarely encountered after this operation. If the patient has had radiation therapy or her breast skin is thin or taut, infection may develop, or in an immediate breast reconstruction some of the skin may die because of poor blood supply, thereby exposing the implant. This complication is managed by removing the implant temporarily and transferring additional tissue to cover the implant or occasionally by resuturing the wound. Breast reconstruction is then started over a few months later; the technique selected at this time is dependent on the individual's situation.

Women who are cigarette smokers can have more difficulty with

healing of the mastectomy skin flaps and experience a higher incidence of infection and exposure of the breast implant or tissue expander
at the time of immediate breast reconstruction. In fact, smoking is a
detriment to any surgical or reconstructive procedure. It reduces blood
flow to the tissues, impairs healing, is associated with increased coughing,
lung complications, and infections, and may severely compromise the
result of any reconstructive attempt. *All smokers are strongly advised to
discontinue smoking for at least 3 weeks and preferably several months
before and after surgery.*

Pain and Recuperation

Most women who select implant reconstruction with available tissue
say that it is not as painful or debilitating as the original mastectomy.
The breast area is somewhat numb after the operation, but this lack of
sensation is a residual effect from the mastectomy. The reconstruction
avoids the armpit area (axilla), so pain in this region and shoulder stiffness are not concerns as they were after the mastectomy.

This operation may be done on an outpatient basis or during a brief
hospitalization of 1 to 2 days. Women recover quickly from this procedure and are usually out of bed the afternoon of the surgery or the
next day and may return to work or normal activity within a week.
The patient may take a tub bath the day after the operation, but the
incision should be kept dry and the dressing intact. Showers may be
resumed 1 to 3 days after the operation if all is going well. Some surgeons place waterproof surgical tapes over the incisions to protect
them and allow the patient to shower the day after the operation. One
to two days after surgery the patient may lift her arms enough to comb
her hair. It is possible to drive a car after 1 to 2 weeks, but the patient
should not take any pain medications or sleeping pills that could impair her alertness and reflexes. Before driving, the woman should attempt turning the wheel while the car is still parked in the garage or
driveway to see if this causes discomfort. It is best to wait 4 to 6 weeks
before gradually resuming upper extremity exercise and sports activities. Although the woman may be feeling fine, she has been inactive
for a period of time and even the muscles not affected by the operation need to be gradually retrained and stretched to regain their sup-
pleness and strength.

Results With Implant Reconstruction

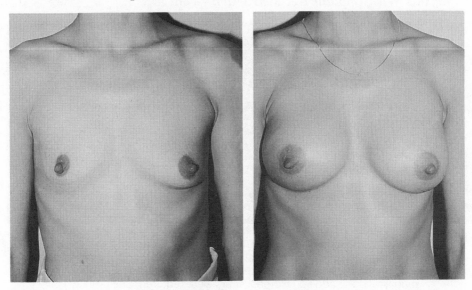

This young woman who wanted fuller breasts with minimal incisions requested breast reconstruction after a partial mastectomy. Implants were placed under the muscle in both breasts to achieve symmetry.

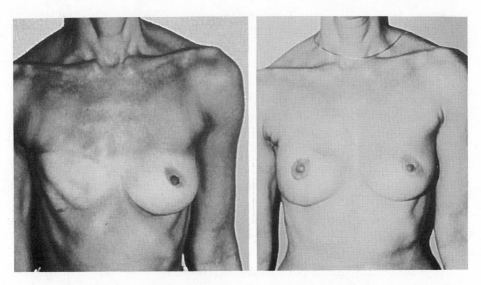

This woman had a modified radical mastectomy. Her breast was reconstructed with intraoperative tissue expansion and immediate implant placement. Her opposite breast was not modified.

Results With Implant Reconstruction—cont'd

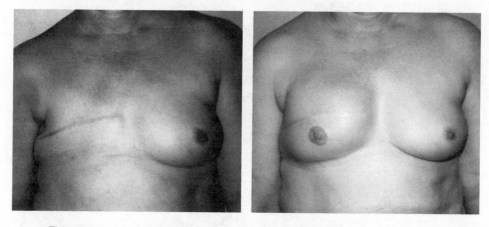

This 42-year-old woman had a right modified radical mastectomy. Her right
breast was reconstructed with a breast implant placed beneath the muscle and
her nipple-areola was reconstructed 3 months later. No opposite breast
modification or additional breast scars were required. She is shown
2 years after breast reconstruction.

Tissue Expansion

Despite tight skin at their mastectomy site, some women prefer to
have simple reconstruction with available tissues rather than a more
complicated flap procedure. For these women, the tissue expansion
method is a good alternative. This is currently the most common type
of breast reconstruction, providing the greatest flexibility in breast size
when a simpler reconstructive approach is desired. With this approach,
the taut skin in the area of the mastectomy is stretched and expanded,
thus avoiding a more complex flap operation and permitting placement of a permanent breast implant of suitable size and shape. Although
this operation is similar to the approach described in the previous section, it differs in the type of implant used and the postoperative management.

Tissue expansion has a number of advantages for the patient and
the reconstructive surgeon. The reconstruction can usually be accomplished without additional breast scars, and the patient can determine
the volume and size of her reconstructed breast. She has input into
decisions about final breast symmetry and the timing of inflation and

second-stage breast reconstruction. This approach is particularly applicable for bilateral breast reconstruction because it permits the woman to determine final breast volume without the tissue restrictions she might encounter if she were depending on donor tissue from a flap from her abdomen, back, or buttocks.

Breast reconstruction with tissue expansion has its drawbacks; it is time intensive, and the woman who is looking for the quickest approach should understand that two or even three procedures may be required. Although the length of hospitalization necessary for the initial placement of the device is not great, the patient requires a number of additional postoperative visits for the actual stretching of the tissues. These office visits and procedures can be inconvenient, require traveling long distances, and interfere with the demands of family and work. The procedure takes longer than breast reconstruction with other techniques, often a matter of months. Even though the desired breast volume is usually attained within a few weeks, additional time is required to complete the reconstruction. For the best results the breast tissue should be overexpanded, the expanded reconstructed breast allowed time to heal, and the breast evaluated for any further adjustments prior to second-stage breast reconstruction when the tissue expander is exchanged for a silicone breast implant or the expander implant is converted to a permanent implant.

Today, most patients having immediate breast reconstruction with available tissue have a temporary expander, a permanent expander implant, or a postoperatively adjustable implant placed rather than a fixed-volume implant. These expandable devices permit a larger breast to be built and adjusted as it is inflated, avoiding the problem of placing an implant that is not symmetric or is initially too large for the tissues and could complicate the healing process.

Surgical Procedure and Postoperative Appearance

Tissue expansion often requires two operations. The first operation normally takes 1 to 2 hours to perform. It may be done under local or general (the most common) anesthesia and may be done on an inpatient or outpatient basis. During the first procedure the surgeon inserts a temporary expander, a permanent expander implant, or a postoperatively adjustable implant through the mastectomy incision or an inframammary incision (as described on p. 219) and positions it above or below the chest wall muscle. The surgeon often manually stretches

Breast Reconstruction With Tissue Expansion

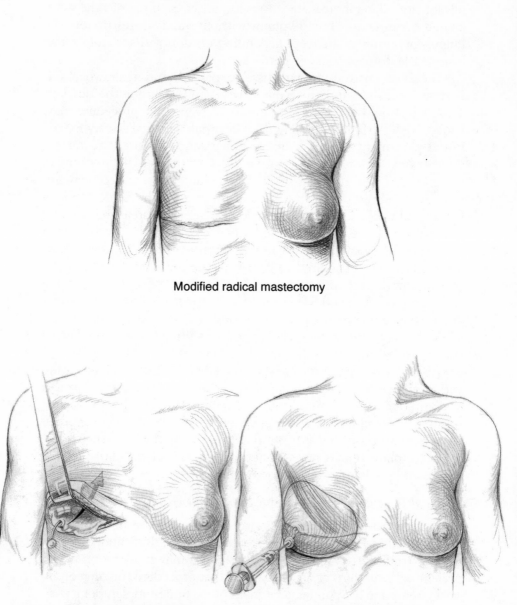

Modified radical mastectomy

Tissue expander inserted
under skin and muscle

Expander inflated

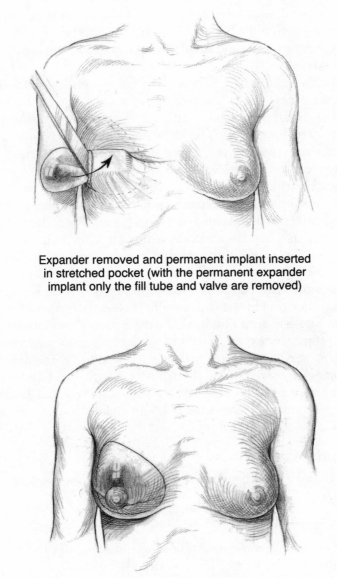

**Expander removed and permanent implant inserted
in stretched pocket (with the permanent expander
implant only the fill tube and valve are removed)**

Nipple-areola reconstructed

the breast skin during this initial operation to permit more rapid expansion later or may use some volume expansion to stretch the overlying skin intraoperatively. He then positions the valve to allow injection of saline solution for enlargement of the implant. In this early postoperative period the breast skin is still tight and the reconstructed breast appears flattened and smaller than the remaining breast on the opposite side.

Once this implant is in place and the valve is positioned under the skin for easy access, the woman schedules visits to the plastic surgeon to have her expander gradually inflated. A typical expansion session lasts from 15 to 30 minutes. The saltwater solution is usually injected through the skin into the valve. The rate of inflation is influenced by the quality of the healing and the tightness and discomfort being experienced by the patient. This gradual enlargement of the implant produces pressure on the woman's skin, causing it to become tense, stretch, and eventually expand to a larger area. Much the same phenomenon occurs when the abdominal skin stretches during pregnancy. This process can be painful for some women, and the volume and timing of the injection and fill process must be individualized. After the breast skin has been distended sufficiently, which is somewhat larger than the other breast (this is called *overexpansion*), and the optimal breast size has been obtained, during a second outpatient procedure the temporary expander will be replaced with a permanent implant or the expander implant will be converted to a permanent fixed-volume implant by removing the fill tube and valve. (Alternatively these can be left in place if future changes are anticipated.) After this second operation the reconstructed breast usually has a more natural appearance.

Postoperative Care

Postoperative care is the same as that described for implant reconstruction on p. 221.

Complications

Capsular contracture, device failure, and implant displacement are all potential problems associated with tissue expanders. The use of textured-surface expanders that adhere to the surrounding tissue has significantly reduced the incidence of breast firmness and implant displacement. The incidence of device failure is greater with tissue expanders than it is with implants because of valve problems, displacement of a remote fill port, inadvertent puncture of the tissue expander during saline inflation, and the possible introduction of bacteria that can lead to infection. If this occurs, the device or the fill port may need to be removed and the wound allowed to heal before it is replaced.

Tissue expansion can lead to thinning of the stretched skin. If the skin at the mastectomy site is already thin, healing problems may occur. To lower the chance of the tissue expander being exposed through this thin skin, the reconstructive surgeon may decide to place the tissue expander under the muscle and fascial layer. As an alternative, he can shift a strip of muscle from the latissimus dorsi (back muscle) to the lower portion of the reconstructed breast at the time of the mastectomy; this seems to reduce the incidence of complications of implant exposure and provides better skin cover over the lower portion of the reconstructed breast. This technique can be performed without additional incisions or scars and without significant functional impairment. (This technique is discussed later in this chapter.)

As with implant reconstruction, women who are cigarette smokers can experience an increased incidence of healing problems after tissue expansion. This potential complication is discussed on p. 223.

Pain and Recuperation

The pain experienced after tissue expansion is similar to that described previously for implant reconstruction. When tissue expansion is done at the time of mastectomy, the patient has additional pain from the stretching of healing tissues, which are undergoing wound contraction. Patients often describe a tight, pulling sensation following inflation. Usually this pain is not severe. If it is, the tissue expansion is terminated temporarily to allow the tissues to heal for a week or two and then resumed. If it is too tight, some saline solution can be removed for a few days. The site for the fill valve is usually in an area where some nerves were removed during the mastectomy and thus is relatively numb.

This operation may be done on an outpatient basis or during a brief hospital stay. If done in the hospital, the usual stay is 1 to 2 days. Recovery from this operation is reasonably quick. The patient can usually return to nonstrenuous activity in 2 to 3 weeks and resume sports in 6 to 8 weeks. All other aspects of recovery are the same as those described earlier on p. 224.

Results With Tissue Expansion

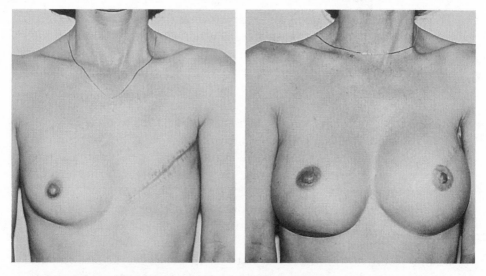

This woman had bilateral mastectomies and immediate breast reconstruction with tissue expander implants placed under the muscle. She is shown 15 months following breast reconstruction.

This woman had breast reconstruction after a modified radical mastectomy. Permanent expander implants were used for reconstruction and augmentation mammaplasty.

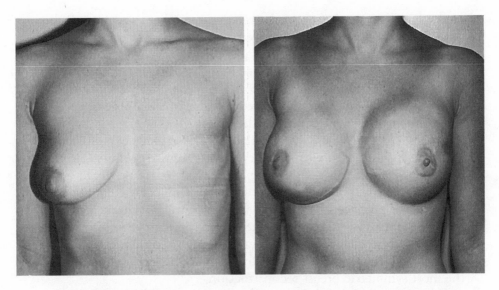

This woman had a modified radical mastectomy on her left breast. When she
was referred for prophylactic mastectomy on her opposite breast, she requested
bilateral breast reconstruction at the time of her mastectomy. Since she wanted
to avoid back or abdominal scars, a flap procedure was not chosen. Her
bilateral breast reconstruction was done with tissue expanders.

When Available Tissue Reconstruction
Is Not the Right Choice

Because reconstruction with available tissues and implants or tissue
expanders is the simplest of breast reconstruction techniques and offers excellent results, you would assume that these techniques would
be the best choice for every patient. Some circumstances, however,
prompt a woman to consider other reconstructive options. For instance,
when her remaining breast is large and she does not want it changed,
reconstruction with these methods will produce breasts of an unequal
size because there will not be enough tissue present to build a large
breast. Although she might be satisfied with the newly reconstructed
breast initially, eventually she will feel lopsided and will probably still
need to wear a prosthesis to make her breasts appear equal in size.
Consequently, unless the normal large breast is reduced to match the
rebuilt breast, reconstruction with the available tissue may not be a
permanent solution for this patient because it will not produce sym-

metric breasts. The experienced surgeon can predict in advance if the other breast will need to be changed or if a flap is needed.

Although silicone breast implants and tissue expanders have a good track record when used for aesthetic and reconstructive breast surgery, some women prefer not to have a foreign material permanently placed in their reconstructed breast. For them, breast reconstruction with their own tissue is the only logical choice.

Nor is reconstruction with available tissue or tissue expansion appropriate for a woman with a radical mastectomy deformity because it does not satisfactorily restore the missing chest wall muscle (pectoralis major muscle), the hollow under the collarbone (infraclavicular hollow), and the fold produced by the arm and breast in the armpit area (anterior axillary fold). Additional tissue must be brought in to reconstruct these areas. For some patients, a combination of additional tissue from the back or the lower abdomen and an implant or expander will offer the most symmetric breast reconstruction.

If a patient has tight, thin, irradiated, or grafted skin, she also may have limited or unsatisfactory results because the skin remaining at the mastectomy site, even with tissue expansion, is insufficient to cover the implant and to provide her with a breast that looks and feels natural. A flap reconstruction technique is a more logical choice for the patient with major skin, muscle, and contour deficiencies. If a woman has had conservative surgery followed by radiation therapy (also called *lumpectomy with irradiation*) and for some reason has to have a completion mastectomy, in all but rare circumstances a flap of the patient's own tissue from the lower abdomen or back is necessary to obtain a satisfactory breast reconstruction.

Sometimes an implant or expander needs to be used in conjunction with a flap. This may be necessary when a woman needs both breasts rebuilt and has insufficient flap tissue or to permit the design of a smaller but necessary flap with a shorter donor scar. For example, a latissimus dorsi flap may be combined with a tissue expander. The flap can then provide muscle or skin and muscle for the reconstruction, and the tissue expander can be used to create a new breast of the correct size. When the latissimus dorsi muscle is being used for immediate breast reconstruction, it can be obtained through the mastectomy incision. A flap of tissue is also used to provide good cover for the breast implant or tissue expander. Sometimes the TRAM flap reconstruction is enhanced with an implant or expander. The newer devices, particularly those which are inflatable and have textured surfaces, are made with thicker outer envelopes; these cause wrinkles and are easily seen and felt through thin skin. If the skin is thin, the result is better if a flap of the patient's own tissue is interposed to provide better cover for the implant.

FLAP RECONSTRUCTION

The use of flaps of muscle or skin and muscle (musculocutaneous) to supplement the tissue remaining after a mastectomy represents a major advance in breast reconstruction. With the newest flap techniques, a woman's breast can now be rebuilt with her own tissue and usually without a breast implant. Furthermore, because the donor sites are often areas of tissue excess such as the lower abdomen or buttocks, these women can receive a full and natural breast that closely resembles the size and shape of their opposite breast. As a benefit, the area from which the donor tissue is taken can sometimes then be contoured to produce a more aesthetic appearance. Now even women with radical mastectomy deformities, radiation injuries, or recurrences after lumpectomy with irradiation requiring a mastectomy can have their deformities filled in and rebuilt.

The three most common sources of tissue for breast reconstruction with the patient's own tissue (autologous) are the lower abdominal wall, the back, and the buttocks. The outer thigh or lateral abdomen can be used, but many women and surgeons find the donor scars objectionable. When the tissue from the abdominal wall or back is used, it is left attached to the blood supply of the muscle beneath it (a musculocutaneous flap). When buttock or thigh tissue is used, microsurgery techniques are necessary to restore the blood supply of the flap by reattaching the vessels supplying this tissue to those in the breast region. Microsurgery can also be used to move a flap of abdominal wall tissue (TRAM flap) for breast reconstruction; however, most surgeons feel that this abdominal tissue can be moved more reliably and expeditiously when it remains attached to its muscle and blood supply. Most surgeons reserve the use of microsurgery for TRAM flap operations for those patients with abdominal scars that preclude the usual TRAM flap, for patients with risk factors that make the free TRAM flap safer, or for patients that prefer the free TRAM flap operation.

All of these flap procedures can cause more blood loss than breast reconstruction with local tissues and implants or expanders. For this reason, the reconstructive surgeon may discuss the possibility of blood transfusions with the patient and recommend that the patient donate her own (autologous) blood before the operation. Her blood is then stored in the blood bank until it is needed. Usually this blood is donated during the month before the operation. For immediate breast reconstruction with a flap, it is usually recommended that 1 to 2 units of the patient's blood be available. This can sometimes necessitate scheduling the operation a few weeks later; this short delay will not lessen the patient's chance of a cure from the breast cancer treatment and can reduce the patient's concern about the possibility of receiving a blood transfusion from the general donor pool.

Reconstruction With the Lower Abdominal (TRAM) Flap

Creation of the breast with a flap of lower abdominal skin and fat over a strip of muscle (rectus abdominis) is a major contribution to breast reconstruction. This operation, developed in the early 1980s, is now the most frequently used flap procedure and provides some of the most attractive and realistic breast reconstructions. This technique allows the surgeon to restore a woman's breast with her own tissues, usually without the need for a silicone breast implant, and at the same time give her a slimmer abdomen. With this approach, the surgeon uses excess abdominal tissue to rebuild the breast after a total mastectomy, modified radical mastectomy, or even radical mastectomy.

The transverse rectus abdominis musculocutaneous flap, also known as the TRAM flap, is recommended for the woman who requires the extra tissue supplied by a flap reconstruction. She prefers a breast reconstruction without a silicone breast implant and is pleased at the prospect of having a "tummy tuck" as a bonus. Sometimes the patient's lower abdominal tissue is insufficient to give a breast of satisfactory volume. This most often occurs with bilateral reconstruction. The patient should discuss her preferences and thoughts with the reconstructive surgeon and get his opinion of whether implants will be needed. As with the other flap operations, this is major surgery and the woman who selects this operation should be in good health. Her tissue is moved a long distance (from the lower abdomen to the chest), and its blood supply must be healthy and sufficient to keep the new tissue for breast reconstruction alive.

It has been found that the TRAM flap blood supply is particularly sensitive and precarious in the overweight woman, the hypertensive woman, the woman who has had radiation therapy, and the woman who is a cigarette smoker. Because cigarette smoking can constrict and narrow blood vessels and precipitate flap failure, the plastic surgeon will insist that the patient avoid cigarettes before and after the operation. Additionally, the surgeon might suggest an exercise program consisting of sit-ups and modified sit-ups for several weeks before surgery to increase blood flow and strengthen her abdominal area. If there is evidence that the blood supply may be impaired from many years of cigarette smoking, another method of breast reconstruction should be selected, either tissue expansion or the latissimus dorsi flap. Microsurgical TRAM flap reconstruction and TRAM flap delay are other strategies to increase blood flow to the TRAM flap tissues. (The TRAM flap delay is discussed in the next section.)

The TRAM flap is not appropriate for every patient. When the woman's abdominal wall is thin or she does not want scars in this region, another procedure should be considered. Women who are cigarette smokers, women who are significantly overweight, women who have had abdominal radiation or who have abdominal scars or have had liposuction, particularly across their upper abdomen, women over 65 years of age, and women with medical problems such as diabetes mellitus or heart disease should strongly consider other techniques.

The TRAM flap is now frequently used for immediate breast reconstruction. An immediate TRAM offers a number of advantages. By combining the mastectomy and the breast reconstruction during one operation, the general surgeon is able to limit the amount of skin removed to only that which is necessary to properly treat the breast cancer. The removed skin is then replaced with the abdominal skin supplied by the TRAM flap. By preserving the remaining breast skin and by restoring the important landmarks of the breast such as the inframammary fold and the lateral breast, immediate breast reconstruction with the TRAM flap creates a natural breast with minimal breast scars. Of course an abdominal wall procedure is necessary to obtain the TRAM flap. When immediate breast reconstruction with the TRAM flap is planned, close cooperation between the general surgeon and the reconstructive surgeon is essential and the patient needs to be fully informed about the specifics of the procedure, possible complications, and the expected recuperation. Usually it is necessary for the patient to donate her own blood so it is available if needed during the procedure.

Surgical Procedure and Postoperative Appearance

TRAM flap breast reconstruction is major surgery and usually takes approximately 3 to 6 hours in the operating room compared to the 1 to 2 hours required for implant or expander reconstruction. This procedure is done under general anesthesia and requires a hospital stay of 5 to 8 days. This operation can only be done once, and the patient should be advised that if the need arises in the future for another breast reconstruction, another technique will have to be used.

Using this reconstructive method the surgeon designs a transverse flap of skin and fat on the middle to lower abdomen. The tissue for the new breast is surgically freed from the abdomen but left attached to a strip of the vertical abdominal wall muscle (the rectus abdominis). Sometimes strips of both rectus abdominus muscles (bipedicle TRAM flap) are used to ensure a better blood supply to the flap. The donor site is closed by bringing the remaining muscles together to restore abdominal wall strength. The scar that is left on the abdomen is similar but may not be quite as low and inconspicuous as the horizontal scar left from an abdominoplasty (tummy tuck), which removes excess abdominal tissue for aesthetic reasons. The flap is then ready for transfer to the chest. In preparation for transfer the plastic surgeon removes the mastectomy scar (if it is in an inconspicuous position) or he creates a new incision that will allow for a more aesthetic reconstruction. The flap is then elevated and transferred to the chest wall area through a tunnel under the upper abdominal skin and extending to the new incision in the breast area. The upper part of the flap is sutured into position to give the best contour for the upper breast area, and the lower portion of the flap is positioned, folded under, and contoured to form a breast mound. The breasts are then checked for symmetry and form with the patient positioned upright, and the flap is carefully stitched in place. If the patient has sufficient excess abdominal fat, there ordinarily is no need for a breast implant.

If the surgeon is concerned preoperatively about the adequacy of the blood supply of the abdominal flap, he may decide on an operative delay. In this approach the operation is sequenced into two procedures. One to two weeks before the definitive flap operation the patient has a minor operation during which the surgeon divides some of the blood vessels going into the lower portion of the TRAM flap. He does this through two short incisions placed in the lower abdomen. Later, during the major operation, these short incisions will be incorporated into the TRAM flap incisions. This so-called delay of the vessels serves to redirect and increase the flap's blood flow and venous drainage and is designed to improve its blood supply and therefore help to ensure flap survival.

After the TRAM flap procedure the plastic surgeon then restores the nipple-areola in a second or third procedure (if a TRAM flap delay has been used) under local anesthesia followed later by a tattoo if additional pigmentation is desirable.

The procedure for immediate TRAM flap reconstruction is similar to that described for the delayed approach, but it does not take as long because the mastectomy has prepared the recipient area and more breast skin can be preserved to help shape the new breast and shorten the mastectomy scar. Results of immediate surgery with this technique have improved dramatically over the past several years. Often a woman's breasts are closely matched after the initial procedure and there is less need to adjust the opposite breast later. However, the woman who decides on an immediate procedure needs to be fully prepared for the donor deformity and scar and the additional breast scars required for placing the TRAM flap. Sometimes the mastectomy and immediate TRAM flap breast reconstruction are delayed for several weeks to enable the woman to have time to donate her blood for future transfusions during the breast reconstruction. The oncologic surgeon should have input in this timing decision. Most oncologic surgeons feel that this short delay has no adverse affect on the patient's outcome.

After this operation the new breast usually has an elliptic pattern of stitches running along the lower breast crease and up toward the nipple area. When done immediately, the skin patch can be smaller and just extend around the area of the areola and sometimes laterally toward the axilla. A donor scar extends across the lower abdomen between the pubic area and umbilicus. In addition, there is often some fullness on the inner portion of the new breast because of the addition of the rectus abdominis muscle, which supplies nourishment to the flap. This fullness usually subsides in the first 2 to 3 months after the operation as the transferred, unexercised muscle becomes thinner. If this fullness persists, if the reconstructed breast is larger than the opposite breast, or if there are other areas of fat accumulation in the lateral or lower abdomen, these areas can be contoured later using liposuction.

Breast Reconstruction With TRAM Flap

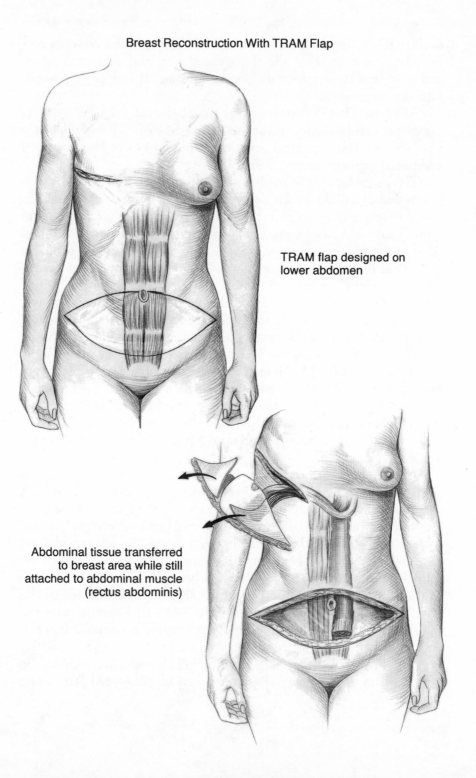

TRAM flap designed on
lower abdomen

Abdominal tissue transferred
to breast area while still
attached to abdominal muscle
(rectus abdominis)

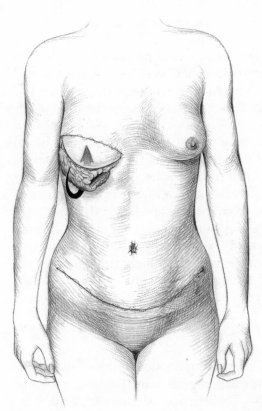

Abdominal tissue fashioned
into breast and lower abdomen
closed as transverse scar

Nipple-areola reconstructed
several months later

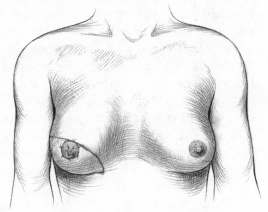

Postoperative Care

Surgical drains are placed in the breast and abdomen for 3 to 4 days after the operation but are usually removed before the patient goes home. The hospital bed is placed in a flexed position to relieve abdominal tension caused by the removal of lower abdominal tissue and muscle during the operation. The patient is usually asked to get out of bed the next day and walk. Even though this can be difficult, it is important for a safe recovery. Activity enhances the blood flow throughout the body and can lower the chance of developing blood clots in the legs, which could travel to the lungs. The reconstructive surgeon may ask the patient to wear support hose or use sequentially compressive stockings for the first few days after the operation to further enhance the blood return from the legs and lessen the chance of deep vein thrombosis. When the patient first gets out of bed, she may notice that she is unable to stand up straight; this is to be expected. It often takes days to weeks for the patient to stand straight, depending on the amount of lower abdominal tissue taken to build the breast. The other specifics of postoperative care are described in the section on implant reconstruction on p. 221.

Complications

Because this is major surgery, there are more possibilities for complications. About 1 in 10 patients experiences some healing problems, resulting in an area of skin loss, fat drainage, or firmness of the fatty tissue on the flap. This hard, thickened tissue can be frightening to a woman because of its resemblance to her original tumor. It sometimes softens in 6 to 18 months. This thickening can be differentiated from a tumor by examination, mammography, and sometimes fine-needle aspiration. Delayed healing or even loss of some or rarely all of the flap because of insufficient blood supply is a potential complication. Sometimes a portion of the skin edge or fat will have a reduced blood supply, causing drainage from the new breast for a few weeks. To avoid this drainage the surgeon may want to remove this strip of tissue as a minor outpatient procedure. If fluid accumulates beneath the abdominal skin, it may need to be aspirated or a small drain placed through the incision to draw off this liquid.

Other less frequently occurring complications include bleeding (hematoma) and infection. If blood accumulates at the operative or donor site, it will need to be drained in a brief trip to the operating room. Antibiotics are frequently used to avoid the problem of infection. The development of venous clots in the legs or pelvic region is a rare but serious complication. These clots can potentially travel to the lungs (pulmonary embolus). This condition is noted less frequently when the operation takes under 4 hours. In addition, the patient should be encouraged to resume some activity right away, actively exercising her leg muscles when she is in bed and getting out of bed and attempting to walk the day after surgery. While she is inactive in bed, compression stockings are recommended.

Since the TRAM flap is obtained from the abdominal wall, there is some chance of a hernia developing. As a preventive measure to strengthen the abdominal wall and reduce the possibility of hernia, the reconstructive surgeon may place a sheet of mesh over the site where the strip of abdominal muscle is removed. This complication is now reported to occur in approximately 2% of patients having this operation. If a hernia develops, mesh may also be used to repair it.

Pain and Recuperation

The TRAM flap operation is potentially more painful and uncomfortable than any of the other methods of breast reconstruction, especially in the abdominal area. Because the surgeon removes a wide strip of lower abdominal tissue during surgery, the abdomen is tight and the woman feels a distinct pull. It may be difficult for the patient to stand upright until the muscle is stretched out again. It can take several days before she is ready to eat, and she may notice that she gets full quickly because the abdomen is tighter. However, as with most operations, each patient has a different tolerance level for pain; some patients take very little if any pain medication, whereas others may experience a great deal of pain and require analgesics for several weeks. The discomfort involved in a TRAM flap has been compared by patients to the pain they experienced after an abdominal hysterectomy or a cesarean section. During the first week after surgery most patients report soreness and pain in the abdominal area; movement is difficult and quite uncomfortable.

The PCA (patient-controlled analgesia) unit is now used to alleviate patient discomfort during hospitalization. This device represents a real advance in the management of pain in the postoperative period. It is safe, provides excellent pain relief, and the patient is in control. The PCA unit is connected to the patient's intravenous tubing, the proper pain-relieving drug and dosage are determined, and the machine is set so that the patient can press a button and administer the pain-relieving medication immediately as she needs it. With this device, the pain medication can also be given much more often than when a nurse administers shots to the patient. (See p. 148 for more information on the PCA.) After about 2 to 3 days the patient's pain is usually controlled with analgesics taken by mouth.

The TRAM flap procedure requires a hospital stay of 5 to 8 days. The patient usually can get out of bed 1 to 2 days after the operation, but it takes another 1 to 2 weeks before she can stand upright. Recuperation is slower with this operation than with the other procedures discussed earlier. Most women resume normal basic activities in 6 to 8 weeks, and they can participate in sports in 3 to 6 months.

Few functional problems exist after transfer of the rectus abdominis muscle. Most patients can return to the same level of activity as they had before the operation. Tests measuring abdominal wall strength after a TRAM flap operation show that patients can experience some residual weakness compared to their preoperative condition. An intensive preoperative and postoperative exercise program helps strengthen the abdominal wall muscles and makes the recovery less difficult. Although sit-ups sometimes may be difficult and women may have to push up when rising from the reclining position, most athletic activities can be continued without difficulty, and many women have returned to tennis, golf, and jogging.

Results With the TRAM Flap

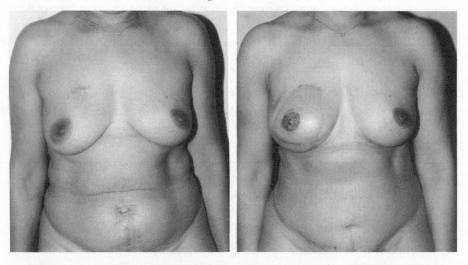

This woman had a modified radical mastectomy followed by immediate TRAM breast reconstruction of her right breast. Three months later liposuction was used to contour her upper abdomen and breast. Her nipple-areola was also reconstructed and later tattooed. She is shown 2 years after her breast reconstruction.

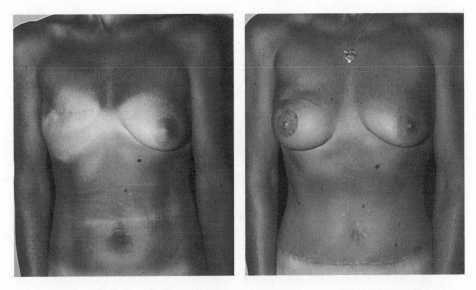

This woman, who had a modified radical mastectomy, requested breast reconstruction with her own tissues. Her right breast was reconstructed with a TRAM flap to match her remaining breast.

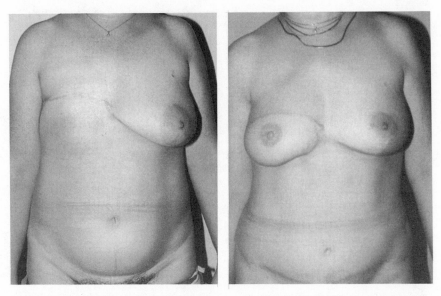

This woman had a right modified radical mastectomy. Her left breast was heavy and her abdomen was flabby. A TRAM flap was used for her right breast reconstruction and a small reduction mammaplasty was performed on her left breast. The patient is shown 2 years later.

Results With the TRAM Flap—cont'd

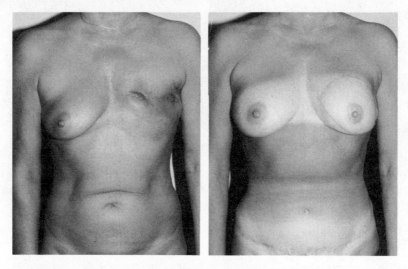

A TRAM flap was used to reconstruct this woman's left modified radical mastectomy deformity, and her right breast was augmented for symmetry. She is shown 15 months after her initial reconstruction.

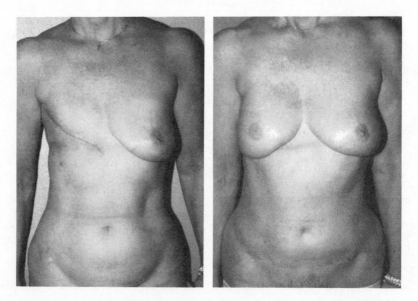

After a right modified radical mastectomy this woman's breast was reconstructed with a TRAM flap; to obtain a better match mastopexy was performed on her left breast. Her result is shown 5 years after breast and nipple-areola reconstruction.

Reconstruction With the Latissimus Dorsi (Back) Flap

A latissimus dorsi flap technique is selected when additional tissue is needed to rebuild mastectomy defects and the TRAM flap is not available or other reasons prevent its use. While some patients can have their breasts rebuilt with the back tissue without a silicone breast implant or expander, many women do not have sufficient excess back tissue and require an implant or permanent expander implant to provide additional volume for the reconstructed breast. In this surgery, skin and muscle or sometimes only muscle from a woman's back is transferred around to the breast area to replace the skin and chest muscle that were removed during a mastectomy. This is a safe, reliable flap with a good blood supply. Because it has a long track record for safety and predictability, many surgeons feel more comfortable recommending it than the other flaps.

The latissimus dorsi flap provides functioning, healthy muscle tissue for covering an implant or expander, for filling the hollow areas beneath the collarbone left by removal of the pectoralis major muscle (a standard part of the radical mastectomy procedure), and for recreating the anterior axillary fold. When additional skin is added to the chest wall area, it also permits the formation of a more naturally shaped, fuller, larger breast than could be created by simple implant placement or tissue expansion. Also the healthy skin added is often thicker and of better quality than the thin expanded skin. This muscle and skin (musculocutaneous) flap is also useful for patients who have skin grafts or very tight or irradiated skin, although the TRAM flap is often the flap of first choice for the woman who has had a mastectomy after radiation therapy. The latissimus dorsi muscle and skin flap can be used after a modified radical mastectomy to eliminate the need to alter the patient's remaining breast if it is too large to match with expansion of the existing tissue. Many women prefer a donor scar on their back or side to a scar on their remaining breast, which would be necessary to adjust it to match the expanded breast reconstruction. In addition, the use of flap tissue provides additional cover and a measure of protection for the breast implant or expander. This is often the case when a woman has immediate breast reconstruction. A strip of the latissimus dorsi muscle can be elevated and brought through the mastectomy incision to provide better cover and safety for the silicone breast implant or tissue expander and to reduce its visibility and palpability; no additional incisions are required.

Sometimes a woman's breast can be reconstructed with the back tissue without a silicone breast implant. This autologous latissimus dorsi flap reconstruction is used when the woman has excess back tissue, especially in her midback, or if she does not have a particularly large breast. In this instance the skin, muscle, and fatty tissue of the back can be brought around to the front and shaped into a breast. Usually this can be done with a single scar across the midback. When there is fullness of the lateral chest wall area, additional skin can be harvested. One of the drawbacks of this approach is that when a large amount of skin and fat are removed from the back, the resulting scar can be unattractive, and the back area from which the flap was taken can appear flatter than the opposite side of the back.

The latissimus dorsi can be used for immediate breast reconstruction either as muscle only (to enhance implant cover) or with some additional skin to replace missing skin. The latissimus dorsi flap is most often used when the reconstructed breast needs to be large or ptotic to match the opposite one, and the patient does not want a TRAM flap or a TRAM flap would pose too much risk and prolonged recovery.

Surgical Procedure and Postoperative Appearance

Reconstruction with the latissimus dorsi flap is a longer, more complex procedure than the techniques using local tissue or tissue expansion. This operation takes between 2 to 4 hours to perform. Since the operation is longer and more painful than simple implant placement, it is done under general anesthesia and hospitalization is required.

When using the latissimus dorsi flap for breast replacement, the plastic surgeon separates the latissimus dorsi muscle from its deep attachments and frees it with its attached skin from the back. This muscle-skin flap is left attached to its nourishing vessel, a main artery in the armpit area that the surgical oncologist saves during the mastectomy. The flap is now ready to be transferred to the chest area. In preparation for this transfer the mastectomy scar is excised or removed (if it is located in an inconspicuous position) or a new, better placed incision is made along the lower outer area where the new breast will be reconstructed. Next the flap is rotated to the front of the chest and passed through a tunnel created high in the underarm so that it extends through to the new incision or to the opening left by the removal of the mastectomy scar. The back donor incision is then closed. The flap is adjusted for the most aesthetic appearance and sutured to the front of the chest; the latissimus dorsi muscle is stitched to the pectoralis major muscle, and back skin is stitched to breast skin to supplement deficient tissue in this area. When an axillary fold is needed, some of the outer layer of skin and a portion of the latissimus dorsi muscle are brought around and stitched out onto the upper arm. This tissue will span from the arm to the chest, thus simulating a new anterior axillary fold. An opening is left in the outer part of the incision for the insertion of a breast implant or tissue expander to provide a breast shape symmetric with the opposite remaining breast. The surgeon positions the expander under the muscle, which provides good cover and permits a more natural reconstruction; he then closes the incision. The nipple-areola is created during a later operation under local anesthesia.

For immediate breast reconstruction, the upper part of the expander is placed under the chest wall muscle (pectoralis major) above and the lower part is covered by the back muscle (latissimus dorsi). When skin is needed, it replaces the skin removed at the time of mastectomy. If necessary, an expander implant is placed to permit accurate postoperative sizing.

The latissimus dorsi reconstruction leaves a donor scar on the patient's back (under her bra line) or on her side (in a diagonal under her upper arm) and additional scars on her breast when the flap is placed into the breast area. The reconstructed breast tends to be somewhat rounder and firmer than the normal breast. In addition, the woman may have a slight bulge under her arm where the latissimus dorsi flap was tunneled through to her chest area. This bulge will shrink with time as the muscle atrophies with inactivity, but it will not completely disappear. This fullness can sometimes be placed in the axillary region to reduce the hollowness after axillary lymph node removal.

Immediate Breast Reconstruction With Latissimus Dorsi Muscle Coverage of Tissue Expander

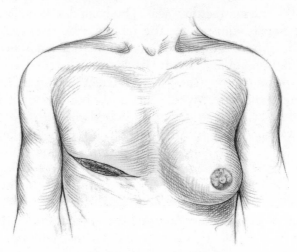

Modified radical mastectomy

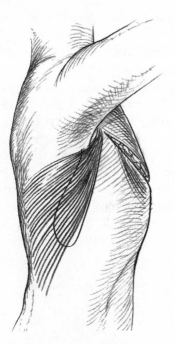

Latissimus dorsi muscle
flap designed on side

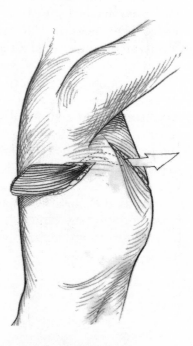

Strip of latissimus muscle
elevated on side of chest

Tissue expander placed under
latissimus dorsi muscle flap

Expander inflated and left in place

Nipple-areola reconstructed
several months later

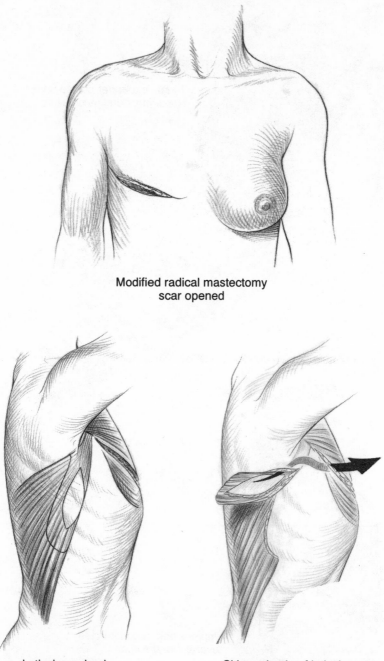

Delayed Breast Reconstruction With Latissimus Dorsi Flap and Tissue Expansion

Modified radical mastectomy
scar opened

Latissimus dorsi
flap designed on side

Skin and strip of latissimus
muscle elevated on
side of chest

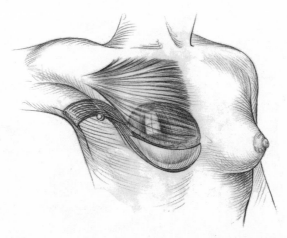

**Skin and muscle supplement deficient tissue in lower
breast area and expander implant restores breast shape**

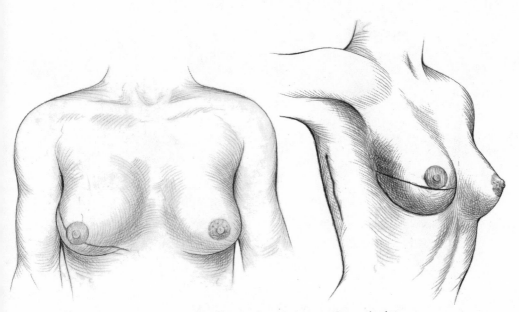

Nipple-areola reconstructed several months later

Breast Reconstruction With Latissimus Dorsi Flap Without an Implant

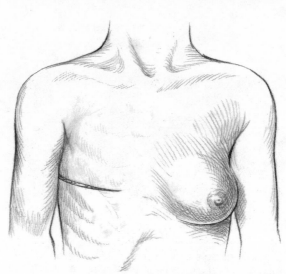

Modified radical mastectomy

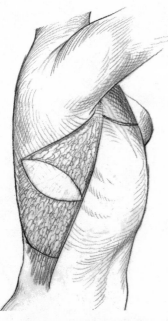

Latissimus dorsi flap
designed on back

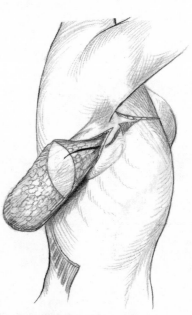

Skin and muscle flap
lifted from back

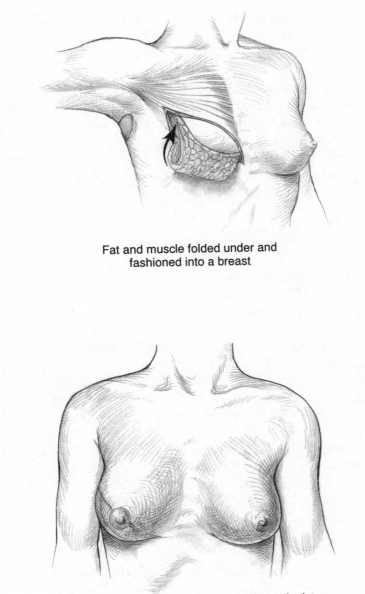

Fat and muscle folded under and
fashioned into a breast

Nipple-areola reconstructed several months later

Postoperative Care

After the operation the plastic surgeon inserts surgical drains into the reconstructed breast and back area to remove excess fluid from the operative site. Patients should be advised to expect significant drainage as a normal part of the recovery process, particularly with this flap. The reconstructive surgeon usually recommends that the back drain remain in place even after the patient goes home and until the drainage is less than an ounce (30 ml) a day. This can sometimes take several weeks to drain. It is advisable for the woman to limit shoulder or arm activity because this tends to increase the fluid. The other specifics of postoperative care such as stitches, dressings, and restrictions on activity are similar to the postoperative instructions provided for patients whose breasts are reconstructed with implants (p. 221).

Complications

Fluid collection in the back area is a common problem after latissimus dorsi flap surgery. Sometimes fluid accumulates after the drains are removed. It usually is reabsorbed by the body and disappears after several weeks. When this fluid buildup becomes uncomfortable, the surgeon may need to drain it with a syringe or reinsert a drain. Blood accumulation (hematoma) in the operative sites of the breast or back is an unusual complication, but if it occurs, it needs to be corrected and the blood removed in the operating room. Infection is also rare, and the surgeon will ordinarily prescribe antibiotics to lessen the chance of infection. Problems with the blood supply to a portion of the latissimus dorsi flap have occurred in about 2% of the operations. These usually have been in women who have had radiation treatments after the mastectomy. When this complication occurs, it may cause a delay in implant placement or the selection of another reconstructive technique. Complete loss of the latissimus dorsi flap because of poor blood supply has been seen in less than 1% of patients. When this occurs, another method of breast reconstruction will be needed.

Pain and Recuperation

This operation is more painful than reconstruction with available tissue. There is normally some pain in the back and underarm area where the flap was taken. The back and arm areas are sore for 2 to 3 weeks; the pain subsides as the arm regains motion. The drains are also usually uncomfortable and occasionally painful, particularly when they are removed. This discomfort is similar to that experienced after a mastectomy.

Hospitalization of 3 to 6 days is required. Recovery time is 3 to 6 weeks to return to work and 2 to 4 months to resume exercise or sports such as aerobics, tennis, and golf. If the woman's anterior axillary fold has been recreated, she needs to avoid strenuous arm activity for 6 to 8 weeks while this area heals.

The latissimus dorsi flap is generally not accompanied by loss of arm and shoulder function even though a muscle has been used. The muscle is still functional. It is simply transferred to the front of the body to provide tissue for rebuilding the breast. Some women report, however, that the muscle transfer makes it more difficult for them to keep their shoulder erect on the side of the muscle transfer. Exercise will help to alleviate but may not totally eliminate this problem.

Results With the Latissimus Dorsi Flap

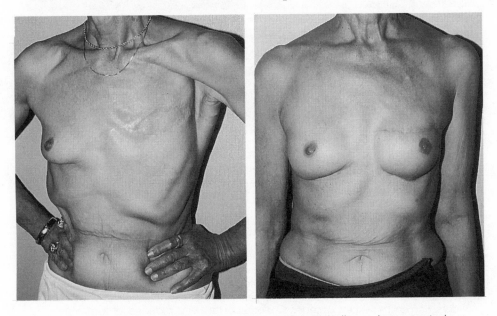

This woman had a radical mastectomy many years earlier and now wanted breast reconstruction with augmentation of her other breast. She had a latissimus dorsi muscle flap with implant placement for reconstruction of her left breast and another implant inserted behind her right breast for augmentation.

Results With the Latissimus Dorsi Flap—cont'd

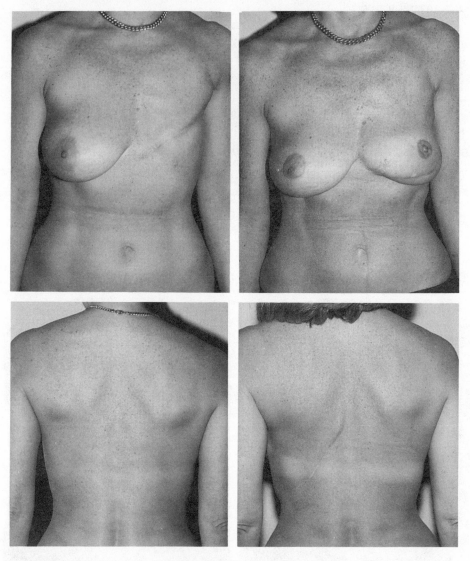

This 42-year-old woman had a left modified radical mastectomy. Since she did
not want a lower abdominal scar, her breast was reconstructed with a latissimus
dorsi flap and a tissue expander. Her other breast was reduced for symmetry.

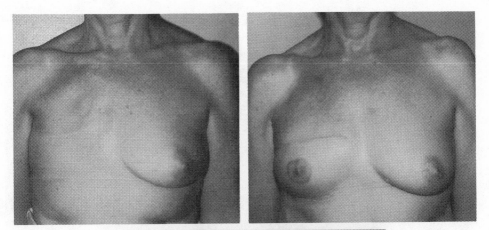

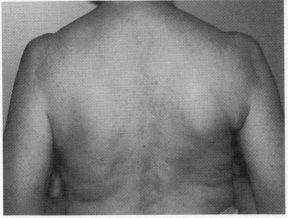

This 54-year-old woman had a right modified radical mastectomy. She did not want a skin island on her reconstructed breast or modification of her opposite breast. Her breast was reconstructed with a latissimus dorsi muscle flap and a tissue expander. Her opposite breast was not modified.

Results With the Latissimus Dorsi Flap—cont'd

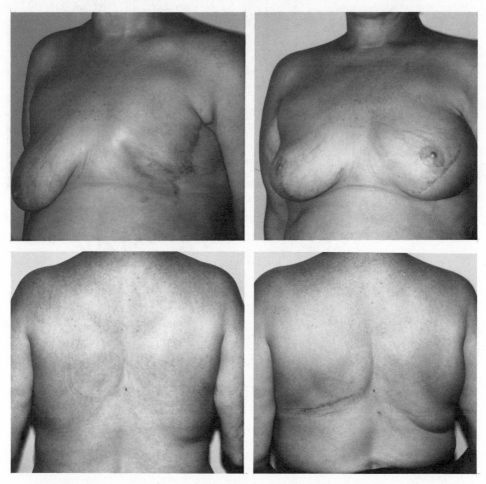

This 48-year-old woman had a modified radical mastectomy. She is shown 2 years following latissimus dorsi flap breast reconstruction with tissue expansion and nipple-areola reconstruction on the left breast and reduction mammaplasty on the right breast.

MICROSURGERY FOR BREAST RECONSTRUCTION

One of the more significant advances in reconstructive surgery during the past 20 years became a reality when surgeons began to suture and repair tiny blood vessels under the magnification of the operating microscope. This skill enables surgeons to move tissues from one part of the body where there is an excess of tissue to a deficient area that needs rebuilding. Because these flaps of autologous tissue (the patient's own body tissue) are separated and *freed* from the donor site and transferred to the new area where the blood vessels are reattached, they are often referred to as *free flaps*. This technique brings added choices to breast reconstruction. The reconstructive surgeon can re- build a woman's breast by transferring her own fully mobilized tissues usually without the need for a breast implant. The most common and popular free flap donor tissues are the TRAM and the buttock skin and muscle (gluteus maximus musculocutaneous) flaps; they provide abundant tissue for a well-contoured reconstructed breast from a donor site that is often enhanced by tissue sculpting. The latissimus dorsi free flap is also a possibility but is used less frequently because abdom- inal and buttock free flaps provide more abundant tissue with more acceptable donor sites for the patient. The upper inner thigh or outer thigh can be used for free flaps, but most patients find the donor site contour and visible scars objectionable.

The freedom and flexibility this procedure offers is balanced in part by the level of surgical support and expertise required. This is the most complex and demanding of all of the reconstructive procedures. It is also prone to more serious complications, takes longer to perform with the attendant risks of greater blood loss, and usually requires a more extended hospitalization and recuperation period than implant or expander breast reconstruction. It is not for the inexperienced surgeon nor the patient who desires a simple, easy route to breast restoration. The patient should fully understand the extensive nature of this operation before she selects it. She needs to be physically and psychologically prepared for the extended convalescence it requires. Even under the best of circumstances, these techniques are not 100% successful. Since the standard pedicled latissimus dorsi flap and TRAM flap have more than 99% reliability, if a free flap is chosen, the surgeon should have a high level of expertise and success with the technique because, if complications of blood flow develop, a reoperation will be needed and the transferred tissue can be lost. The patient should have an idea of the surgeon's success rate with this operation before choosing it.

Immediate TRAM free flap reconstruction has some advantages over delayed free flap reconstruction. Because the oncologic surgeon exposes the vessels for suture of the free flap during the axillary dissection, they are readily available to be sutured to the tissue moved from the lower abdomen.

For microsurgery to be successful, a woman should be healthy and have normal blood vessels. Excess scarring and radiation to these vessels may reduce the chance of a successful result. Patients with radiation damage to the chest wall and patients in whom previous flaps have failed are prime candidates for free flap breast reconstruction, as are women in whom the traditional pedicled TRAM or latissimus dorsi flap is unavailable or inadequate. This would include women with abdominal scarring that precludes the TRAM flap or patients in whom the nerve and blood supply to the latissimus dorsi muscle has been severed or the area damaged by radiation. It is also crucially important for a woman who desires this technique to find a skilled microsurgeon experienced in performing microsurgical breast reconstruction with an equally skillful and experienced breast management team.

The TRAM Free Flap

The TRAM flap is usually the first choice when additional tissue is needed for breast reconstruction. Sometimes the TRAM flap cannot be transferred safely in the usual manner, that is, by moving the lower abdominal tissue to the breast region while maintaining its blood supply within the strips of the rectus abdominis muscle. When the abdominal wall is scarred or when the upper abdominal vessels are judged not to have sufficient blood supply to keep the lower abdominal tissues alive, as in the woman with a long-standing history of cigarette smoking or the woman who is overweight with evidence of diminished flow from the vessels from the upper abdominal muscle (rectus abdominis), then a TRAM free flap is indicated.

Surgical Procedure and Postoperative Appearance

Reconstruction with the TRAM free flap is a major operation and takes approximately 3 to 8 hours in the operating room, on some occasions even longer! This operation is done under general anesthesia and requires a hospital stay. As with the pedicled TRAM flap, this operation can only be done once, and the patient should be advised that if another breast reconstruction is needed at a later date, another technique and tissue source will have to be used. The TRAM free flap is designed on the lower abdomen, a bit lower than the design used for the standard TRAM flap. After the flap from the lower abdomen is transferred to the breast region, the vessels in the lower portion of the abdominal flap are sutured into the blood vessels of the armpit region. The chest wall is prepared by removing and reopening the mastectomy incision (if it is in an inconspicuous position) or creating a new incision that will permit a more aesthetic reconstruction. The incision is extended into the underarm or a separate incision is made to permit access to the vessels in that area for microsurgical hookup. The flap is then transferred to the chest wall area. The highly technical hookup of the small vessels of the flap to the breast region is performed under the magnification of the operating microscope.

After the vessels have been connected and checked, the transferred muscle is firmly sutured to the underlying chest wall tissue. The overlying skin and fatty tissue is shaped and inset to form a breast mound to match the other breast. The breasts are checked for symmetry and shape and the flap is stitched into place. The nipple-areola reconstruction is performed in a second or a third procedure, depending on the amount of contouring that still needs to be done to the reconstructed breast.

Microsurgery can also be combined with the pedicled TRAM flap. This has been called the *supercharged* or *turbo* TRAM flap. With this procedure the lower blood vessels along with a strip of lower abdominal muscle are transferred for the reconstruction, and these blood vessels are hooked into the blood vessels of the underarm. Sometimes just suturing a vein or artery in conjunction with a standard TRAM flap is adequate for this supercharged approach. The results of this procedure are similar to those of the traditional TRAM flap with its pedicle intact.

The operation for an *immediate* breast reconstruction with a *TRAM free flap* is basically the same as that described for the delayed TRAM free flap reconstruction. Technically it is an easier operation because the axillary vessels are already freed up and there is no scarring. Results of this procedure are quite acceptable, but as with the immediate pedicled TRAM flap, the woman must be fully prepared for the donor deformity and scar and the additional breast scars required for placing the TRAM flap. Again, some delay in the immediate surgery

Breast Reconstruction With TRAM Free Flap

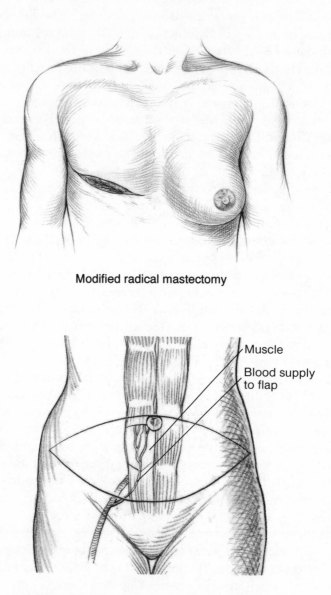

Modified radical mastectomy

Muscle

Blood supply
to flap

TRAM free flap designed on lower abdomen

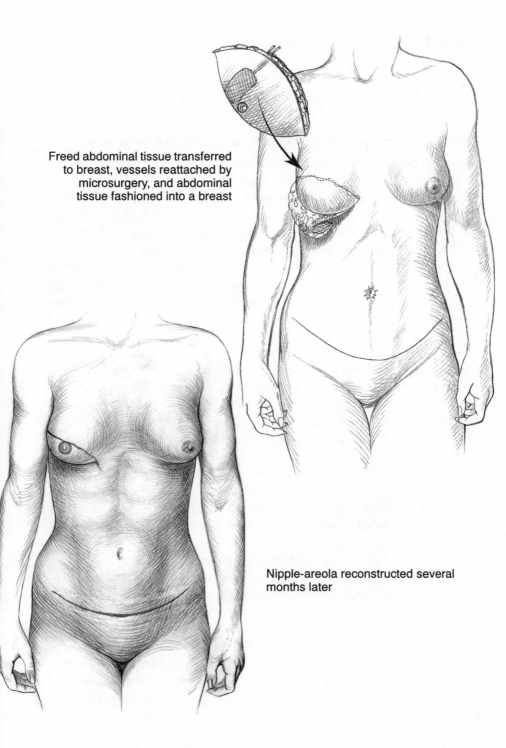

Freed abdominal tissue transferred to breast, vessels reattached by microsurgery, and abdominal tissue fashioned into a breast

Nipple-areola reconstructed several months later

might be required to enable the woman to donate blood for this procedure.

The description of the scars and postoperative appearance for a free TRAM flap is similar to that described on p. 239 for the standard pedicle TRAM flap.

Postoperative Care, Complications, and Pain and Recuperation

As with the standard TRAM flap, drains are placed in the breast and abdominal areas for 3 to 4 days after the operation. The drains are usually removed before the patient leaves the hospital and after the antibiotics have been discontinued. Sometimes the donor defects accumulate serum and may need to be drained during a subsequent office visit after the patient has been released from the hospital. Antibiotics are administered to all patients undergoing microsurgical breast reconstruction for the first few days postoperatively. Cigarette smoking and environmental tobacco smoke are prohibited during the postoperative period.

A primary concern of the reconstructive surgeon in the postoperative period after a TRAM free flap is that the vessels are open and the transferred tissue is maintaining a good blood supply. The color, blood supply, and temperature of the flap are carefully monitored postoperatively. The blood supply to the flap can be assessed by checking the blood flow with needlesticks into the flap. If it is determined that the flow to the flap has stopped, this necessitates an immediate return to the operating room to reexplore the vessels and repair the problem.

The potential for blood clots in the leg may be somewhat greater with microsurgical reconstruction because of the length of this operation and the dissection is nearer the veins in the pelvis. To protect the transferred vessels the patient's upper extremity movements are restricted for 5 to 6 days after the operation.

A hospital stay of 6 to 8 days is required. The patient usually can get out of bed 1 to 2 days after the operation, but it takes several weeks before she can stand upright. Most women resume normal basic activities in 6 to 8 weeks, and they can participate in sports in 3 to 6 months. All other aspects of postoperative care, potential complications, and recuperation for the TRAM free flap are similar to those described for the standard TRAM flap on pp. 242-244 and implant reconstruction on pp. 221-224. However, since the muscle is removed with the TRAM free flap, there is usually less abdominal pain.

Results With the TRAM Free Flap

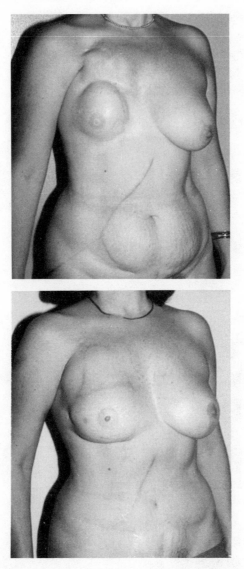

Five years earlier this 43-year-old woman had her right modified radical mastectomy deformity reconstructed using a breast implant. Breast firmness and asymmetry developed over time. Previous abdominal scars precluded a standard TRAM flap breast reconstruction. Her breast was therefore rebuilt with a TRAM free flap. She is shown 4 years after her breast reconstruction.

Results With the TRAM Free Flap—cont'd

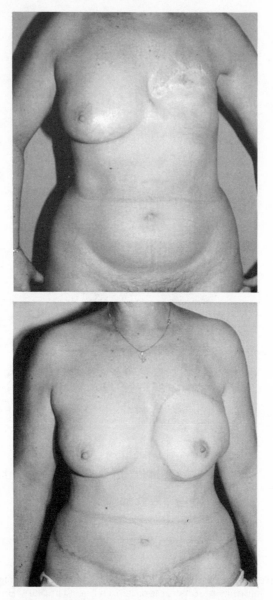

This 54-year-old woman had a modified radical mastectomy of her left breast. Because she was a heavy smoker a standard TRAM flap reconstruction was ruled out. Her result is shown 1 year after TRAM free flap breast reconstruction.

The Gluteus Maximus Free Flap

When the TRAM flap is unavailable or of insufficient size, the tissue for the breast reconstruction can be supplied by transferring a portion of the buttock skin and muscle to the breast region and resuturing the vessels of the buttock tissue to the vessels in the axilla or in the midchest region under the ribs. The buttock skin and muscle can be taken from either the midportion of the buttock (superior gluteus free flap) or more often from the lower buttock crease (inferior gluteus free flap). The advantage of using the lower crease is that this is the region of the most excess tissue. Removal of the tissue from the lower buttocks can actually reduce and flatten a large buttock, and the scar can be placed in the crease where it is less obvious and can be covered by a woman's undergarments. In addition, the vessels of the lower gluteus flap are often better suited for microsurgical hookup.

Surgical Procedure and Postoperative Appearance

Patients selected for this technique must be healthy and able to undergo a procedure that takes a minimum of 4 to 8 hours and possibly longer. This operation is done under general anesthesia and requires hospitalization. The success of the operation depends on the excellent technique of the microsurgeon along with the artistic design and shaping of the buttocks into the new breast.

The surgeon designs an elliptic flap along the buttock crease, either along the fold, where the buttocks meets the thigh, or slightly higher, depending on where the greatest concentration of fatty tissue is located and on the quality of the vessels. The flap of skin, fat, and a small portion of the gluteus muscle is obtained along with the small blood vessels going into the muscle that nourish the tissue. The flap is then transferred to the chest wall, where the mastectomy incision has been opened and extended and the recipient vessels have been located. Next, the flap is connected to the vessels in the underarm or occasionally in the midchest region using microvascular techniques performed under the operating microscope. The vessels and flap are checked to ensure that there is good blood flow. Then the transferred muscle is sutured to the underlying chest wall and the flap of skin and fat is shaped and inset to match the opposite breast. During a second procedure it is sometimes necessary to further improve the breast shape and to contour both buttock and hip regions using additional surgical revisions and/or liposuction.

Breast Reconstruction With Gluteus Maximus Free Flap

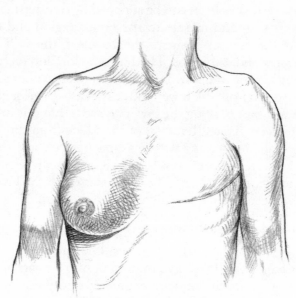

Modified radical mastectomy

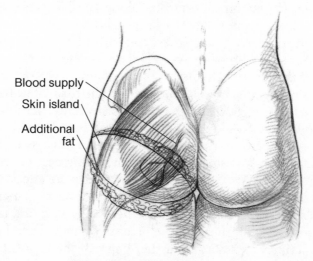

Blood supply

Skin island

Additional
fat

Gluteus maximus free flap designed on buttock

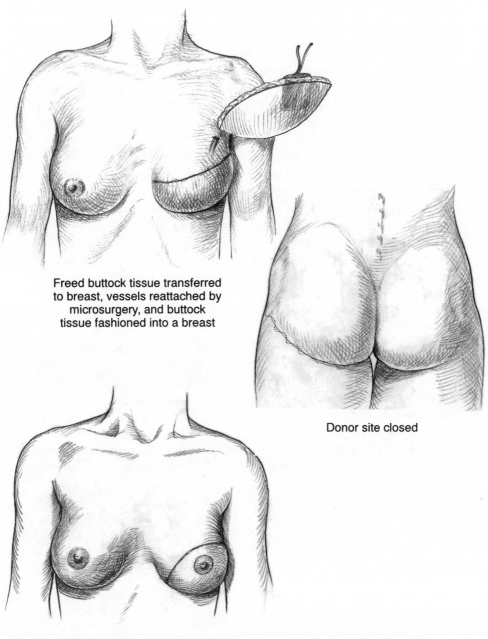

Freed buttock tissue transferred
to breast, vessels reattached by
microsurgery, and buttock
tissue fashioned into a breast

Donor site closed

Nipple-areola reconstructed
several months later

The procedure for the immediate gluteus flap is similar to that described for the delayed gluteus free flap. This procedure is not performed as frequently for immediate breast reconstruction because of the additional time requirements and because the TRAM flap is usually considered a better alternative for free flap reconstruction.

After this operation the rebuilt breast usually has an elliptic pattern of stitches running along the lower breast crease and up toward the nipple area. When done immediately, similar to the immediate TRAM flap, the skin patch can be smaller and just extend around the areola and toward the underarm area. When used to replace implants, the entire gluteus free flap is buried beneath the breast skin. The resulting donor scar is across the lower crease of the buttocks or across the midportion of the buttock. It is usually hidden by the patient's underpants.

Postoperative Care

Drains remain in the buttock and breast for 3 to 4 days after the operation. The breast drain is usually removed before the patient leaves the hospital, and the buttock drain is left in place until the fluid loss is less than 1 ounce (30 ml) per day. This may take several weeks. The reconstructive surgeon avoids removing the drain too early because fluid accumulation (seroma) would require aspiration or replacement of the drain. To protect the transferred vessels the patient's upper extremity movements are restricted for 5 to 6 days after the operation. Antibiotics are administered for the first 4 days postoperatively. Cigarette smoking and environmental tobacco smoke are prohibited during the postoperative period. All other aspects of postoperative care are similar to those described on p. 266 for the TRAM free flap, p. 242 for the pedicle TRAM flap, and p. 221 for implant reconstruction.

Complications

There is a risk that the blood flow into the transferred buttock tissue that forms the new breast will fail or occlude. If this occurs, the surgeon will need to reoperate to restore the blood flow. Because a nerve in the back of the leg has to be divided with the buttock flap, a portion of the back part of the thigh is numb after this operation. This nerve can also develop a sensitive swelling (neuroma), which could necessitate another operation. The accumulation of fluid in the buttocks can require drainage either intermittently with a syringe and needle or by replacement of the drain. Antibiotics are usually prescribed in the postoperative period, and it is unusual for an infection to develop after the operation. For a fuller discussion of potential complications, see pp. 242 and 246.

Pain and Recuperation

Since the donor site is in the buttock region, after the operation the patient will have to lie supine or on her opposite side. The pain and discomfort from this operation are usually not as severe as that experienced with the TRAM flap but more than that experienced after breast reconstruction with implants and expanders. The PCA unit is used to relieve the postoperative pain. To alleviate pressure on the buttock area where the flap was taken some surgeons use a low air loss type of bed. Pain in sitting can be relieved by using an inflatable donut pillow for the first few weeks after surgery. As with other free flap breast reconstructions, care is taken to monitor the flap after surgery to ascertain that there is good blood flow to the transferred tissue.

A hospital stay of 6 to 8 days is required. The patient gets out of bed the following day. Most women resume normal basic activities in 6 to 8 weeks, and they can participate in sports in 3 to 6 months.

Results With the Gluteus Maximus Free Flap

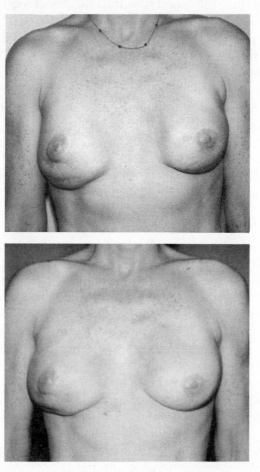

This 39-year-old woman requested bilateral flap breast reconstruction because she was dissatisfied with the results of her previous implant reconstruction. She is shown 6 months following reconstruction with lower gluteus maximus free flaps.

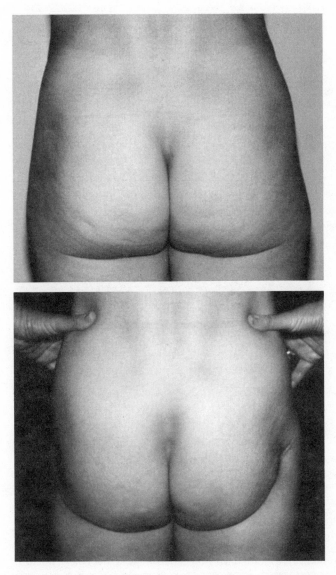

The buttocks region is seen before and after the procedure.

Results With the Gluteus Maximus Free Flap—cont'd

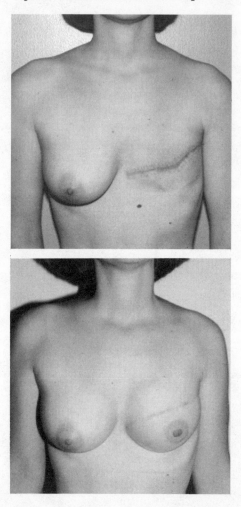

This 24-year-old patient had a modified radical mastectomy on her left breast. She wanted a breast reconstruction to match her unmodified opposite breast. Since her lower abdomen was thin, scarred, and irradiated, an abdominal flap could not be used. The patient did not want a back scar. She is shown 18 months after an inferior gluteus maximus free flap.

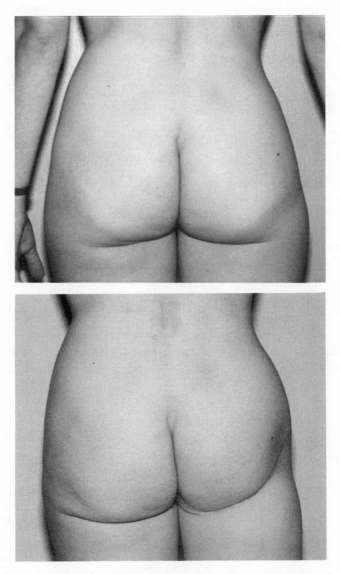

Her donor scar is located in the right buttock crease. Her opposite buttock was suctioned at the time of the nipple reconstruction.

FOLLOW-UP OPERATIONS

While it would be ideal for breast reconstruction to be completed in one operation, thereby creating a superbly shaped, symmetric breast, in practice this is expecting too much. The usual breast reconstruction can often be enhanced with a second refining procedure. At this time the scars can sometimes be improved, excess tissue can be removed or deficient tissue supplemented, and if necessary, an implant can be inserted. Reconstruction of the nipple-areola is usually accomplished during this second operation. (A detailed explanation of nipple-areola restoration is provided in Chapter 16.)

Proper timing for the second operation to place the nipple-areola should be determined once the breast appearance after the first operation is evaluated; the woman's breasts should look as similar as possible. If they are not symmetric, the surgeon may need to modify the size, shape, and position of the reconstructed breast, either before or at the time he creates the nipple-areola. The need for a second operation does not indicate that the first procedure was a failure. The second operation presents the woman and her doctor with an opportunity to obtain the best possible result.

When a significant modification of the reconstructed breast is necessary at the time of the second operation, it is best that the nipple-areola reconstruction be delayed until a third procedure to ensure that it is accurately positioned on a stable breast reconstruction.

The timing of the second operation is also determined by the need for additional treatment such as chemotherapy. This is particularly true for the patient who has immediate breast reconstruction and then discovers that she requires chemotherapy. Her second operation should usually be delayed until chemotherapy is completed. It is wise to wait at least 2 to 3 months after chemotherapy for the woman to feel her best and her general metabolism, particularly her blood count, to return to normal. Because of unforeseen complications such as unpredictable healing or an especially radical defect, sometimes additional operations are necessary in addition to the two procedures.

A common secondary operation after implant or expander reconstruction requires the replacement of one implant with another to improve the breast contour, size, or position. The new implant is inserted through the incisions that are already present. Conditions of recovery are similar to those described for the initial implant placement (p. 224), but pain and recovery time are frequently less than for the initial procedure. If capsular contracture persists after several operations, the implant can be replaced with the fatty tissue from the lower abdominal area, a TRAM flap.

After a TRAM flap reconstruction it is often necessary to shape the breasts further, especially in the lower inner area where the muscle is transferred. The patient's overall body contour can also be improved at the second operation with some finishing touches. These include liposuction of the reconstructed breast if it is larger in some areas than the opposite breast. The abdominal wall and hips may also be recontoured with liposuction to give a more aesthetic appearance. Similar corrections may be needed after the gluteus free flap to contour the breast or the buttocks and hip area so that they are symmetric. When there is not enough tissue to create the ideal size breast reconstruction or the breast lacks projection, an implant or expander can be inserted at the time of the second procedure. Many women, however, who choose these procedures do so to avoid implants and prefer the flatness to the use of a foreign material in their breast. Sometimes thickened areas of fat occur in the reconstructed breast after flap surgery; when this happens, these areas may need to be excised or biopsied both to confirm their diagnosis and to remove them.

• • •

Today the woman requesting breast reconstruction and the plastic surgeon performing this operation have a number of options to choose from. Local tissue reconstruction with implants and expanders and reconstruction with abdominal, back, and buttock flaps are all means of restoring women's breasts. A woman's personal needs and the specifics of her deformity dictate which procedures are more suitable than others. It is very important for the woman to communicate her desires for this surgery to her plastic surgeon so they can examine the different procedures together and decide on the simplest and most reliable operation that can meet these expectations.

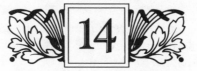

WHAT TO DO ABOUT THE OTHER BREAST: AESTHETIC BREAST CORRECTIONS

After losing one breast to mastectomy, a woman finds that her remaining breast assumes a special importance to her. It is a reminder of the breast she lost and a symbol of her once un-scarred chest. She fears the development of a second tumor in her breast, but she also is protective of this lone survivor, not wanting to alter or touch it unless she has no choice.

When a woman contemplates breast reconstruction, her feelings about her remaining breast must be thoroughly discussed with her plastic surgeon since this will affect the type of reconstructive procedure she chooses and ultimately the success of her operation. Both she and her doctor are understandably concerned about the development of a new tumor in the remaining breast, and this possibility should be discussed with the general surgeon. Because the remaining breast will be used as a model for reconstructing the new breast, it must be carefully evaluated. If its appearance is difficult to match, the plastic surgeon may suggest an aesthetic surgical procedure to alter it. Then the woman has to decide whether she is comfortable with this suggestion.

Most women having a breast restored want to avoid an operation on their remaining breast; in fact, some women absolutely refuse to submit to any surgery, which always entails some scarring. Usually these women were happy with their breast appearance before the tumor developed, and under ordinary circumstances, they would not have changed their breasts in any way. Therefore they want a reconstructive approach that will leave their surviving breast untouched, but will still produce a balanced, aesthetic result. If a woman's remaining breast is of an average size (B- or C-cup brassiere) and the skin at the mastectomy site is not particularly tight, then reconstruction with an expander or implant will be sufficient to match her breast without performing any surgery (see p. 214). If a woman does not want her existing breast changed and it is relatively large or sags (ptotic) or the tissues at the mastectomy site are tight or irradiated, the missing breast will usually have to be rebuilt with a flap of extra tissue from her lower abdomen or from her back or buttocks, resulting in additional scars in one of these locations. This is also the case for the woman who wants her breast built with her own tissues and prefers not to have a silicone breast implant for breast reconstruction.

Sometimes the size or shape of the remaining breast cannot be easily duplicated. With newer techniques for reconstructive surgery, however, this does not happen as often as it once did. Now breast reconstruction techniques can frequently match the other breast. Thus aesthetic alterations of the other breast are not as essential for obtaining symmetry and become more of a positive option for the woman who wishes to incorporate an aesthetic breast alteration into her breast reconstruction. In those instances when symmetry is difficult to achieve, the woman may be willing to consider an operation on her opposite breast if it will ultimately produce breasts that more closely resemble each other. An operation on her remaining breast is preferable to feeling lopsided after her reconstruction and perhaps even having to wear a prosthesis. In this situation the plastic surgeon uses one of the procedures developed for aesthetic breast surgery to augment, reduce, or lift her other breast. The final decision for breast size is made by the woman herself, and she needs to clearly explain her expectations to her plastic surgeon before undergoing breast reconstruction.

BREAST AUGMENTATION

If the woman's existing breast is small and flattened, she may want to consider having it enlarged to make it fuller and rounder. Then her reconstructed breast can be created to resemble this larger breast. This is particularly true if her breast reconstruction will be done with an implant or expander; implantable devices currently on the market come in a limited number of shapes and sizes and tend to produce breasts that are round and full. It is therefore difficult to rebuild breasts to match natural breasts that are small, flat, and droopy. Breast augmentation is a relatively simple procedure; however, it does require

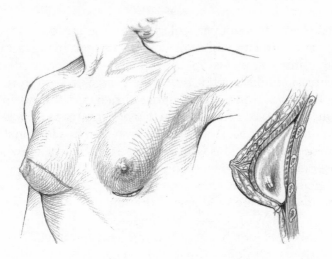

Breast augmentation with implant placed under muscle

a breast implant or expander, usually a silicone envelope filled with saline solution. As with any operation, the patient should be fully informed about the benefits and risks of implant surgery before choosing this option. (See Chapters 11 and 13 for detailed information on implant surgery.)

To perform this operation the surgeon makes an incision, usually under the breast, in the axilla, or sometimes around the lower portion of the areola, and inserts a breast implant behind the breast tissue and muscle layer, thereby enlarging the breast shape. It is then easier for the plastic surgeon to copy this larger and fuller breast contour.

Breast augmentation may serve a psychological as well as an aesthetic need, giving a woman a boost in self-confidence during a time when she needs an emotional lift. Fears that breast augmentation will hide the development of a new tumor are unwarranted. Because the implant is placed behind a woman's breast and muscle layer, it does not cover her breast tissue, which still can be accurately and effectively checked for the development of any lumps or tumors. Mammograms also may be taken, and even a breast biopsy can be done without disturbing the breast implant. Some have expressed concern that a breast implant can impair mammography, whereas many mammographers feel that with appropriate views the breast can be imaged satisfactorily. (See Chapters 11 and 13 for detailed information on implants and expanders.)

Result

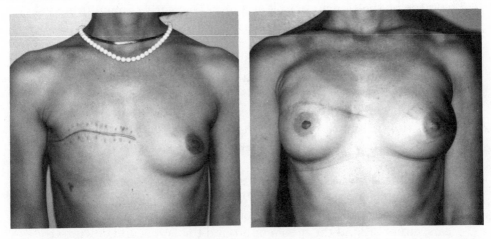

This 30-year-old patient had a right modified radical mastectomy. She requested implant reconstruction of her right breast and augmentation of her opposite breast. Both procedures were done on an outpatient basis at her request.

BREAST REDUCTION

When the woman's remaining breast is large, she may need to have it reduced and lifted if the rebuilt breast is to match it. A reduction also may make the reconstruction easier to perform because less tissue will be needed for the new breast. Many women with large, heavy breasts are only too willing to consider having their normal breast reduced to allow them to feel more comfortable and balanced and to mitigate functional problems caused by large breasts. In addition, tissue removed during a breast reduction is checked for tumors, and this information helps the surgeon assess this breast's tumor status. Current breast reduction techniques are very reliable and have a high level of patient satisfaction and acceptance. A baseline mammogram is recommended before a reduction mammoplasty and 6 to 12 months after the operation.

The plastic surgeon does not want to reduce a woman's breast too much; he must know what size to make the breast because, above all, he does not want her to feel as if she is losing another breast. Therefore the expected size of her reduced breast must be carefully explained and the woman must understand how it will look before the reduction of the remaining breast is done. The decision for final breast size should be made by the woman herself and must be clearly communicated to her plastic surgeon. To avoid overreduction it may be necessary for the surgeon to perform an extra reconstructive operation later to expand the remaining breast tissue. By reducing a woman's existing breast the plastic surgeon may be able to rebuild her missing breast without a flap procedure; however, a flap should be used if the woman is worried that her breasts will be too small. Most women with a full breast requiring a reduction will have better long-term symmetry if the breast reconstruction is done with a flap of tissue either from the abdomen, back, or buttocks.

The incisions used for breast reduction result in permanent scars that resemble an upside-down T. When only a small or moderate reduction is needed, newer reduction techniques can produce shorter scars, either around the areola or around the areola and down to the inframammary fold. Breast function is also a consideration during reduction mammaplasty. The nipple ducts are left intact to permit future breast feeding. Even though there may be temporary numbness after this procedure, breast sensation is usually not permanently affected. It is possible, however, that nipple-areola sensation can be decreased permanently.

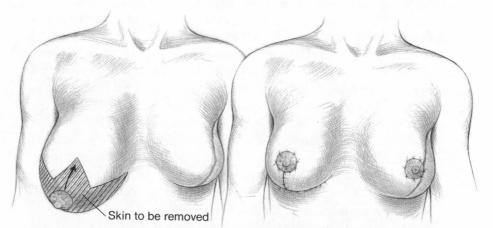

Reduction of the other breast to obtain symmetry with the reconstructed breast

During this procedure the surgeon removes the excess breast tissue to reshape the breast to a smaller size. Extra skin is excised and the final skin closure leaves a scar around the nipple, down to the crease below the breast, and in a line in the crease. With smaller or moderate reductions the scar will just circle the areola or it will circle the areola and extend to the inframammary crease. These scars are easily covered when a brassiere is worn. As with all scars, they are often red for the first months after the operation but will usually fade and lighten after 1 to 2 years.

During the postoperative period the reduced breast is often somewhat swollen and firm. The patient may also note decreased sensation in the breast and nipple-areola. The sensation usually returns during the first few months after the operation. As the sensation returns, the nerves may have heightened sensitivity, occasionally accompanied by shooting pains. When this occurs, the patient is instructed to massage her breast with different textures of cloth and during a bath or shower to use different water temperatures on her breast so that the sensory response can return to normal.

Result

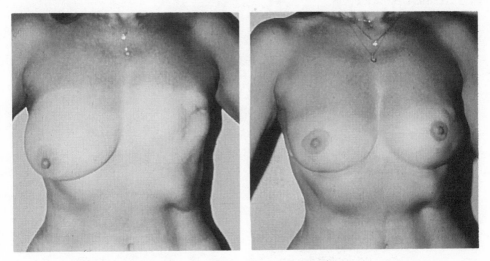

This woman had a modified radical mastectomy. She wanted her large opposite breast reduced and a smaller breast reconstructed to match. She had implant breast reconstruction on the left and a reduction of the other breast.

BREAST LIFT (MASTOPEXY)

If the opposite breast is of reasonable size but sags because of excess skin, the surgeon may find that the skin remaining after the mastectomy is insufficient to stretch to match this sagging breast. In this case the plastic surgeon may suggest a breast lift, or mastopexy, for the remaining breast. Many women are pleased with the prospect of altering their drooping breasts to give them a fuller, more uplifted, youthful appearance.

With a mastopexy, the surgeon moves the nipple-areola upward on the breast to a new position and removes the skin below the nipple and just above the lower breast crease. The incisions are placed in a position similar to those used for a breast reduction and are sometimes even shorter. When the breast does not sag very much, the operation can be done with only a scar around the areola or with one around the areola and down to the inframammary fold.

Many women have considerable flatness in the upper breast region. Simply lifting the breast will not restore fullness to this area. It is best done with a breast implant. For the woman whose other breast is being reconstructed with an implant or expander implant, insertion of an implant in the normal breast is often a good means of providing the best balance.

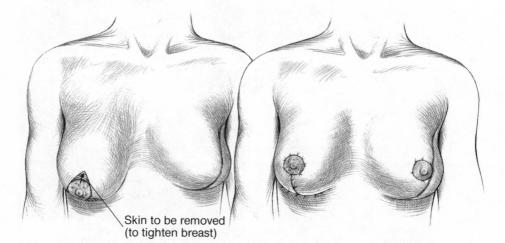

Skin to be removed
(to tighten breast)

Mastopexy (breast lift) of the other breast to obtain symmetry with the reconstructed breast

Result

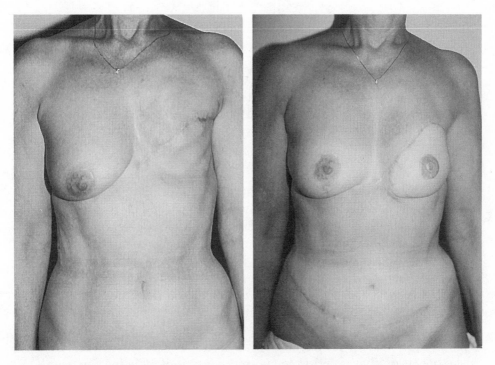

This woman had a modified radical mastectomy. She had breast reconstruction with a TRAM flap and her left breast was lifted for symmetry.

• • •

Frequently the reconstructive surgeon can modify the remaining breast and reconstruct the missing breast shape during one operation. The new breast then can be built to match the existing breast. When there is some question about the necessity for changing the remaining breast or when the woman has doubts about this surgery, it should not be modified at the time of the breast reconstruction. In this case only the missing breast should be restored during the initial operation. Then, later, after the results of surgery are evaluated, a decision can be made about whether the natural breast should be changed or left alone.

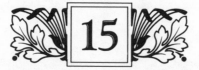

PREVENTIVE MASTECTOMY
FOR THE WOMAN AT RISK

M any women live in constant fear of developing breast cancer. Some of these women have witnessed the suffering and even death of mothers and sisters from this disease; others have themselves fallen victim to breast cancer. The American Cancer Society statistics reporting the growing incidence of breast cancer in U.S. women further adds to their fears. Realizing that they are in a high-risk category for developing a malignancy, these women are often terrified by this possibility. Understandably, some women seek a way of preventing this disease before it occurs.

A preventive (prophylactic) mastectomy with reconstruction is an operation that is performed with the intent of reducing a woman's risk of developing breast cancer by removing most of her breast tissue and then rebuilding her breasts. By its very nature this preventive surgery is controversial and often raises more questions than it answers. The decision to have this operation with the goal of preventing breast cancer also involves removing a healthy breast that may never develop a malignancy. The crucial question is whether this operation actually prevents cancer and whether other nonsurgical treatments could accomplish the same purpose.* Unfortunately, there are no clear-cut answers. Some cancer surgeons are skeptical about the efficacy of this

*The National Institute of Health (NIH) is currently conducting a large study to determine if breast cancer in high-risk women can be prevented with tamoxifen. If the results of this study prove tamoxifen to be an effective prophylactic treatment, this may obviate the need for preventive mastectomy. (See Chapter 6 for more information on these clinical trials.)

surgery. They believe that many prophylactic mastectomies are un-necessary. As one renowned surgeon has stated, "The decision whether to perform a prophylactic mastectomy is difficult for the patient and surgeon because diagnostic methods for cancer are still inadequate and there are no certain methods for preventing cancer."

Others ask why a mastectomy is done to prevent a cancer that can be treated with conservative surgery and irradiation if it does occur. If you wait for cancer to develop, however, there is always the possibil-ity that it may have already spread systemically.

Only a woman in a high-risk category with more than one risk factor present should even consider prophylactic mastectomy. Further-more, the motivation for this operation should be based on her level of concern over cancer. Is she terrorized by her fears of malignancy and subsequent death or can she be reassured that her breasts can be care-fully and adequately monitored without surgery? Most women at high risk are managed by careful evaluation by their physician, breast self-examination, mammograms, and biopsies of any suspicious breast areas (Chapters 3, 4, and 5). (The use of fine-needle aspiration is de-creasing the need for open biopsy of these suspicious breast masses.) Women need to be fully informed about their risks and their options. An operation, however, is usually not recommended. Finally, if a preventive mastectomy is considered, the specifics of the operation should be understood—a prophylactic mastectomy is major surgery. Afterward, the reconstructed breasts have less feeling than normal breasts, their appearance often is not as attractive, and complications may develop that require additional operations. Physicians are un-derstandably circumspect about an operation that can decrease the aesthetic and functional aspects of a woman's breasts while not ab-solutely guaranteeing that it will prevent breast cancer. A decision to have a prophylactic mastectomy should only be reached after an extremely careful discussion by the woman, her physicians, and her surgeons. She needs to have her doctors explain her risk status and the full ramifications of this operation, both positive and negative. She also needs to discuss this operation with others with whom she is intimate. Finally, input from other physicians involved in her care and second opinions from other surgeons are recommended to ensure that this option is weighed as carefully as possible before she makes a final decision for or against it.

HIGH-RISK FACTORS FOR DEVELOPING BREAST CANCER

Three main factors are believed to contribute to an increased risk of breast cancer. Many women fit into at least one of these categories, but that does not mean that they will necessarily develop breast cancer and thus should have their breasts removed. What they do need is good information about their risk status, particularly those women who fit into any of the three high-risk categories.

Family History in a Mother or Sister

A woman's lifetime risk of developing a breast cancer is about 12%. When a close relative such as a mother, sister, or daughter develops the tumor before menopause, the risk increases by a factor of 2 to around 20% to 25%. When a woman's mother or sister develops bilateral cancer before menopause, her risk of developing a breast cancer some time during her lifetime increases to about 50%.

Previous Personal History of Breast Cancer

If cancer develops in one breast, the chance of a new cancer occurring in her other breast increases. For women over 50, the risk is about 4% for their remaining years, and for those under 50, the risk is approximately 14% over the rest of their lives. If several cancerous areas are found in the first breast, the risk to the second breast is greater. These risks are further increased if the woman who had one breast cancer also has a family history, especially if her mother or a sister had this disease and particularly if it occurred before menopause. In addition, those women who have a small tumor that has not spread to the lymph nodes are more likely to live longer and therefore are at risk of developing a second tumor for a longer period of time. The pathologist's report on the first breast cancer can suggest an increased risk for the remaining breast. For instance, if the changes of LCIS (lobular carcinoma in situ) are noted, the patient's risk for another tumor increases by a factor of 2 to 3. The risk of this happening is about 1% for each year of life. If a woman develops breast cancer before the age of 40, the chance that she will develop another cancer in her opposite breast is somewhat increased.

Advanced Age

Although recent statistics suggest that more younger women are now affected by breast cancer, the overall incidence rises with age. About

85% of breast cancers are clinically detected in patients over 45 years old. Advances in mammography have made it easier to detect early breast cancer in women whose breasts are less dense after age 50.

RELATIVE RISK FACTORS

Women in the following categories have a *slightly* increased risk of breast cancer:
• History of breast cancer in maternal or paternal grandmother, father's sister, or mother's sister
• Excessive exposure to radiation, particularly before age 20 (Currently used diagnostic x-ray examinations [even cumulatively] do not reach these levels.)
• Early menarche (beginning of menstruation)
• Birth of first baby after age 30
• Never having borne children (nulliparity)
• Late menopause
• Obesity
• History of some types of fibrocystic changes
• High-fat diet
• Use of estrogen supplements or estrogen replacement therapy
(For the convenience of our readers a similar, slightly more detailed discussion of risk factors is also included in Chapter 6.)

PROPHYLACTIC MASTECTOMY AND RECONSTRUCTION: WHAT TO EXPECT

The objective of a prophylactic mastectomy (also called a "total" mastectomy and subcutaneous mastectomy) is to remove as much glandular breast tissue as possible while preserving the skin covering of the breast so that the breast may be reconstructed to an attractive appearance. Because breast tissue is close to the skin, its removal can sometimes impair the blood supply to the skin and nipple-areola. The surgeon usually will request that the patient refrain from smoking cigarettes a few days or weeks before the operation and for at least 1 week after surgery to prevent any further compromise of the blood supply.

Heavy cigarette smoking causes the small vessels in the skin to constrict, thus creating further changes in the skin, possible scarring or loss of the nipple-areola, or implant exposure that will require its removal. Women who smoke are at great risk for developing lung cancer; it seems illogical for these same women to undergo prophylactic breast removal because of their fear of breast cancer while continuing to smoke and risk lung cancer. Furthermore, smoking increases the possibility of complications after prophylactic mastectomy. In reviewing patients with major complications after prophylactic mastectomy, the common link and contributing cause of these complications is cigarette smoking.

When the breast is of normal size, the nipple-areola skin can be left on the breast after the breast tissue beneath the nipple is removed. Some surgeons and patients, however, prefer to remove the nipple-areola during preventive mastectomy. The surgeon then reconstructs the breast with the woman's own tissue or by placing an implant or expander implant under the pectoralis major muscle layer (reconstruction with available tissue, see p. 214). This muscle cover will help to ensure that the implant remains soft and does not become exposed through the skin. Experience with the textured-surface implants and expanders indicates that they provide equally soft results regardless of whether they are positioned under the remaining skin or muscle; however, for patients with thin skin cover, the implant's contour and folds can be seen and felt through the thin skin and so it is best placed under the muscle. If the patient is concerned about using breast implants and still requests prophylactic mastectomy, breast reconstruction with bilateral TRAM flaps can be considered. Autologous tissue is a good alternative for these women who decide to remove their breasts out of fear of cancer and do not want to use a foreign material that might be a source of further anxiety. If the woman's breast is large and pendulous, it will require either a flap reconstruction (Chapter 13) to provide sufficient fill for the remaining breast skin or modification of the remaining breast skin so that the breast appears smaller and more uplifted. In the latter case the plastic surgeon temporarily removes the nipple-areola and excises the breast tissue and ducts from beneath it. Then he replaces the nipple-areola as a graft in the proper position on the newly reconstructed breast.

After the surgeon removes the breast tissue, he uses one of the methods described in Chapter 13 to reconstruct the breast. The prophylactic mastectomy and the subsequent reconstruction usually are performed in one operation (as described for immediate breast reconstruction), even though some surgeons advise delaying the reconstruction for a few days to months. Delaying breast reconstruction after prophylactic mastectomy is recommended routinely by some surgeons and others delay it only for the patient with increased risk factors such as cigarette smoking or breast scars from previous breast biopsies, which could compromise the primary healing of the skin and lead to postoperative complications.

WHERE ARE THE INCISIONS PLACED AND DO THEY SHOW?

A number of incisions can be used for preventive mastectomy, and the patient should discuss these variations with her surgeon. Some surgeons remove the tissue through an opening in the crease beneath the breast. This incision produces the least obvious scar. Another option is to use a second axillary incision in additional to the one at the inframanimary fold. Other surgeons have difficulty gaining access to the upper axillary breast tissue through this approach and use an incision lateral to the areola. Sometimes this incision is extended over the nipple to elevate it when the breast sags.

The presence of biopsy scars can influence the safety and position of the prophylactic mastectomy incisions. When the biopsy scars are relatively long, the prophylactic mastectomy can often be done through these scars, thus avoiding additional breast incisions and causing less risk of some of the breast skin not surviving. When the breasts are large or there is excessive breast skin, the surgeon removes the extra skin from below the nipple-areola and just above the crease, leaving an inverted T scar, or through the middle of the breast, leaving a scar going through the midportion of the breast. The woman considering prophylactic mastectomy who has larger breasts that also need to be lifted or made smaller should know that she has an increased chance of having problems and complications from the operation. The nipple-areola skin often has to be taken off from the low position on the breast and either grafted to its new position or reconstructed at a later operation. Removal of a larger amount of breast tissue and the need for larger skin flaps also increase the risk that the skin will heal poorly. In some cases the breast implant used for reconstruction may have to be removed and replaced a few months later.

WHAT IF A BREAST CANCER IS FOUND AT THE TIME OF A PROPHYLACTIC MASTECTOMY?

The breasts should be carefully evaluated for breast cancer at the time the decision is made to have a prophylactic mastectomy. Occasionally, either during the operation or later after the pathologist evaluates the tissues removed by the mastectomy, a breast cancer is found. Because of this possibility, the prophylactic mastectomy should be done as a total mastectomy with breast tissue removed according to recognized cancer treatment guidelines. However, to determine if the breast cancer has spread, an axillary dissection with removal of the axillary lymph nodes may still be needed to provide more information about the stage of the tumor and the advisability of chemotherapy or hormonal therapy. These possibilities should be considered prior to prophylactic mastectomy and an agreement reached as to how to proceed should breast cancer be found. If cancer is discovered during the prophylactic operation, the axillary lymph nodes can be removed in the same procedure. If found later by the pathologist, a secondary axillary lymph node removal may be necessary. If the breast cancer is found near a preserved nipple-areola, it can be removed during a subsequent operation.

HOW WILL MY BREAST LOOK AFTER A PROPHYLACTIC MASTECTOMY AND RECONSTRUCTION?

Breasts reconstructed with insertion of a breast implant under the muscle after prophylactic mastectomy are usually not as soft, sensitive, or mobile as natural breasts. Scars from the operation will be visible, and the recreated breasts often will not exhibit the flow and mobility of natural breasts. They are also flatter and do not have normal conical projection in the area under the areola since the tissue in this area has been removed. This flat appearance often improves during the first few weeks after the operation.

When prophylactic mastectomy is followed by breast reconstruction with the patient's own tissues, the appearance and feel of her breasts are more natural, but she must also endure a more involved flap procedure that usually takes tissue from the lower abdominal wall and leaves an abdominoplasty scar in addition to the breast scars. Breasts reconstructed with autologous tissue often develop better sensation than those reconstructed with implants. Up to 70% of these autologous breast reconstructions demonstrate some sensation. The unique sensitivity associated with the nipple-areola is not restored with any of the currently used methods of breast reconstruction.

Despite the limitations of reconstruction performed after a prophylactic mastectomy, women having this procedure usually are satisfied with the decision to have the operation because their main purpose for having this surgery has been accomplished: they have reduced their worry about their high-risk status.

The woman considering prophylactic mastectomy must be aware that even though only one operation is planned, additional procedures may be needed to correct asymmetry, treat a complication from the initial procedure, or to improve breast appearance if it does not meet the patient's expectations for size or shape.

Results

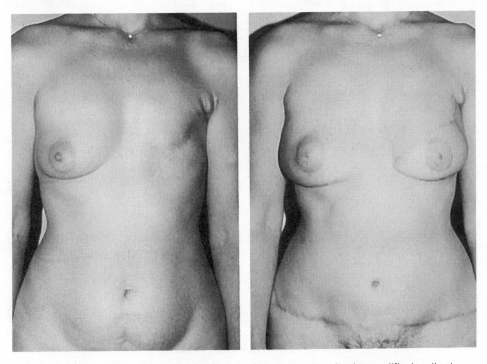

This woman with a strong family history of breast cancer had a modified radical mastectomy several years earlier. Because of her fear she later had a left prophylactic mastectomy and bilateral TRAM flap reconstruction.

Results—cont'd

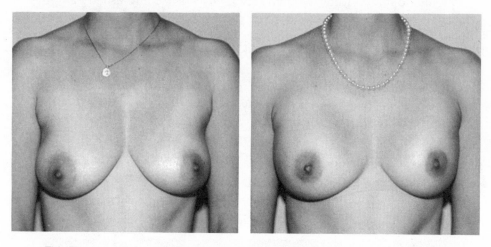

This 34-year-old woman lived in constant fear of breast cancer because her mother and 38-year-old sister both had premenopausal breast cancer. She had bilateral prophylactic mastectomies and immediate reconstruction with implants.

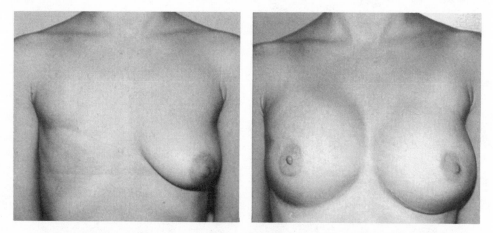

This 34-year-old woman had a prior mastectomy and a family history of breast cancer. Terrified at the prospect of developing breast cancer in her other breast, she had a left prophylactic mastectomy with nipple-areola preservation and immediate reconstruction with tissue expansion. Her right breast was also reconstructed with the same method at that time and her right nipple-areola was rebuilt several months later. The result is shown 1 year following breast reconstruction.

PROS AND CONS OF PREVENTIVE MASTECTOMY AND RECONSTRUCTION

Although recent advances in technique have made a prophylactic mastectomy and reconstruction more aesthetically predictable, serious complications do still occur. To help her make a more informed objective decision the woman needs to question her surgeon about the positive and negative aspects of this procedure.

Pros

- Decreases the fear of breast cancer by removing most of the breast tissue.
- Decreases the risk of breast cancer. The effectiveness of this preventive surgery remains a source of controversy. There is no definitive evidence to prove that a prophylactic mastectomy reduces a woman's risk of getting cancer, even though any tumors occurring in the thin layer of breast tissue remaining after this procedure are usually easier to detect while they are quite small. Available reports do indicate, however, that the incidence of subsequent breast cancer is very low (less than 1%) after prophylactic mastectomy in women initially determined to be at high risk of developing breast cancer.
- Reduces painful symptoms caused by fibrocystic breast changes; however, breast pain alone should not be the primary indication for the operation. There are many other reasons for breast pain, and these are not improved by prophylactic mastectomy. In fact, some additional pain is always a possibility whenever a breast operation or any operation is performed.

Cons

- As with any major surgical procedure, there are risks from general anesthesia and complications of bleeding infection, skin loss, nipple loss, capsular contracture, and implant loss. Additional abdominal complications can occur if a TRAM flap is used for breast reconstruction. Correction of these problems often requires additional operations.
- Frequently does not produce a reconstructed breast that is as attractive as the original breast. There are permanent scars and a lack of normal breast flow and projection. Additional operations may be needed to improve the appearance of the breasts after prophylactic mastectomy and immediate breast reconstruction.

- Results in decreased sensation or loss of sensation in the reconstructed breast, especially the nipple-areola, because of the division of the sensory nerves when the breast is removed. Even though breast sensation does not return, the woman's breasts may feel uncomfortable, even painful.
- Often requires more than one procedure to achieve the best result or manage complications.
- Still leaves a small percentage of breast tissue as a potential site of breast cancer.

A woman's decision for a preventive mastectomy and reconstruction requires input from the general surgeon and other members of the breast management team. These specialists can advise her concerning her particular risks of developing breast cancer as well the normal, expected results of a prophylactic mastectomy for a woman with her type of breasts. She needs to be examined and counseled by at least two physicians who can evaluate her risk factors and their implications for her future health status. Preventive mastectomy is not an emergency procedure. If there is a suspicious breast mass or indication that breast cancer is present, this question should be resolved before a decision is made for prophylactic mastectomy. Most women at high risk are monitored most effectively by breast self-examination and regular physician examinations and mammograms. Some are now participating in clinical trials to assess the benefits of tamoxifen as a prophylactic treatment. A woman should carefully consider all of her options and all aspects of her situation with the greatest of care before a final decision is made for preventive surgery.

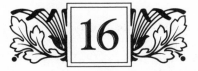

CREATING A NIPPLE-AREOLA

When a woman has her breast reconstructed, she also must decide whether she wants her nipple and areola (the circular pigmented area surrounding the nipple) reconstructed. Some women only desire to have their breast shape restored so that they feel balanced and symmetric. For them, the nipple-areola is of little consequence. To others, however, a nipple-areola is an important component of reconstructive surgery. This represents the finishing touch that makes their breasts look and feel more natural.

In interviews and surveys with women who had breast reconstruction we discovered an interesting correlation between the success of the initial procedure to build the breast and the woman's subsequent desire for a nipple. When the rebuilt breast does not meet her aesthetic desires, she usually does not want her nipple restored because it merely emphasizes a poor result. The attitude of these women is "enough is enough," and they are content to be able to fill out a bra. Women who have satisfactory aesthetic results frequently have the opposite reaction. They want a nipple-areola reconstruction as the final phase of their operation to create a more natural breast appearance and to provide a good match with their breasts. The creation of the nipple-areola seems to complete a rehabilitation program for them. As one woman explained, "It becomes the icing on the cake; it is not absolutely necessary, but it is so beautiful when it's there."

Although reconstruction of the breast and nipple-areola is possible during one operation, the best results are obtained when the ideal breast shape is achieved first. Most plastic surgeons prefer to wait a few months after the first operation or after tissue expansion has been completed until the newly created breast is stable and symmetric with the remaining breast. Then the plastic surgeon and patient can more accurately determine the proper position, size, and projection of the nipple-areola. It is important for the woman to participate in this decision-making process. Once the nipple has been built, it is very difficult to change its position later. She is going to have to live with it and it should look right to her. Unless additional corrections are needed on the reconstructed breast, the actual reconstruction often can be done on an outpatient basis under local anesthesia.

Significant advances have been made in nipple-areola reconstruction techniques during the past few years, and there are a number of new techniques for women to choose from. It is now possible to rebuild a woman's nipple with tissue already present at the site of the new nipple-areola on her reconstructed breast. The areola can also be created with excess skin at the lateral portion of the mastectomy scar, or if the patient had a TRAM flap breast reconstruction, it can be grafted from excess tissue at the end of the abdominal scar. The color of the nipple-areola is defined a few months later with a tattoo. The circular area of the areola can also be simulated with a tattoo of the approximate color and size to match the opposite areola without the need for taking a skin graft to form the areola.

These new techniques are often more appealing to women than previous approaches that created the nipple and areola from two different types of tissue transferred from other areas of a woman's body. These older methods are still used for some patients when appropriate, and they continue to give excellent results. The newer methods, however, are simpler, frequently less painful, and are often preferred because they seem to fit in more readily with most women's active life-styles.

NIPPLE RECONSTRUCTION

When a woman chooses to have her nipple reconstructed, she does so for aesthetic reasons, to enhance the appearance of her reconstructed breast and to make it more symmetric with her remaining breast. Projection seems to be a key issue with many women who elect to have their nipples reconstructed; they want the freedom to wear T-shirts and swimsuits without being self-consciousness that one nipple is more prominent than the other. A woman should not decide to create a nipple for sensation or for milk production potential; these functions are impossible for the reconstructed breast.

There are presently two primary methods of nipple reconstruction that use local tissue at the site of the future nipple-areola to build the new nipple—the *skate flap* and the *C-V flap* (thus named because the

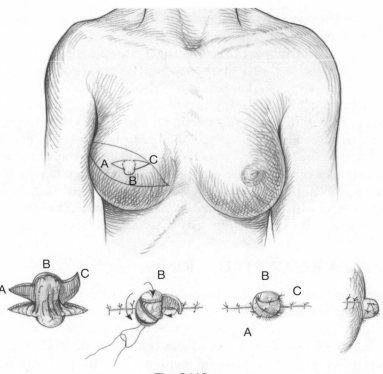

The C-V flap

design of the flap resembles two V's connected by a C). With these techniques, a layer of skin and fat on the reconstructed breast is shifted to the center of what will be the future nipple-areola area and formed into a nipple. The skin is used to create the nipple and the underlying fat is used to add bulk, fullness, and permanent shape. The skate flap uses much of the skin at the site of the future areola for the nipple reconstruction, and a graft of skin taken from another site such as the outer portion of the mastectomy scar is then used for the areola reconstruction. With the C-V flap, not as much local tissue is used and consequently it may not produce as large and projecting a nipple as the skate flap. Advantageously, the donor site for the C-V flap can be closed with two short scars; therefore an areola graft is not always necessary with the C-V flap operation. A tattoo can be done later for nipple color and areola reconstruction.

Although a nice-sized nipple can be created from breast skin, often its color is not dark enough to match the remaining nipple. In this case a tattoo provides a better color match. (See later discussion on tattooing.)

The opposite nipple can also be used for nipple reconstruction but is not a frequently chosen method today. It is often not acceptable to either the patient or her husband, and other sources of tissue for nipple reconstruction are selected. When the remaining nipple is very large and projecting, however, this method is still the best way to create a nipple that is symmetric in size, color, and texture. With this technique, a portion of the lower part or end of the remaining nipple is used for the nipple reconstruction so that the donor area of the normal nipple is not significantly changed or scarred. This donor area usually heals in 1 to 2 weeks without any numbness and little pain. After the nipple has healed, it does not lose its sensitivity or feeling.

AREOLA RECONSTRUCTION

Methods for recreating the areola range from simple tattooing to the more complex graft techniques. The decision as to which technique is appropriate depends on a patient's life-style and preferences.

Some women do not care if the color is exact; they want the simplest, safest, and least painful method for creating a semblance of an areola. Tattooing, which may not always produce a realistic result, may be the solution that these woman desire. Although the texture and projection of the natural areola will be lacking, the color match of a tattooed areola can be quite good and an areola graft is not needed. Many women appreciate the convenience of this approach.

When local breast skin is used for the nipple reconstruction, the tissue for the areola graft is usually taken from the lateral portion of the mastectomy scar or the lateral portion of the abdominal scar if the woman had a TRAM flap. This technique is very acceptable to most women and it avoids additional scars; it is also very effectively used in combination with the skate flap. The mastectomy scar and the excess skin at the lateral end of the scar can often be improved when the areolar graft is removed. Since this area is usually numb from the mastectomy, little pain is experienced during the taking (harvesting) of the graft or afterwards. The main drawback is that the skin graft is not pigmented, and although it will appear pink during the initial weeks to months after grafting, it usually fades and a tattoo may be necessary to obtain a better color match.

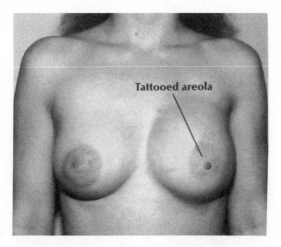

Tattoo without areola grafting was satisfactory
for this woman who preferred a simple,
nonsurgical procedure that produced a
semblance of an areola.

A graft of tissue from the upper inner thigh is another means of reconstructing the areola, but this technique involves a painful donor site and has become unpopular with the advent of the newer, less painful techniques just described. Although this method is not preferred by most patients, it still produces excellent results and is still used for some patients. The tissue obtained from this area is pigmented and usually provides a good match with the opposite areola without the need for an areola tattoo. A round areola skin graft is removed from the upper thigh, and the remaining thigh skin is brought together as a thin scar line in this crease; this scar is practically invisible when healed and does not show, even in a bathing suit. The groin area is usually painful after this procedure and will feel tender for about 2 weeks.

Once the areolar graft has been obtained, the actual placement of the new areola onto the breast area can be accomplished. If the upper inner thigh graft has been used, a very thin circular layer of surface skin needs to be removed first to make room for this new areola. (In the skate or C-V flap operation this skin layer has already been removed to build the nipple.) The areola skin graft is then positioned on this area.

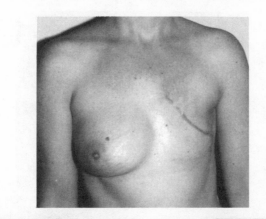

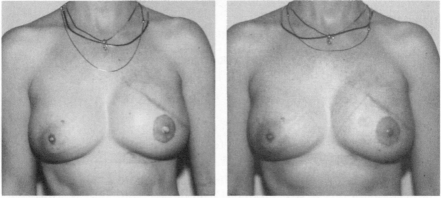

This patient had nipple-areola reconstruction with local skin used for nipple reconstruction and an areola graft taken from the lateral end of the mastectomy scar. Her nipple-areola was tattooed 2 months later.

NIPPLE-AREOLA TATTOO

Many times the color of a nipple and areola created from breast skin is not dark enough to match the remaining nipple-areola. In this case a tattoo provides a better color match. A tattoo is the most direct and permanent method for pigmenting the reconstructed nipple-areola. It is also effective, as discussed earlier, in creating the appearance of an areola for the woman who does not want to have another surgical procedure or for a woman whose opposite areola is so large that it is not practical to reconstruct a matching areola using a skin graft. The plastic surgeon uses tattooing to create a pigmented circle to match the other areola without resorting to a large skin graft.

Many plastic surgeons who do breast reconstruction can perform the tattoo in their office as an outpatient procedure or can arrange to have the tattoo done by a qualified professional. The procedure is quite easy. The patient participates in determining the proper color for the new nipple-areola. The natural nipple-areola has a wide spectrum of colors, and the best color match is achieved by blending the pigments.

A local anesthetic is often used prior to tattooing. The tattoo device is then dipped in the pigment and placed into the outer layers of skin. The pigment is applied until the areola and nipple have been uniformly tattooed. Slightly darker pigments are used for the nipple tattoo. The area is a little raw for a few days after the procedure. An antibiotic ointment is used to keep it moist. If a woman's skin tones have a lot of yellow, the match may not be as close. Newer pigments are providing better matches for these individuals. Over the next few weeks to months the tattooed nipple-areola may look darker than the color selected; however, with time it fades, usually to an acceptable color. The woman should be warned that the tattooed nipple-areola will initially appear much darker than the natural one so that she will not be unnecessarily alarmed. Even so, some women are disturbed by the early disparity in color and are anxious for the color to fade so that it matches the remaining nipple-areola and does not stand out "like a beacon."

• • •

To protect the nipple and areola after surgery a protective dressing is taped over the nipple and stabilized with surgical tapes. The reconstructed nipple-areola tends to be dry after surgery; the application of a moisturizing cream can improve this condition.

Although the creation of a nipple-areola is not an essential component of a breast reconstruction, it can add a touch of realism to the result. By creating a nipple-areola on a woman's new breast a surgeon can transform her surgically created mound into a natural and aesthetic breast form.

BREAST CANCER AND ITS EFFECT ON RELATIONSHIPS

WHAT WOMEN WANT: MALE SUPPORT

"It is always hard on the man. He stands there, outside, and he sees all of the problems down the road. He is both frightened to death and threatened. But the patient, somewhere along the way, comes to terms with herself because she has no choice."

These words express the feelings of one breast cancer patient as she reflected on the predicaments that this disease creates for men and women. Her statement typifies the type of answers that we received when we surveyed women about this topic. Drawing on the responses of over 500 women who had mastectomies, we have summarized their feelings and thoughts about the problems they encountered in their relationships as a result of their breast cancer. Issues addressed include the response to diagnosis, recovery from mastectomy, the male reaction to mastectomy, issues of intimacy and sexual relationships, common fears of the mastectomy patient, and male support for breast reconstruction. Although there are no prescribed rules for a man to follow under these circumstances, many of the women we surveyed had suggestions about what had been most helpful for them. This chapter incorporates these suggestions. In addition to information gleaned from our questionnaire, we have also included a short section written by a general surgeon on the topic of the patient-surgeon relationship.

Facing the Diagnosis

The discovery of breast cancer provokes many fears in a couple and these fears need to be shared. Both are worried about the prognosis of cancer and its effect on their future life together. They worry about possible treatment options and the effects of chemotherapy, radiation treatment, or surgery. Their concerns may not surface immediately, however, since there seems to be a tendency for couples to hide true feelings behind a cheerful, "make the best of it" facade. These true feelings can be damaging to a relationship if they are not brought into the open and examined. All of the women we contacted believed in and stressed the need for open and honest communication. As one woman said, "I asked my husband if he could allow me to feel what I was feeling, and I would try to allow him his feelings. I didn't want pity. I just wanted him to listen when I talked because it was a release to say how I was feeling." Women also stressed the importance of physical closeness and contact accompanying this communication process. The value of hugging and holding was mentioned in virtually all of our surveys and interviews. One woman expressed this feeling most poignantly when she said, "Sometimes when the words wouldn't come, he would just hold me, hug me, stroke me, and I would cry. That was real communication. Even though he told me he loved me, and I loved hearing it, his touch revealed all I needed to know. The physical closeness made me feel loved and accepted. Hugging makes a big difference."

Women emphasized the ameliorative effects of talking about their problems with someone else. It was crucial to have someone close to share the burden. Sometimes they just needed someone to listen to them and to hold them without "trying to make things right." As one woman explained, "During the tears, the anger, the insecurity, the fear, the ups and the downs, there is really no need to give advice or try to cheer a woman up. A man just needs to allow her to have all of these feelings and be understanding, even if none of these feelings make sense. More than anything else a man needs to listen to a woman's feelings, her fears, her hopes without judging or trying to 'fix' things." Another woman wrote, "There is no way that anybody can really understand what you are feeling when you have cancer, unless that person has experienced it himself. What can you say to someone, 'I'm sorry?' Sometimes you just need somebody to talk to in a one-way conversation. Men can help us by just letting us get upset and release some of the tension."

The time between the diagnosis of breast cancer and the selection of treatment is a tense one for both a man and a woman. For a man, the fear of his loved one's death from cancer usually far overshadows her possible breast loss. Understandably, his priority is the woman's health and survival. It is important, however, for him to acknowledge her concerns and be careful not to minimize her attachment to her breasts. Together they need to define their priorities and investigate her therapy options.

The first priority is for the woman to get the best care for her tumor. She often feels confused and depressed by all that is happening to her. By accompanying her to medical consultations a man can actively demonstrate his concern and help a woman to focus on the issues being discussed. Together they can learn about and critically evaluate the various treatment options. Most of the couples we interviewed had taken the time to inform themselves about breast cancer and about breast reconstruction. They had read articles and books on these topics, attended lectures, and even seen movies and slide presentations. They agreed that this process helped them cope and also gave them a better understanding of what the future held. Repeatedly, in both our surveys and in our discussions with men and women, couples stressed the beneficial value of this educational process. As one man related, "By learning about my girlfriend's cancer we at least were able to understand our choices and make some decisions based on knowledge instead of fear. I actually think it brought us closer together."

The Patient-Surgeon Relationship
ROGER S. FOSTER, Jr., M.D.

It is normal for a woman diagnosed with breast cancer to react to her disease and to the surgeon responsible for her treatment with mixed emotions. Feelings of desperation, rage, and hopelessness may coexist with feelings of courage, hope, and determination. She may be angry with fate, God, or even herself. Some of her resentment will naturally focus on her surgeon. Frequently he is the messenger delivering the bad news about her cancer and her prognosis. Furthermore, his treatments inflict pain, create scars, and may deform her body, all good reasons for her to react negatively. In addition to these negative feelings, however, most women also experience positive feelings for their surgeons. Because a woman is dependent on her surgeon, having entrusted her life and body to him, she feels vulnerable and exposed. She needs to reassure herself that his skills are great and that he is a particularly sensitive and caring individual, personally interested in her welfare. Her intense feelings about her cancer and its treatment may lead her to attribute laudatory qualities to her surgeon that are really more reflective of her emotional needs than of the actual character of the surgeon himself.

These conflicting emotions of resentment and admiration are dif-ficult to deal with, particularly for an already stressed woman trying to cope with a life-threatening disease. Her strong feelings are not wrong, but it helps if both the woman, her loved ones, and her surgeon are able to recognize these feelings for what they are. Her anger and hostility should not be personalized by the surgeon and taken as an affront. Similarly, a woman should not feel guilty about experiencing these negative reactions. Perhaps the surgeon has been lacking in tact and diplomacy. Maybe his people skills need some polishing. Even so, a woman and her loved ones need to understand that her anger is not necessarily attributable to the surgeon's personality. Much of her rage is situational, a reaction to circumstances beyond her control. The positive feelings of affection and even adulation that she may devel-op for her surgeon should also be recognized as situational in nature and should not be misinterpreted by the woman experiencing them or the man who cares about her. The patient's affection or even "love" for her cancer surgeon or plastic surgeon is not the same as the love she may feel for a husband or significant other, where reciprocity of af-fection is expected. Even though a man may experience moments of jealousy or resentment because of his loved one's seeming transfer-ence of affection to her doctor, he should realize that with time and recovery this affection as well as the anger she feels toward her doctor will diminish and she will view her relationship with him from a bet-ter perspective.

Recovery From Mastectomy

After a mastectomy a woman commonly experiences a period of "peak" stress as she attempts to recover from the physical and psy-chological effects of this operation. Her physical recuperation usually takes 2 to 3 months but may be prolonged if chemotherapy or radia-tion therapy is necessary. At this time she may be weak, tired, irritable, and possibly ill from the treatments. Lifting a vacuum cleaner or carry-ing groceries might be too much strain for her, and she may need some-one to assume some of her physical responsibilities until she feels better. A man's attitude when helping is crucial. Women stressed the importance of a man offering assistance willingly and not begrudg-ingly so that the woman does not "feel needy or as if she is nagging him to help her." Many women said that their arms felt sore and stiff for the first few weeks after surgery, and they appreciated having someone accompany them on trips to the doctor so that they did not have to worry about driving the car and possibly straining themselves. It also was helpful when a man could assist with some of the organizational and parenting responsibilities of the household, seeing to the children's appointments and schedules, attending recitals and athletic events, paying bills, arranging for repairmen, and filling in when necessary. As one woman explained, "My man was there when I needed him most, yet we were thousands of miles apart physically during portions of my treatment. He cared for our children and his phone calls were sufficient to help me through." By doing the heavy cleaning, driving the carpools, or doing the grocery shopping a man can provide very positive support for a woman during her recovery.

There is a delicate balance between willingly assisting a woman until her strength returns and actually doing everything for her. Most women we surveyed appreciated the physical assistance men provided them during their initial recuperation, but they were quick to resist any attempts to take over. Even though some of the men that we interviewed felt that they could best help their wives by relieving them of all worries and responsibilities, their wives did not agree. Most women were uncomfortable with this treatment. "Don't put us on pedestals. Help us, if we need help, but don't cure one thing and start something else. We do not want to be treated as invalids." Getting back into the mainstream of life seemed to be the focus for most of the women we surveyed. They actively feared being left out of life. They wanted to feel useful and to participate as they always had. They did not want people to "whisper and tiptoe around them."

Reactions to a Woman's Changed Physical Appearance

A man's response to her changed physical appearance worries the woman who has had a mastectomy. Above all, she fears his expressing shock at her missing breast. Many women worry that they will appear less feminine and lovable. Fearing rejection, they desire physical attention, love, and continued reassurance of their desirability. As one woman explained, "No woman is less feminine or intelligent or attractive because she has had a mastectomy, but sometimes it helps to be reminded."

The problem of how to react to a woman's altered appearance is not an easy one. In some cases the woman cannot adjust to her missing breast and does not want the man to see her. Some of the women we surveyed are "still dressing in the closet so no one sees them." Some have never shown their scars to their husbands or boyfriends, worried that they will be disgusted at what they see. Some even avoid intimate relationships and possible exposure of their scarred chests. In other cases the woman is willing to show her missing breast to her loved one and allow him to help her change bandages, rub ointment on her scar, or reassure her that she still looks okay. Many of the women responding to us suggested that problems could be avoided if the scar were seen as soon as possible after surgery. One woman wrote that many of her worries had been eliminated because she and her boyfriend had viewed the scar together in the hospital in the presence of her doctor. They shared the shock together, recovered from it, and went on to concentrate on other matters.

Although many of the women we contacted felt that men were usually supportive of women cancer patients, not all of the stories we heard were positive. Some relationships ended. Divorces occurred both after the mastectomy and after breast reconstruction. Some men could not adjust to their wife or girlfriend's changed physical appearance or to her status as a cancer victim. They "could not handle the tumor" or stand to "look at her lopsided chest with a breast on one side and a long red scar on the other." Others could not cope with the added responsibility of worrying about a life-threatening illness. Some men found that the woman in their lives had changed and now had difficulty relating to her. They tired of "hearing about her cancer" and found her so inwardly directed after this experience that they did not feel that she could talk about anything else.

The missing breast itself, however, did not seem to be the actual cause of divorce after a mastectomy. Sometimes it inhibited a woman sexually and made a man more timid in his sexual approaches, but these inhibitions were often overcome with time. Interestingly, both men and women seemed to agree that divorces or breakups after a mastectomy were usually the culmination of a long history of problems that had previously existed between a couple. These men were temporarily supportive through surgery and recovery, but then when the fear of death had subsided and life returned to its status quo, the old unhappiness was evident again and often the relationship ended. Marriages or relationships that were strong before the surgery became even stronger afterward.

Intimacy and Sexual Relationships

Romance and intimacy is another sensitive area for women after mastectomy and even sometimes after breast reconstruction. Worried about how their changed appearance will affect their sexual relationship with a man, these women, no matter how close to their husbands or boyfriends, express fears of rejection. Men also have concerns; they worry about making the wrong moves, saying the wrong things, or pushing a woman before she is ready. Most of the women we surveyed desired a return to normal sexual relations as soon as possible. Keeping an element of romance in a relationship was very important to all of the women and men we interviewed. It helped them infuse a feeling of normality into their relationship. As one woman candidly explained, "Even though I was missing a breast, I still wanted to be treated as a sexy and romantic woman. I wanted to be flirted with. I wanted him to do romantic things to help me to feel loving and sensual. I wanted my man to touch my body, to tenderly caress me, and to look at me in such a way that I knew it didn't make any difference to him. As a woman I needed to know that I was still sexually attractive."

Many of the women we spoke to also agreed that women will differ in their readiness for intimacy and a man should "take the lead from the woman and try to encourage but not to rush sex." That cautionary note also applies to the woman who has had breast reconstruction. As one woman advised, "I think that men should not expect sex too quickly after a woman has had reconstruction. Women need some time to recuperate. They still feel protective of their bodies. I know that I still protect my body and breasts during intercourse." Obviously this is a problematic situation; a man straddles a line between expressing his affection too forcefully or remaining aloof and standoffish. Each couple needs to work out their own individual method of relating and dealing with questions of intimacy; they need to talk about these problems and understand them.

The value of foreplay and afterplay was frequently reinforced by women as they divulged their personal desires in lovemaking. Many felt that a man should initially be more gentle and stroking, and this caring should continue. "He should not pull away physically after orgasm but should tenderly embrace her and tell her he loves her." A man should not be afraid to touch the woman as he did before. Stroking during lovemaking and after was judged vitally important for a woman's self-esteem both before and after reconstruction. "My husband of 30 years was and is fantastic. He didn't care if I had reconstruction or not. In fact, my new breast is caressed as lovingly as the old one." One woman suggested the need for a man "to learn new sexual techniques to help a woman achieve arousal." As she explained, "With the loss of a breast and even after reconstruction, a major hot spot is irrevocably gone and all of the sexual sensitivity that accompanies it. Breasts are a 'turn on.' You lose that after a mastectomy and reconstruction does not fully restore it. You can't get that special sexual sensitivity back; there is a numbness now where you used to feel titillation. You need a good relationship with your sexual partner to compensate for this loss. And sometimes you need to be creative."

For the single woman involved in dating, her missing breast presents special problems, particularly in deciding how to inform a suitor when a more intimate relationship is desired. Most women feel that a straightforward approach is probably the best. Numerous scenarios were described in which the woman sat the man down and explained about her changed physical appearance and what it meant. Generally, men accept this news far better than women anticipate, sometimes even better than the women themselves. As one woman revealed, "The worst part of having a mastectomy is that you just don't feel feminine. My male friend didn't make me feel that way; those feelings were self-inflicted. The first time we made love I didn't want to expose myself and I was terribly self-conscious. He just said, 'It doesn't matter to me,' but I said, 'It matters to me.' I always wore a nightgown. I just couldn't do it without it." Many of the single women we spoke to said that they were self-conscious about having the man see them totally undressed or in full light. One woman explained how she "always had a nightgown on and the room was always darkened." Some women, although not as many, even expressed feelings of embarrassment after reconstruction because of their scars, the telltale signs that they had surgery. As one young girl revealed, "For a long time I wore a shirt to bed or I took it off in the dark, but he was patient with me until I reached a point where I didn't feel self-conscious."

Learning to relate intimately is not always easy for a couple under the best of circumstances; after a mastectomy, with or without reconstruction, it is particularly challenging. This is a very emotional time for a woman, and in many ways she feels that her femininity and her self-esteem are on the line. Patience and understanding are required of a man, and she in turn must be willing to communicate her feelings and fears to her partner in order to reach a level of comfort and fulfillment.

A Woman's Fears

Understandably, the mastectomy patient has many questions and fears to cope with. Knowing about her doubts sometimes helps a man to be more sensitive to them. One woman poignantly summarized these worries when she sent us a series of questions that she felt needed to be answered:

• How can I face my husband or male friend?
• Will sex ever be the same?
• Will I be afraid for him to touch me?
• How will I feel about myself?
• Will I be the same person?
• Will I have the same outlook on life?
• Will my sex life be affected?
• Knowing that my husband fell in love with my body as well as me, how will he feel about my body now?
• After I get a prosthesis, will people look at me and wonder which breast was cut off?
• Will people pity me, feel sorry for me?
• If I seek reconstruction, will people think I am vain and self-centered?

Support for Breast Reconstruction

When a woman decides that she wants to have her breast reconstructed, she often looks to a man for encouragement for this important decision. Frequently, in our surveys, women explained that despite their strong personal motivation for reconstruction, they still needed a man's emotional support. They wanted to be reassured that reconstruction was okay and that they were not being vain or selfish because they desired more surgery to restore their missing breasts.

Some men will resist the idea of breast reconstruction, hoping to shield their loved ones from additional pain, operative risk, and hospitalization. Judging from our questionnaires, we found this initial negative male reaction to be very common. Most of these men felt that the woman had suffered enough and they wanted to get on with life. Most of the women we surveyed understood these male concerns but felt that if a woman's commitment for reconstruction were strong, a man should respect her desires and encourage her.* Unlike the mastectomy, breast reconstruction was regarded as positive surgery meant to restore what the mastectomy removed. As one woman explained, "It is important for a man to support a woman's decision about breast reconstruction because it is her body, her feelings, her life. He should avoid making decisions for her. She needs to feel that she is in control."

*Most plastic surgeons are pleased to see a man accompany a woman for a consultation about breast reconstruction. His presence usually indicates that she is not alone in her decision and has someone to support her.

A woman may not be as pleased with her new breast immediately after breast reconstruction as she had anticipated. It will not fully resemble the original breast and will bear a scar and feel numb to the touch. At this stage of her recovery she is extremely sensitive and vulnerable to criticism. She does not want to hear that her new breast is not as nice as her normal breast; she cannot tolerate negative comments or criticism of her appearance.

The man's role in dealing with a woman's breast cancer experience is a difficult one. It requires sensitivity and understanding of the great loss that many women feel when treatment of their cancer results in the loss of their breasts. If a woman seeks breast reconstruction, his support helps to enhance this experience and contributes to her rehabilitation. It is not easy being a man in this situation. If he encourages her too much, she might feel that he is unhappy with her appearance and does not love her for herself. If he is negative, she might feel misunderstood and unhappy because he doesn't realize how important this surgery is to her. Finding a middle ground and playing the role of supporting player may be the best position he can take; a man needs to listen to a woman's concerns, communicate with her, and try to understand her desires. His attitude and assistance can have a beneficial effect and can contribute to a woman's return to good feelings about herself, about him, and about the future.

THE MAN'S ROLE: TWO STORIES

The following two interviews further investigate the man's role in the breast cancer experience. George Johnson and Bill Jones describe their concerns about cancer and mastectomy, their apprehensions about reconstructive breast surgery, and their suggestions for other men experiencing similar situations.

George Johnson

Jenny's lump was discovered 1½ years ago during her regular checkup. Her mammogram revealed a possible mass within her breast that had not shown up on her physical examination. She had three other biopsies before, but they had always been benign. When she entered the hospital, the doctor told us that this lump might be cancerous and a decision needed to be made about therapy: whether to go ahead and have a frozen-section biopsy and do a mastectomy right away or come back later for treatment. Her physician also informed her of other treatment options, including breast reconstruction.

When cancer was diagnosed, it was her decision to have the mastectomy immediately. I had mixed feelings about having it done right then, but I wanted her to do what was really best for her. She seemed determined to get it over with, so the surgeon went ahead and removed her breast at that time.

After surgery the doctor reassured us that the cancer had been caught early, before it had spread, and Jenny would not have any more problems. Knowing that she didn't need chemotherapy was a relief, but we were still anxious because her sister had recently died from cancer. Her death created more concern on both our parts. Now, when Jenny has any kind of problem, no matter how minor, cancer is the first thought that comes to mind because it is apparently in the family and has been present all along.

I tried to be supportive after the mastectomy. I must admit that I was distressed by seeing her body with only one breast on one side and a huge scar on the other side. She takes such pride in her appearance that I hated for her to have this done to her. It was painful for me to look at her and know that she was unhappy. The mastectomy had little effect on our relationship. Initially, maybe, there was some constraint there, particularly in lovemaking, but it was quickly overcome. There really was no problem.

When a couple confronts this type of trying situation, it's important for them to have a deep love for each other, and obviously, after 35 years of marriage, Jenny and I have this feeling. Coping with breast cancer and a mastectomy might be more difficult for a couple who has only been married for a few years because they wouldn't be sure of each other and would be uncertain about what the future would hold for them. I would also think that cancer and mastectomy would be more traumatic for a younger individual because of the sexual implications. If people love each other, however, no matter what their ages or the length of their relationship, they will talk about their problems and try to help each other. If a man leaves a woman over a mastectomy, there wasn't much love there in the first place.

My wife was not happy with her appearance after her mastectomy. She felt that she did not look right in clothes, even though with a prosthesis an observer cannot tell the difference. But I could tell she felt uncomfortable. When she put on a bathing suit, she would stretch and pull it to make it cover more of her body. Just by looking at her expression I could see how displeased she was because she felt her deformity was noticeable. I tried to reassure her that she looked just as good as she always did, which she did. I felt she looked fine in her clothes, but I don't think she really believed me. Her prosthesis was also uncomfortable and she complained about it. The inconvenience of the prosthesis probably speeded up her decision to have reconstruction. Emotionally, I could tell that she just didn't feel right. She was not satisfied with the way she looked.

I believe that my wife had already made up her mind to have breast reconstruction even before she had her mastectomy. Almost immediately after she came home from the hospital she started talking about reconstruction and reading about it. We really hadn't discussed this topic before. To get more information Jenny and I talked with a physician friend of ours who lived in Virginia. At that time he did not recommend more surgery. He was not really sold on breast reconstruction, and he did not suggest that she have it done. But I could tell before the end of our conversation with him that Jenny really wanted this surgery.

I had mixed feelings about breast reconstruction, but I did not make any suggestions one way or the other. My feelings were somewhat negative because I worried that she wanted this done for my benefit. I also didn't want her to undergo any more surgery with its pain and discomfort. I felt that she had suffered enough. I gradually changed my mind as she helped me to realize that she actually was enthusiastic about this operation and she wanted it for herself and not for me. After I understood her determination to have breast reconstruction, I got on her side 100%.

If a man feels that reconstruction will make his wife or friend feel happier or as if she were more of a woman, then he should encourage her, be supportive, and go along with her wishes. That's really all he can do because she will have to make the decision herself, if this is what she wants done. He needs to talk to her about her needs and really listen to what she has to say. If anything, reconstruction might enhance their relationship. If a husband is totally against reconstruction and discourages his wife from having it done, their relationship might suffer. Once he sees that she is determined to proceed with this operation and that it will make her happy, he should encourage and help her.

In order to learn more about reconstruction, Jenny secured a number of pamphlets, and we read them together to understand the nature of the surgery and the various types of reconstructive procedures. Some of this material was really graphic and showed exactly what the plastic surgeon would be doing and how the new breast would look. It's important for a man and woman to get literature before reconstruction and decide what will be done. They also need to consult with a surgeon together and determine what procedures will be used and what the expected recovery period and restriction on activity will be.

After much research, Jenny got our friend in Virginia to check with a well-known surgeon who could suggest a plastic surgeon for breast reconstruction. We also got a local recommendation for a plastic surgeon. Both doctors recommended the same plastic surgeon, so we felt very comfortable because his name had come up twice. This vote of confidence was particularly reassuring for Jenny. She made the decision to have reconstruction and set up an appointment for us to go interview this plastic surgeon.

Needless to say, we were very impressed with him. He seemed concerned for her and interested in doing what she wanted. His first question to us when we came in for the visit was, "Well, what do you want to talk about?" This is really how the conversation started. We discussed our interview at great length, later, and I don't think we could have been more pleased with him. He is a gentle person and did not try to push us in any way. After meeting with him, Jenny went ahead and made the necessary arrangements to have the plastic surgery done.

Her breast was reconstructed with a flap of tissue from her back. It was called a latissimus dorsi flap reconstruction. She also had surgery on her other breast. My wife is at high risk for developing another breast cancer. Over the years she has had breast biopsies for lumps in both of her breasts and these biopsies have been very anxiety provoking for us. Our plastic surgeon knew of Jenny's cancer status and suggested that when he reconstructed her left breast he also remove the mass of tissue inside her right breast and replace it with an implant. He felt that this operation might prevent the recurrence of cancer. Jenny decided to have this preventive surgery to help alleviate some of her preoccupation with cancer.

Jenny also had a nipple-areola created as a second procedure. She wanted her breast to be complete. Knowing my wife, I don't think that she would have been satisfied without going the full way and having a nipple put on. She has been delighted with it and so have I.

After reconstruction her recovery was rapid, with no complications. Initially, she could not drive for 2 weeks, but the inconvenience to me was minimal. There were times when I had to chauffeur her somewhere, and I assumed responsibility for certain chores around the house that she could not do physically, but none of this was a problem. A man should plan on offering some extra help during this time.

Jenny's physical condition contributed to her speedy recovery as much as anything. She is conscientious about taking care of herself and has always been in very good shape. She was this way before any problems developed and is even more so now that she has had reconstructive surgery. I think she looks great. Until she healed completely, she was limited initially in what she could do with her arms. Now she is fully recovered and participates in aerobic exercises twice a week. She was never confined much. I think she was determined to recover quickly because she knew that I did not originally want her to have this surgery, and she was trying to prove something to me.

Breast reconstruction has totally changed Jenny's attitude about herself and her appearance. It makes me feel good to see how pleased she is with herself. For all practical purposes, she is just like she always was before she started having trouble. She is active now with the American Cancer Society as a Reach to Recovery volunteer. She visits and counsels other women about her experiences. She is grateful because her surgery was so successful, and she wants to reassure women who have had mastectomies or who are considering reconstruction that everything will turn out okay.

Her friends around her age and even younger are all interested in her reconstruction. During our vacation with some other couples the girls got together and they had show and tell. They wanted to see her breast, even though none of them have had breast cancer. One of our friends who lives in Nebraska and might need to have a mastectomy is very interested in Jenny's experiences. Our friends can hardly believe that she went through what she did, because she looks so good. They are impressed with the results, with her great attitude, and, I daresay, that anyone who does not know that she had the surgery *would not know*. There is no way.

I give my wife credit. She changed my attitude about reconstruction. I really think it's something special now.

There is one final point I didn't touch on that might be interesting for people to know, and it has to do with a person's age and what makes you "too old." When Jenny wanted to have this surgery, nobody discouraged her necessarily, but I think there was some feeling, "Why go through with this at your age?" She was 54 years old, and they felt that if she were younger, say in her twenties or thirties, that this would be fine, but at her age, why bother? But that is not so. She is still just as much of a woman as she was when she was 20, and I hope women considering reconstruction will keep this in mind. If you are over 50, so what! Forget about your age; it really doesn't matter. Do it for yourself if it makes you feel good. My wife did and it has done wonders for her and for us.

Bill Jones

Diane and I were on a trip when she mentioned that something was going wrong with her breast; her nipple was receding. As soon as we got back, she called the doctor, who told her to come in immediately for a mammogram. That is how he detected her cancer. He didn't inform her about her disease while she was still in his office. Instead, he waited until she was home and then he called. I answered the phone, but the doctor asked for Diane and he just told her: "Diane, you have cancer. You had better see a surgeon." He was so rude. He just said it over the telephone; at that time I wanted to kill him.

When Diane developed cancer, we regarded it as our cancer; it was a family problem. We were shocked and didn't know what to do or where to go. The haste in which we had to act was traumatic, not only for me, but for her. We needed to find a surgeon and then endure the ordeal of another examination and confirmation that it truly was cancer.

We didn't know that there were any alternatives other than a mastectomy; nobody informed us about other treatments. We went from the gynecologist to the surgeon and that was it: no options, just surgery. Like sheep, we followed.

Diane did not want to have an operation; she did not want to lose her breast. She was really tearful before we went to the hospital for surgery. It was very difficult for me because I don't like to see my wife cry. She did not want to go to the hospital, and we didn't get there until 8 P.M., when we were supposed to be there at 4 P.M. We put it off as long as possible. She had a mastectomy 1 week after discovering that she had breast cancer.

During the operation the surgeon first biopsied the lesion to determine if it were malignant. When the results came back positive, he apologized and said he would have to remove her breast. He did a mastectomy and removed her breast and the lymph nodes in her armpit area. After the operation, Diane had a difficult time coming back from the anesthesia; we almost lost her. She did not want to live and would not come to. She went to surgery at 6 A.M., but she didn't get back to the room until 6 P.M.

When Diane finally got back to the hospital room, she wouldn't look at me or speak to me. Then we learned that her cancer had spread and she would require chemotherapy. That was another blow to us. At that time Diane was training to be an elder in the church, and the first thing she said was, "I will not be an elder. I will not go through all of that. I cannot stand it now with this operation and the chemotherapy." The only demand I made of her at this time was that she continue with her efforts to become an elder. I wanted her to have a goal to work toward and not to give up hope. Our minister came to visit and was very supportive; he said, "I'll teach you a minute a day, *but you will be an elder.*" His efforts and my insistence represented hope and support from me and from the clergy. I kept telling her, "Don't get mad at God because he did not have anything to do with this." I was trying to fight these feelings myself, and I kept telling her that cancer was just one of those things that we could not do anything about, other than what we were told to do by professionals.

The American Cancer Society had as much to do with getting Diane out of the hospital after her mastectomy as anything else. They sent a volunteer to visit her when she was in the hospital. I still become tearful when I realize that this big organization would take the time and effort to send a volunteer, a woman who had a mastectomy, to visit us just to make us feel better and to demonstrate that people cared about us. They let us know that if we needed help, we could make a phone call and it was available. I think that initial visit got Diane interested in support groups. At first, she wasn't happy because this lady from the American Cancer Society was coming. Diane kept saying, "I don't want to see her. She's just going to tell me that I am going to die in 2 years, and personally I don't want to hear it." Miss Saunders, however, was well trained and she really helped. She was not at all what Diane had expected. By the time she had left she had raised Diane's spirits so much that my wife was like a different person when I reentered the room. As Diane put it, "Miss Saunders has been through as much as I have. That means a lot to me, knowing that someone else has had similar experiences. She had cancer 3 years ago and just look at her; you would never know it!"

Diane had to undergo chemotherapy, and she resisted it. Every week she would say, "I'm not going to take it anymore." One of the reasons I went with her each time was to make sure that she went. I also had to watch her at home because she needed to take pills, and I worried that she would flush them; I didn't want that to happen. She had a terrible time with chemotherapy; she was nauseous all of the time. She wanted something to help her with the nausea, and we even considered getting some marijuana through the hospital. But I really didn't want her to take any more drugs, and our oncologist gave her medicine that helped her control the tension in her stomach so that she could continue to eat.

While she was on chemotherapy we started noting questions to ask the oncologist during our visits. Diane would ask, "Am I supposed to feel that way? Am I supposed to feel dizzy? Is it strange that I wake up in the middle of the night with nightmares?" We questioned everything that was happening to Diane and asked the doctor to provide us with answers. Then Diane developed arthritic pain, and even though she exercised her left arm, it became almost frozen on her. The oncologist had to refer us to a physical therapist to help her with exercises. Some of the oncology medicine was also beneficial in relieving her arthritic pain. All of her problems seemed to manifest themselves at the same time.

Then came the hair. It was not bad enough to have a sore arm and a breast removed, now her hair fell out. Fortunately, she had wigs that she had used before, and she started wearing them; they helped a great deal. She also got a good prosthesis, which made her feel a little bit more together.

After her operation, Diane did not want anybody to see her. When we were in public, she imagined that everyone was looking at her and that they knew she had a breast removed. She was fearful that I hadn't seen the scar, even though I had looked at it every day. In fact, I insisted on seeing her scar right after her operation. I even helped massage it with vitamin E formula that one of the surgeons had recommended. She would tell me, "You don't even want to look at me." That was difficult for me to handle. I had seen her and I did touch her and look at her; I just tried not to make a big deal of it because I knew how she felt. We finally worked through those feelings to what I thought was a better situation. But apparently, as I would discover later when we discussed breast reconstruction, these worries were still in the back of her mind and she feared that I hadn't accepted her mastectomy.

Our sex life was very bad. Diane was really turned off and the chemotherapy drugs didn't help. The seriousness of the situation relieved me from worrying about sex. Sex was painful for Diane, and even though she wanted to participate, she was remorseful and unhappy when we were intimate. I think we came through that experience all right, without any scars or mental damage, because we did not make an issue of it.

I never made an invalid out of Diane; that would have depressed her more. I tried to be supportive, but I still insisted that she do things on her own. I wanted her to return to normal as soon as possible; that was probably the most supportive thing I could do. If a man wants to help a woman in this situation, he needs to return to their life-style before the mastectomy. He should remember what he did before the woman got sick, whether it is a slap on the fanny or whatever, and continue those activities. If you socialize, get out there as quickly as you can; get back into the bridge club, back on the golf course, go to church, whatever is your normal style. Let people know. That is what we did. We did not have a closed door in our home.

Our church is our life and it's our social life as well. Consequently, there were many people wanting to know what they could do, how to help. I decided that I would monitor all of this activity. If Diane wanted to talk, then it was fine, and I would tell people. If she didn't want to talk, that was all right also, and I warned them that Diane would explain to them exactly how she felt. That is one way I supported my wife. I told her, "It is okay if you don't want to talk about your cancer all the time. Every conversation cannot be about cancer, and you don't want to tell it over and over again." Anyway, I put the word out so Diane did not feel guilty telling people, "I'm sorry, but I really don't feel like talking about it today." There were no hard feelings and they just talked about something else. A husband has to control that. He can handle phone calls; sometimes a woman is upset and doesn't even want to talk to her husband, let alone somebody else who is saying, "Why you poor thing" or "God bless you." She doesn't need that additional emotional stress, and it helps to remove any unnecessary conversation.

If there are children involved, they should know what is happening. I have seen situations where children can't accept their mother's cancer. They don't even want to talk about it, because the father did not say "Hey, we have a family problem, and we need to discuss it." This sharing is needed before a woman has surgery. The whole story has to be told: "Your mom is going to come home; she is going in the hospital to have an operation to save her life." Let the kids feel a part of it, and then they will be more supportive. They have a right to be included. Then they can tell people at school and confide in their friends and they don't have to hear it from others. The involvement of the entire family, in-laws, children, husband, sisters, is all important. Everyone needs to be informed and be told about the prognosis. Once they know the facts, the mystique disappears and they can handle the problems better. You can't cope with something that you don't know anything about.

After 3 months of chemotherapy, Diane told me that she wanted to join a self-help group. I was really surprised, and I told her that I didn't think we needed any group. But she said, "Well, I do. I'm depressed." I thought she was doing okay. Evidently, she covered it very well. I had tried to cheer her up. I like to cook so I tried to please her palate. We tried to make life exactly the way it was before, but my efforts weren't really totally successful. Evidently, she needed something more.

The support group we joined had just started; it was only 3 or 4 months old. When we joined, they needed a secretary and Diane volunteered. Knowing she was having chemotherapy, I worried if she could handle this responsibility, but I let her do it. I figured I could help her if she didn't feel right. It wasn't that hard anyway because I can type, send out postcards, and make phone calls. Her work with the group inspired her and she started thinking about others. That is the benefit of self-help groups. We recover from depression when we begin to think about others. You go there for your own self, but you are aiding others and that in turn brings about help for you. Psychologically, it did wonders for her.

Before Diane developed cancer, we planned a trip to Europe. When her chemotherapy was almost over, we decided (if everything was okay) that we would still go on our vacation. It was a goal we set. If her blood count were normal and she didn't miss her treatments, then we would make the trip. It worked out beautifully. She got through chemotherapy and we were in Europe 2 weeks later. We were scared to death because we didn't know if she would be strong enough. We were in a tour group of 40 people, and they were going to castles and mausoleums and everywhere; I just called time out when I felt it was necessary and we would sit down. Some days we would stay in the hotel and be on our own for the day. She accepted that very well. It was a

15-day trip and it was a part of her rehabilitation, a reward for all of the problems of losing her hair. Her hair was beginning to come back then, and she felt better the second it started to appear. She didn't lose it all, but she lost enough to make her feel very badly.

By the time we returned from our trip, Diane was talking about breast reconstruction. I told her that it was not necessary for me; I was still fearful because of her last operation. I did not want her to go through major surgery. She'd already had two major operations (an earlier hysterectomy) and I did not want her to have to go under anesthesia again. She kept talking about it though, and then one day she said, "I have made an appointment with a plastic surgeon who is going to reconstruct my breast." When I asked Diane what her general surgeon thought about reconstruction, she told me that he advised her to wait another year because he was worried that we could cover up a recurrence. I decided to ask Diane's oncologist (a woman) for her opinion. I asked her publicly during our self-help group meeting. "Dr. Worth, why does Diane have to feel that she needs reconstruction? Isn't it dangerous?" The doctor's answer really startled me. She said, "I'll tell you, Bill. Let her have the operation; it's her body." Afterward I started thinking about what Dr. Worth said, and I realized that she gave me a pretty darn good answer. If Diane felt that she needed reconstruction to feel whole, by golly, she should have it. It was not my decision to make. Why should I tell her to feel badly for the rest of her life? It wouldn't make her live any longer anyway. With the help of breast reconstruction, maybe she could live happier. So the die was cast at that meeting.

Next, Diane and I went to see a plastic surgeon. We interviewed him, and he told us what he was going to do. Frankly, we fell in love with him. Plastic surgeons are different from other surgeons; they are building something, not taking it away. It must be harder for other surgeons to have a relationship with their patients. It must be horrible for these doctors to remove a breast, and I guess they protect themselves from getting too close to this hurt. A plastic surgeon puts you back to your normal self again, or as close to that as he can. So it is a happy event, and he wants to build you up and help you emotionally.

I have never seen my wife so excited about the thought of surgery. Just being whole again was all she talked about. Because of her attitude, I became increasingly enthusiastic about her breast reconstruction. Her actual operation went very smoothly. She recovered quickly and in 6 months her scars had started to fade.

Diane needed reconstruction for her final rehabilitation. She has been a happier person since she had her breast restored. The sad times that we had before are gone. She likes to wear a sundress now and work in the garden. She doesn't have to feel awkward anymore or worry that people are staring at her. The first thing she said after her reconstructive surgery was, "Now I can dress and put on my face like I used to without being upset when I look in the mirror. Before, when I saw myself, I thought, 'I look like a little boy.'" To me she always looked beautiful.

Our sex life has also improved; everything is easier and more relaxed. She is back to normal, and she says that she feels whole again. We have a full life again, and we have gone back to doing everything that we did before. I didn't realize that we had stopped doing things, but apparently she had put restrictions on herself. With breast reconstruction, she is her old self again, filled with enthusiasm. Her zest for life has returned. Reconstruction was the icing on the cake for Diane. It put back what surgery took away and completed her rehabilitation.

Diane was 53 when she decided to have her breast reconstructed. Her age had nothing to do with her decision. Women who are 60 and 70 years old are having it done, and their enthusiasm is great. Some of these women never even considered reconstruction for 15 years and then they say, "You mean I can have my breast reconstructed now, after all this time? I just may do that. I have often thought about it." It's amazing, but their mastectomy deformities still bother them. They are not rehabilitated. Age is not important, and a woman should consider breast reconstruction if it makes her feel better.

Reconstruction has allowed Diane to forget her cancer and focus on other aspects of her life. The cancer experience has produced a great desire in her to help others. Now she is spending 30 to 40 hours a week in volunteer work and I have become involved with it also.

We have formed a self-help group for mastectomy patients; it meets in our home and boyfriends or husbands are invited to come. Many times I'll take the men in the yard and we will talk. One man that I talked to was having trouble because of his wife's anger. He didn't know how to talk to her. Everything he said seemed to make her angry or volatile. We discussed it. It was beneficial for him just to unburden himself. Men need to talk; they also need to express their feelings. I told him that it was all right for his wife to cry; it was all right for her to be angry. She needs time to work through her emotions.

I reminded him that if he and his wife had a normal relationship, she had probably fretted with him before. Yes, as he thought about it, she had been a bit that way all of her life. Once he thought through it, he felt better and it eased the situation for him. Many of the boyfriends who come seem to be well adjusted and just want to support their girlfriends. I think that kind of support is really beautiful.

When our self-help group meets each time, we sit in a circle and each person tells why he or she is there: to provide support or to fill a need. Then we get involved in conversation. Someone will say, "I have a problem: I'm gaining too much weight" or "What can I do about nausea?" The conversation gets pretty personal. Soon, if anyone has any inhibitions, they are forgotten. By the time a lady tells you that her breast was cut off, it's pretty easy to talk about your feelings.

It seems to me that in many of these groups, half of the ladies are divorced. Sometimes it's during the divorce process that they develop cancer. I've often wondered if the stress produced from the divorce contributes to the cancer showing up at that crucial time. I do know that cancer strengthens a marriage or breaks it apart. Some men just can't handle cancer and they move on, even if there are children involved. They aren't very supportive.

Cancer produces some terrible strains on individuals and on relationships. Divorces sometimes occur because neither the man nor the woman can handle the word "cancer" and the man runs because he doesn't know what to do about it; he might even think he is going to catch it. That type of ignorance is still out there. Some men also don't like the deformity. To them the exterior, the physical, is so important.

People need to be informed about cancer and the importance of self-help groups. Women with breast cancer need the camaraderie of other people experiencing similar problems. That is how you build bridges. You may come to a meeting and find some other person who lives close to you, and you develop a friendship. You can have lunch together and then you have a buddy to depend on. This person can help you get back into the mainstream and can contribute to your rehabilitation.

Through our experiences, Diane and I have come to appreciate the importance of learning about your options. Today, mastectomy is not considered the only treatment for breast cancer; lumpectomy and irradiation is also an option, and chemotherapy is given for shorter periods. There are many positive choices possible for ladies; breast reconstruction is one of them. It is important to remember, however, that even though the choices exist, women are not always aware of them. They need to know the possibility of recurrence and the chances for survival. They should understand the different options for treatment and rehabilitation and know which treatments promise the best chances for survival for each individual patient.

Maybe, when cancer is discovered, a doctor could tell his patients about support groups. Tell them about the American Cancer Society and Reach to Recovery. Let women know what is available. Most women don't realize the type of assistance that the American Cancer Society provides; there are people available who will drive them to chemotherapy and help them get their medication. Women need to know that there are organizations that will stand behind them. This information needs to come from the professionals, and doctors need to acquaint themselves with what is available in the community for their patients. Once a woman is out of the hospital, she is on her own, and she needs some assistance. If doctors want to be helpful, they should encourage their patients to seek help from others. The patient needs to say to the doctor, "Well, Doctor, now that I am through with surgery, what should I do?" Then it is the obligation of the doctor to be able to tell her.

HOW COUPLES RELATE

The final interview in this chapter is with a young, unmarried couple: Scott Meyers and Sheila Andrews. Together, they relive their experiences from the diagnosis of Sheila's cancer, through her mastectomy and chemotherapy, to her present decision to have her breast reconstructed. Discussing the problems that a couple faces when the woman develops breast cancer, they offer insight into the various methods they have used to help them cope with this disease and the trauma associated with it.

Sheila Andrews and Scott Meyers

Sheila: It all started when I went to my gynecologist for what I thought was a cyst, nothing big. When he checked me and said, "I want you to see someone else," the alarm went off. He assured me that it was nothing to worry about, but when I wanted to wait a month to make the appointment, he wouldn't let me; he insisted I go the next week. I went to see the surgeon that he recommended; he did a needle biopsy and said he would call me in a few days with the results. When I didn't hear from him, I called his office because I was getting anxious. It was the day of our Thanksgiving dinner at work. I asked the nurse for the results, and she gave the phone to the doctor who asked me to come in to talk to him. I said, "No, that is worse than you telling me right now, over the telephone. Tell me now, and then I will come in later today and we can talk." He told me that the lump was malignant. My head was spinning from the news; I felt as if I were in another world. I was just 30, recently divorced with a teenage daughter, and I had no idea that it would be cancer. There was no breast cancer in my family. I was trying to get myself together, so I went into a private office to cry. I was hysterical . . . and then I thought about Scott.

Scott and I had only been going together for 3 months, and we were very new into our relationship. All of a sudden, I was finding out that I had cancer and not only did I have to cope with that, I had to deal with trying to tell someone who I had only known for a short while. I called him on the phone and told him.

Scott: After I got off the phone from talking with Sheila, I fell apart. When I managed to pull myself together, I picked Sheila up from work and we went for a drive. Cancer was something that I had never dealt with or been exposed to before. I'd never known anyone that had it; it was all new to me. I was scared for her, not knowing what she was going to have to experience. Ours was a new relationship at the time and I didn't know how this was going to affect it and really how I felt about it. I don't know that Sheila knew either. Neither one of us was aware of what was going to happen in the next few months, or even the next year. It was a matter of waiting, talking to doctors, and slowly finding out.

Sheila: When I went to see the doctor, he told me that he was going to put me in the hospital and schedule surgery. Before doing the mastectomy, he would do another biopsy while I was under anesthesia. He had all the consent forms ready for me to sign, because he felt that it was better for me to sign the papers ahead of time so he would not have to wake me to confirm that I had cancer. I signed the papers and went in blindly. I just said, "Yes, yes, yes." I did not know anything.

After I knew that I had to have a mastectomy, Scott and I were just wasted. Saturday night, before I was to go into the hospital, we went through several bottles of champagne, drowning our sorrows. We decided to have a going-away party for my breast. We put on music, got loud and crazy, and poured a bottle of champagne over my breast. Scott kissed it goodbye. It was a wild thing to do, but it made us feel better. Now that I am thinking about reconstruction, I guess we will probably have to christen the new one, too, when I get it. It will be like having a new boat, only I'll be getting a new breast.

    That night we just lay in each other's arms and cried half the night. We hardly said anything. We just got everything out, all the tears that might have been held back. We cried and cried and cried.

Scott: It is essential to be open with each other. You just can't keep your feelings hidden. From a man's perspective, you need to express yourself. You can't be afraid to cry. If you can't cry about this, what can you cry about?

Sheila: I was terrified before surgery. I broke out in hives and went white. I had never had an operation in my life. The only time I was in the hospital was when I had a baby, 13 years earlier. I never had a sick day. This was the first time I had been sick, and that really threw me. It had been such a little problem.

    I went to the hospital a week later and when I woke up I did not have a breast. It was that fast. They did a modified radical mastectomy, and I didn't even know what a modified radical was. At that time I didn't know anything. The only thing I knew was what I was told; I put my entire life in the hands of a doctor that I had never met before, and I said, "Just do what you have to do."

Scott: I don't think I thought so much about the mastectomy or her losing a part of her body. I just wanted to see her recover her health. My main concern was her survival.

Sheila: After surgery the doctor told me that my cancer had spread; I had three positive lymph nodes. I was in stage II of my breast cancer, which I didn't understand. Then he started talking about chemotherapy, and that was another whole trip. Everything you hear about chemotherapy is devastating, and all of a sudden, the focus wasn't on losing my breast, but it was on chemotherapy. I thought, "God, how am I going to survive this?" Then the oncology nurse talked to me and gave me brochures on chemotherapy. All of this time when I was in the hospital, Scott took care of my daughter and ran my house. He did all of the cleaning.

Scott: I did all of the housework. There were some habits formed there that are very hard to break.

Sheila: I have a high tolerance for pain, probably abnormally high. The evening of my surgery I took no pain killers, and by the time I was released from the hospital, I was reaching over my head. I was determined to block out what had happened to me. "You know," I said, "there is not a damn thing wrong with me. Life will resume as normal." In fact, I ran the vacuum cleaner when I got home, just to prove that nothing was going to stop me. I caught the wrath of God when Scott got home and found that I had vacuumed the bedroom. After that scene, I just gave up vacuuming forevermore.

Scott: That was a good example of her proving to the world that she wasn't sick. I said, "Don't prove it to me, and don't prove it to the world either. You don't need to be vacuuming this house. You don't need to have that attitude." We talked about that for a long time.

I was asking myself many questions during this period, and I was questioning many values. I had to go back and think about the way I regarded Sheila before she developed cancer. I had to determine how I felt and then ask myself why I should feel any different now. I mean, I love this woman, and at the time I decided that I would see her through this experience, just because of my feelings for her; I didn't think they should change because she had this disease. If anything, this experience probably strengthened my feelings for her in helping me give her the support that she needed.

Sheila: He helped me cope with my problems all the way through. The day after surgery, he said, "Okay, let's see what we are dealing with." He just opened my gown and looked down and said, "Uh, huh." I was the one who looked at my scarred chest and passed out. All he did was go, "Uh, huh, okay." He changed my bandages when I got home and rubbed lotion on my scar, even when I couldn't do it. He helped me with my bra, he helped me get dressed, he did everything for me. I was never embarrassed or ashamed in front of him.

Scott: It didn't bother me at all. It was just something she had to go through. I knew she didn't want it; who would? I certainly didn't enjoy it, but we had to live with it. I'm also not a squeamish person. Scars don't really bother me. I wanted to see her scar, not merely from curiosity, but from a real interest in her.

I also knew that she was worried about how I would feel about her body, but it really didn't affect our sex life. We had sex the day after she came home from the hospital. I was worried about hurting her, sure, but it worked out just fine.

Sheila: Even though Scott never made me feel ashamed, I was self-conscious about my body, and I probably still feel some self-consciousness. It's hard, even now, to have a romantic candlelight dinner, put on a beautiful gown, and have one side totally flat. Whether you like it or not, breasts are very, very important in sex and in the way you present yourself. I'm sure they also affect the way he looks at me. He says it doesn't bother him, and it probably bothers me a lot more than it does him. It is tiresome, looking down there and seeing no cleavage.

You have to realize that I had only been with Scott for 3 months when this occurred. There were still many things I didn't know about him. We became very close, immediately, but I still wasn't completely comfortable. Even now, there are times when I am shy about the way I look, and I have a hard time dealing with it. I'll tell him, "Kill the lights; I'm coming to bed." I know that is absurd. You would think that your feelings are somehow attached to your eyesight. But, when you are missing a breast, there is definite comfort in darkness.

When I went back to see my surgeon after I had been released from the hospital, I had many questions for him. I wanted to know about the chemotherapy: Who would administer it and would it be done in his office or in the hospital? He referred me to the university hospital and to a whole new set of specialists. That scared me. I didn't know these people, and I didn't know what to expect from them. He gave me names of the doctors at the hospital and handed me my pathology report in a sealed envelope.

I went home and immediately ripped open the report and read through it. I came to the part that said, "Prognosis: poor" and I went bing! I had no business reading that report. I didn't know what I was reading and I did not know how to interpret it. It scared the hell out of me.

Scott: We both read through the pathology report, but I didn't understand most of it, only words here and there. At the bottom, it read: "Prognosis: condition poor." That, everyone can read; it was black and white and simple language. It was also very difficult to take. We had both just been through her surgery and were trying to remain positive. Then to have something like that come along is demoralizing. It is like having someone tell you that all of your effort is not worth shit; it doesn't matter what you do, because this is the way it is.

Sheila: Six weeks after my surgery I went to the hospital to see the doctors about chemotherapy. They told me that the type of cancer I had was poorly differentiated and had a high recurrence rate.

That was another blow. I went into a rage. I cursed them and screamed, "Bullshit. You are not telling me that I am dying. I am only 30 years old. I have a daughter and my own house. For the first time in my life, after a terrible marriage, I have a man that I really love; I have everything to live for: a new job, a new relationship, a child, everything." I really fought it, and I've continued to fight it. I have bad moods, but I am not going to let it get me.

Scott: I think the chemotherapy was even more of an adjustment for Sheila than the surgery itself. Chemotherapy required a great deal of patience and understanding from me and from everyone around Sheila, especially her daughter. The drugs affected her poorly. She was moody and short-fused. She had a temper and she cried all of the time. She stayed in bed a lot. I could deal with that and her daughter handled it well. Her daughter showed real understanding and patience for her mother and what she was enduring; I think she knew that Sheila was not always going to act that way and there would be an end to it. We were all relieved when the chemotherapy was over. It really pushed everyone to the maximum. I had to keep telling myself that the drugs were making her react the way she was. She said many dumb things during that time. I think her logic and reasoning were not as clear as they normally were, and she was very emotional.

Sheila: You go through so many emotions with cancer, and chemotherapy does trigger those emotions. You are high at one moment and then lower than a snake the next. My moods were up and down. I don't think I was really rational for many of the things that I did or said. I wasn't altogether there and I wasn't in control all of the time. Despite my actions and the way life was treating me, Scott moved in with me during my chemotherapy. I really knew he loved me if he could move in at that time.

Chemotherapy was terrible for me. I had very long, luscious blonde hair, and after the first chemotherapy treatment, it started coming out in handfuls. During the second week I had big clumps of hair falling out of my head. I made an appointment to see wigs, and they matched me with several long, blonde wigs. Soon, I was practically bald. I looked like Bozo the Clown; I had a strip of hair running along the edges of my scalp. I not only lost the hair on my head, but I also lost the rest of my body hair, every bit, from head to toe. I still had a few eyelashes, but my eyebrows were almost nonexistent. I had to wear a lot of makeup to look normal. I also gained 18 pounds on chemotherapy, which I am having a hard time losing. So, besides being bald, not getting into my clothes, and losing a breast, I kept saying, "What is next?" It is a tremendous amount to deal with.

Scott: Hair loss was traumatic for Sheila. She seemed to have an enormous amount to cope with, and it was sometimes hard for me to help her.

Sheila: With a breast, you can camouflage your loss, but with hair loss, what can you do? I mean, I couldn't wear wigs to bed. Talk about romance. He had to look at this woman who had one breast and was bald as a billiard ball. "Oh my God, I looked like I just stepped out of a circus." We can laugh now, but at the time there were many tears. Finally, all this hair was falling out and he made the ultimate decision. He said, "Sheila, you are clogging all of the drains. I have to cut off every bit of your hair because it is falling out, and it is getting all over your clothes. Let's just get it over with once and for all." I said, "Okay," and he got the scissors and just snipped off the rest; that was probably the best thing he ever did. He just got rid of it, and I stopped worrying about it falling out.

Scott: There were times when I needed someone to confide in. I have one or two close friends that I can talk to, but they didn't really understand what was happening.

Sheila: We often talked about our relationship. In fact, there were times when we weren't sure that it would last. It had nothing to do with my cancer; it was just his own feelings. He has other commitments; he goes to school, he works, and he loves to travel. It's hard to commit yourself to a woman who has cancer, who is going through chemotherapy, and who has a 13-year-old daughter and a house. That's a lot to ask of anyone. He had to be absolutely sure how he felt about me before he made any kind of commitment to me.

Scott: I needed to work through my own feelings and think about my life. I thought about how I felt about Sheila before surgery and before she had cancer. I had to decide what I was feeling now. I had to confront myself: "Am I staying with this woman because I pity her or because I love her?" There were times when I really couldn't answer that question. Finally, I decided that if I left I would never know, and if I stayed, I would have to be very careful about why I stayed. I decided that I wanted to stay. I love her and I wanted to give her 100% of my support and love and see her through this experience. If there were anything that I could do to help her, I would do it. That meant taking care of her, her surroundings, and her daughter. It meant providing moral support and letting her know that she was going to get through this okay. I was determined to keep as optimistic an attitude as I could and to show some strength for her.

Sheila: He was always planning for the future. That was important for me because when all of this first happened, I didn't take any interest in the house or even in balancing the checkbook. I owned my own house, and we talked about painting it. But I would say things like, "Why should I paint this damn place if I am going to die? Why should I buy anything?" I didn't want to buy anything: clothes, furniture, paint, anything. Why should I, if I weren't going to be able to enjoy it in 6 months? Toward the end of my chemotherapy, many of these feelings disappeared; we repainted the house, and I started buying clothes again.

Scott: She started living a normal life again. She joined a support group through the American Cancer Society and she started taking dancing lessons. By remembering that there were other things that she needed to do with her life, she began to get out again and not let this hold her back.

Sheila: You can allow yourself to get depressed and let everyone feel sorry for you. It's easy to have a sad face and then people will say, "Oh, I'm so sorry." I didn't want that crap. I just wanted to be happy and to laugh. Scott and I had funny experiences and we tried to keep our sense of humor. Our laughter has helped me survive this experience. When I go to my support group, I tell people about the funny things that happen. Like the time I forgot to put the toilet seat down and my wig fell in. I had to shake it out, wash it, and hang it out in the sun to dry. Then I realized that I couldn't go anywhere because I was bald, my other wig was being fixed, and I only had this one. You must laugh at things like that.

Scott: I wanted to take her to a loud dance studio in town, with her dressed like the lady in "Star Trek." She wouldn't have it.

Sheila: He wanted to dress me in silver tights and makeup. He wanted me to be a Trekkie. He told me it would be the chance of a lifetime.

Actually, we did have fun with it. We went to a Kenny Loggins concert in June and I was still pretty bald at the time. I had ⅛ inch of hair all over my head, so I decided to dress in style. I bought myself a bright lavender headband and put on a black jumpsuit with high heels and makeup. I wore lavender and black jewelry, earrings that were as big as my head, and beads. I didn't wear my wig. We went to the concert and people did double and triple takes. I'm sure they were talking about that bald woman. "A good-looking man like that with a bald woman, yuck!" It was really interesting. The women made derogatory comments about my head, but the men seemed to be complimentary. It was very, very strange. If they had only known why I looked the way I did.

Getting involved with support groups has also helped me to adjust. Women need to know that there are self-help groups available and that we are not alone. The American Cancer Society has a number of these groups going. Reach to Recovery is one and I am now a volunteer. I'm also in another support group that meets once a month and we swap stories about our experiences. It's one of those meetings where you can cry, especially with the women who have just come out of it. We cry, we hold each other, we laugh. You can face a lot of things together.

One of the women in our group just had a recurrence. She had her surgery the same time I did, and she was just getting ready for her yearly checkup when they found an inoperable mass in her chest. She only has 6 months to live. You have to learn that when you are working closely with people, not everyone is going to make it and that's hard to take. I had to come to grips with that reality this month with her.

We share everything in these meetings. We talk about sex and looks and feelings. Many of these women are single and are dating. They ask, "How do you tell a man that you've had this surgery? Maybe you've only gone out with him two or three times, and it gets to a point where you might end up in bed. What do you do then?" That's a problem that you need to broach and you need to know what to do. Even with Scott it was difficult for me because I was still self-conscious.

I learned about breast reconstruction in my support group. One of the women had it done and she told me about her plastic surgeon. I had no idea that there were any alternatives. My surgeon never said anything about reconstruction. After I heard about it though, halfway through my chemotherapy, I started asking doctors at the hospital about breast reconstruction, and they said, "Go for it." They were very supportive. But they also told me that I would have to wait until the chemotherapy was over. Then they said, "Do it. You're young and you want your breast back. It would be a great thing for your mental attitude."

Scott: I really didn't like the idea of her doing it. I'm not comfortable with it. I don't want her going into an operating room again. We have talked about it quite a bit, and I am concerned because I feel that she is doing this entirely for me, and there is no need.

Sheila: Probably he is right to a certain extent. I am doing this partly for him, but it is also for me. I think that if I have breast reconstruction, I'll feel better about myself and the way that I look. After a mastectomy, every time that you look at yourself in the mirror, it's a reminder of cancer. Personally, I don't feel I have cancer anymore; I really don't. It's something I had to deal with at the time, but now it is time to go ahead and get my breast reconstructed and stop worrying about it. I don't want to look down any more and see that there is a breast missing. I miss wearing regular bathing suits and nice lingerie. Actually, the more I think about it, the more I realize that I am doing it for myself. It is to help me forget this disease.

I like to sleep on my stomach, but with a missing breast this position becomes awkward and off balance. I am also uncomfortable with my prosthesis. I'm an accountant, and just moving my arm to the calculator makes the prosthesis rub; it bothers me. The first thing I do when I get home from work is kick off my shoes and throw out my prosthesis.

In my mind, I made a commitment to investigate breast reconstruction the minute I heard that it was a possibility. I decided that I wanted it if I could have it.

I was really scared when I went to see the plastic surgeon. The first time he saw me, he told me to take off my clothes so he could take some photos. He got out his camera and took about 20 pictures of every angle of my breast. He was also taking pictures of my stomach and my hips. Meanwhile, I'm thinking, "Oh my God. Blackmail." I felt like I was posing for *Playboy*. But he needed those pictures to decide what to do, and he said that with the weight I had gained during chemotherapy and after having had a child, he felt an abdominal flap was the best operation for me. You see, I don't have an 18-year-old stomach anymore, and yet my remaining breast has a nice size and shape. If I had this flap surgery, he wouldn't have to touch my opposite breast. He felt he could get the best match for my breast with an abdominal flap reconstruction; and I would be more pleased with it, knowing that I could get rid of my stomach and also get a breast to match my remaining breast.

I had to think a long time about having this operation. Not only am I going in for more surgery, but I am having a major operation; this is the most complicated form of reconstruction. It is a big deal to decide. When you have cancer, you don't have a choice. You go into the hospital, and you get surgery. I'm going into a major operation that is by choice and that is hard. I am saying, "Okay, Doc, I'm going to let you rearrange my entire body and I'm putting it in your hands." If I didn't trust my plastic surgeon, I wouldn't be able to say that. It shows you how much faith I have in him. I am saying, "Do your best. I totally trust you with my life."

Scott: She isn't making this decision based on ignorance, however. Since her mastectomy, we've taken time to learn about reconstruction.

Sheila: Several weeks ago we invited a girl over to our house. She had this same operation by another surgeon, and we wanted to see somebody else's work. She came over 8 weeks after her surgery and she showed Scott and me her breast. She just stripped down and said, "Okay, this is what I look like." It was nice seeing another breast. When you go into this, you have to understand that your body is never going to look exactly the same as it did before. There are going to be some concessions. There are going to be some scars; I will have a scar across my stomach. My main concern is my appearance in clothes; now I will be able to wear a bra and will not have to wear a prosthesis. I will be able to fill something out again.

Scott: I'm still having problems with her having more surgery. It's another operation and it worries me. But if it's going to help her psychologically and improve her self-image, then I want her to have it. It has to be important to her.

Sheila: I am looking forward to breast reconstruction. I am not interested in having a nipple-areola put on right now; it's not a priority for me. I've heard that it is an uncomfortable procedure, and I told my plastic surgeon that I will wait until he perfects things a little better. I can always go in later and have it put on. I'm not in a hurry. No one would really see the nipple, except Scott. If I feel deprived, I can probably just cut out brown construction paper and stick it on.

I want to be able to wear a normal bathing suit this summer. In fact, the night before my surgery I'm meeting my plastic surgeon at the hospital with my bathing suit. It has a French cut to the legs, and instead of a straight line cut across my abdomen, he is going to give me a "happy face" scar so that I can still wear this suit. I'm going to try on my suit for him so he can plan my scars to fall in the right area. Women don't understand that the scar doesn't have to extend straight from hip to hip; it can be curved up. It's nice to know that even these details can be individualized.

Women need to know about breast reconstruction and about the different options for cancer treatment. They need this information before it happens to them. Every woman should be informed about breast cancer. She should know about mastectomies and reconstruction before she has to worry about them. I went into this experience so ignorant. I just said, "Do what you want." I didn't know anything. I didn't know that there were alternatives; I didn't know that there was breast reconstruction. I think if women knew about reconstruction and knew the results, they might not be so hesitant to go in if they felt a lump. I really think that detection is the key, and knowledge about alternatives and treatment will encourage women to report problems as soon as they discover them.

Scott: I agree with Sheila 100%. I think women should be educated. They should know their options, and they should get involved in them. Once you've experienced what we have experienced, you learn to be happy and to make the most of life. You learn that one of the most effective ways of coping with a situation like this is by remaining positive.

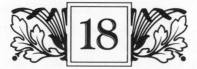

THIRTEEN WOMEN TELL
THEIR STORIES

Women are the inspiration behind this book; their voices permeate our writing. Many of these women have been transformed by the specter of breast cancer and have shared their thoughts and feelings to help make this book a reality. Their input has been invaluable and their sensitivity and generosity are reflected in the stories they have to tell. Following are 13 stories of women who had mastectomies for breast cancer and sought breast reconstruction. These 13 new interviews replace the original eight published in the first edition of this book. As difficult as it was to leave those eight stories behind, it was also a necessity. Procedures for breast reconstruction have improved over the past 10 years, and we wanted our readers to benefit from others' experiences with the latest technical advances. Although the narrators of these stories may have changed, we have tried to retain the spirit behind the interviews and capture the courage and honesty typical of all of these women. Interestingly, as we compare the original interviews with the more recent ones, many of the same phrases, comments, fears, and emotions are echoed. The operative details may differ, but the concerns remain surprisingly constant. Most striking is the similarity of responses given to questions probing women's reactions to breast cancer, motivations for seeking breast reconstruction, and satisfaction with this operation. We have also been impressed that over the years women have become better informed about breast cancer and its treatment, and increasingly they have become their own health advocates. As in the previous edition, we have altered names and personal details to protect the privacy of these women.

From the many taped interviews, we have purposely selected those women who underwent different reconstructive procedures, some immediately after mastectomy and others delayed until various times after surgery, to give you some idea of the reconstructive possibilities available and the potential benefits and problems. These women range in age from 29 to 60 years and represent diverse social, cultural, professional, and family backgrounds. We have included single women, widowed and divorced women, and married women with and without children. The questions asked each woman were varied in the interest of providing a wider coverage of topics. Thus one interview focuses on the issue of self-image for the woman seeking breast restoration; another examines the problem of explaining breast cancer to children, and still another explores the predicaments that a single woman with a mastectomy faces when dating. Certain subjects, however, are dealt with in each dialogue, including reasons for deciding on breast reconstruction, timing of reconstructive surgery, pain and recuperation after reconstruction, physical and psychological results of reconstructive surgery, and benefits and limitations of reconstructive surgery. An attempt has been made to present an honest, balanced discussion of this option so that women contemplating breast reconstruction will have a realistic understanding of what this surgery offers. The implant controversy has complicated the decisions a woman must make. The intense publicity surrounding the FDA investigation left women with lingering questions about these devices. We wanted to determine their level of concern and how it affected their choices. Thus specific questions were directed to women who chose implant surgery about their satisfaction with this reconstructive approach, any problems they had experienced, and fears generated. Because the female half of this writing team did the firsthand interviewing to facilitate a free and candid discussion, these stories and the questions and observations are presented in the first person.

We begin with Sandra whose medical background and profession gave her an unusual insight into the life-threatening disease that abruptly altered her life and reshaped her perspective.

SANDRA: YOU JUST NEVER THINK IT IS GOING TO BE YOU

"I was standing in the room undressed from the waist up. The technologist came in with my film, and I held it up to the light. I took one look at it, and I saw the breast cancer. I just stood there, and I thought to myself, I have breast cancer. I cannot believe this; I never thought it would happen to me. I have breast cancer. I was almost paralyzed, and I said to her, 'I have breast cancer!' She said, 'You can't know that.' But I knew.

"I got dressed quickly, ran to my office to get my old films, and banged on Jill's door. She is the other mammographer I work with. I banged on her door and I said, 'Jill, get over to the breast center. I have breast cancer!' I ran back over to the center and then I just collapsed and cried while she looked at the films. I kept thinking to myself, and saying over and over again, 'You just never think it is going to be you.' "

Interviewing Sandra is an electrifying experience; she is animated and intense, and I sense that she has already anticipated my questions and formulated answers long before I pose them. At 40 Sandra is a slender, energetic brunette whose straight shiny hair bounces as she talks. She has a busy career, a happy marriage, and three young children. As a radiologist at one of the country's leading medical centers, Sandra spends her working days interpreting breast x-ray films for other women. She is more knowledgeable about breast cancer than most women and has ready access to some of the leading specialists in this field.

As she speaks of that day 2 years ago when she diagnosed her own breast cancer, she is still overwhelmed by a sense of disbelief. A biopsy several days later confirmed her diagnosis. Drawing on her knowledge of breast cancer, she carefully planned her own therapy, choosing to have bilateral mastectomies: a modified radical mastectomy to treat the cancer in her left breast and a prophylactic mastectomy on her right breast. Although cancer had not yet been detected in her right breast, she knew that her odds of developing a new cancer in her opposite breast were good, and she preferred to have both breasts removed rather than live with the fear of a more serious cancer. She also knew about breast reconstruction and felt that her chances for breast symmetry would be improved if both breasts were reconstructed simultaneously. Because her cancer was localized, she did not have chemotherapy.

Six months after her cancer surgery Sandra had bilateral breast reconstruction. Her decisions about breast reconstruction were made with the same care and intelligence that she had applied to her cancer therapy. She interviewed four different plastic surgeons and explored the surgical options for breast restoration. She chose the plastic surgeon and the reconstructive approach that would achieve her personal goals. Although she originally considered a TRAM flap, a major reconstructive procedure, she eventually selected a much simpler technique, intraoperative expansion with implant placement. This approach required less recovery time, promised good results, and allowed her to get back to living a normal life in the shortest period of time. Her story is a compelling one.

Did the fact that you were a physician make it easier for you to deal with your breast cancer and your decisions about treatment?

Most women have to go through a learning phase first. They start out knowing nothing about breast cancer and suddenly they are diagnosed with it. They struggle with weighing one expert's opinion and recommendation against another; they don't know what to expect next. I knew all that. I was one step ahead of where other women would be. I was trying to guess the pathology, to see whether I had an invasive cancer. I knew exactly what I wanted to know: the good prognostic signs and the bad prognostic signs. I wanted to move as quickly as possible to find out my prognosis. I wanted to know exactly how far along my cancer was, how big it was, and whether there was invasion so that I could feel comfortable with what I had to face. This waiting period was not easy for me, perhaps because I knew so much. It was one of the most intense experiences that I have ever been through. I was anxious every waking moment; I barely slept until I knew my pathology. At one point I was so tense that I just wanted to cry as loud as I could. But I knew that the kids would hear me and want to know what was wrong. So Bob took them to McDonald's and then I just cried and cried. I felt much better after that. It is amazing how crying can make you feel better. The unknown, the waiting was very tough for me. Once I knew the pathology I was fine and it was not difficult for me to make a decision about therapy.

How did your family react?

I called my husband right away. I said, "Bob, I just had a mammogram and I have breast cancer, but I don't think I am going to die from it." He was totally speechless, then almost hysterical. We didn't tell the children until after the diagnosis was made.

How did you tell your children?

The biopsy report was back on Monday and I was in the hospital having my cancer surgery by Thursday. I didn't waste any time because I knew what I wanted. We told the children on Wednesday night. We sat down in the family room, Bob and myself and these three little boys. They knew this was a big deal because we were having a family conference. Before we said anything, Jonathan, the little one, said, "Okay, who's dying?" Bob and I looked at each other. We thought we had kept a good secret. We tried not to let them know, but they knew anyway; they could sense the tension. We said nobody is dying. Then Bob said that I had a mammogram and Jonathan said, "And you have breast cancer, right?" He knows that mammograms are to find breast cancer. And so we said yes. We told them that there were good kinds of cancer and bad kinds of cancer. Lung cancer, for example, is a bad kind of cancer; breast cancer can be bad or good, but I had a good kind and we expected that I would be cured of it if we took care of it right. I was going to go into the hospital to have surgery to get rid of the cancer. That would be the end of it. They wanted to know if I was going to get new breasts. I said yes, but at a later time.

They wanted reassurance. They wanted to know if I was going to die? How long was I going to be in the hospital? We told them that I would go into the hospital and the doctor would take my breasts off and that would take care of the problem. I also told them that they would have to help out after I came home from the hospital since I wouldn't be feeling well for a while. I would be home for a month and that was good, because I wouldn't be working and they would get to see me a lot. They would have to be very patient and easy on me and soon I would be strong and feeling well again and that would be the end of it.

Why did you choose a mastectomy over a lumpectomy with irradiation?

I was diagnosed with intraductal carcinoma of the comedo type. Because this type of cancer tends to have a higher recurrence rate, it doesn't do as well with lumpectomy and radiation therapy as it does with mastectomy, especially if the margins of the resected tumor are positive. Even before I knew that the margins were positive, I elected to have mastectomy because I didn't want to take a chance or worry about the possibility of local recurrence. My decision was also influenced by the fact that this tumor has an excellent prognosis if the whole thing is removed.

Why did you choose a prophylactic mastectomy to remove the tissue from the normal breast before any diagnosis of cancer?

I know, realistically, that people who have had one breast cancer are at higher risk for developing another breast cancer in the other breast. I wanted to minimize the chance of developing a worse lesion on the other side. This lesion that I had was theoretically curable or highly curable. Why take the risk 5 years from now of developing an invasive cancer in the other breast that might become systemic and threaten my life? That was a compelling reason for me. As it turns out, the prophylactic mastectomy was a smart move. When they removed the opposite breast and biopsied it, it showed atypical hyperplasia, a high-risk lesion. That meant I had quite a significant risk of developing breast cancer on the other side.

The fact that I am a mammographer also factored into my decision. I see women with breast cancer and I see women with second breast cancers all the time. I just couldn't have it on my mind. I wanted to do it and get it over with. I didn't want to wait year after year to see if I was going to get a second breast cancer. I also see many women with breast reconstruction. I know how difficult it is for a plastic surgeon to make the reconstructed breast and the original breast look symmetric. To me it wasn't a big deal to have the other breast removed. I wanted my breasts to match, and I wanted to minimize my chance of having a second breast cancer. So I decided to have both breasts removed and then to let a plastic surgeon reconstruct both at the same time to make them symmetric.

How long did it take you to recover from your mastectomies?

In 4 weeks I was back at work and able to function. I couldn't move my arms very well, but I could drive a car; I certainly could read films. I was glad to be back because I could interact with people. I worked part-time for a few weeks. After 2 months I was back in full swing, although not feeling completely well yet. That took about 3 months.

Did you join any kind of support group?

I didn't really need a support group; I desperately needed people; there's no question about it. I needed the support of people in my daily life. I needed them to visit me, to call me, to be solicitous, to stroke me, and to tell me they were hoping that I recovered. I had lots of support from the people that I work with. They relieved me of any clinical responsibility; I wasn't forced into stressful situations. That's the most people can do for you. It helps enormously to have people tell you that they are thinking about you and wishing for the best.

How did your husband help you cope with this experience? Was he supportive?

He helped me by listening, taking me everywhere I needed to go, and not making any demands on me. He totally relieved me of responsibility for the kids. He interfaced with them because he knew that it would be difficult for me and they would sense my anxiety. As it turns out, they sensed it anyway. He did whatever he could for me. After all, there wasn't anything much he could do.

Why did you decide to have your breasts reconstructed?

I had my breasts reconstructed for convenience, for my own self-esteem, and to look good again in clothes, whether or not I looked perfect in the nude. I wasn't after the perfect cosmetic result. I was annoyed with wearing prostheses. It is difficult to get comfortable prostheses, especially after a bilateral mastectomy. I got the smallest size that I could find, so they were as light as possible. Despite my efforts, they were hot and heavy and they didn't feel natural. If I wanted to go on a trip, I had to worry about how I was going to pack all this stuff; it was not convenient at all. I bought bilateral prostheses that cost over $600 ($300 apiece, plus the price of the bras, a swimsuit, etc.), and I wore them five times in 6 months. A friend of mine said, "Sandra, if you're so uncomfortable in those prostheses, don't wear them. Everybody that knows you, knows that you don't have any breasts, and we don't care. The people that don't know you, don't know if you were flat-chested before or what. Just don't wear them." So I didn't.

I walked around flat-chested for 6 months because I was symmetric and could get away with it. I did not wear my prostheses, and I felt perfectly fine and comfortable, except that I looked absolutely dreadful in clothes. There is no way that you can get clothes to drape on you; women's clothes are not made for a total flat-chested look. And we are talking about more than the normal flat-chested appearance of a woman with small breasts. With a bilateral mastectomy there is actually less subcutaneous tissue in front. I decided that I wanted to look more natural and normal and feel good about myself and the way I looked—not necessarily at home, in the nude, but in clothes to walk around every day of my life. I did not want to wear prostheses to accomplish that purpose.

Was it difficult to face more surgery after you had just had your mastectomies?

Yes it was. I hurt and I was uncomfortable for so long. You can't sleep very well when you have bilateral mastectomies. I was flat on my back; I could not roll over in bed for 6 weeks. I was just trying to get better. I wanted desperately to be able to hug my children again and to cuddle them; they needed me to be able to do that. And I really didn't want to hurt again. I was also very tired for at least 3 months. I am a fast-moving person who likes to accomplish a lot of things in a day, so it was very annoying to me to spend 3 months dragging around. The prospect of giving up another few months of my life was not appealing. Actually, it was the experience of recuperating from the initial surgery that helped me decide what type of reconstructive method I was going to select. I wanted breast reconstruction, but I also wanted to minimize the time I had to spend recuperating.

Did your husband support your decision to have breast reconstruction?

My husband did not want me to have reconstruction. He said, "You've been uncomfortable enough. Why would you want to have any more surgery?" He made it perfectly clear that if it was for him, not to do it. It didn't matter to him. He didn't care. But I told him that it was really for me. I didn't want to wear prostheses. I wanted to feel comfortable in clothes without having to wear a harness (that's what it feels like). It was entirely for me and not for him. Then he accepted my decision and was supportive.

If you were interested in minimizing your recovery period, why didn't you have immediate breast reconstruction at the time of your cancer surgery?

I investigated that possibility before I had my mastectomies. I consulted with a plastic surgeon about immediate reconstruction. I decided against it primarily because the surgeon could not guarantee that I would not need blood. My surgeon assured me that he had done bilateral mastectomies for years and never had required a transfusion just for mastectomies alone, but he couldn't guarantee that I wouldn't require blood if I had bilateral reconstruction on top of that. Getting blood these days is risky. If I needed a transfusion for my reconstruction, I wanted to bank my own blood. I did not want anyone else's blood. So that was the primary factor that influenced my decision-making process. In addition, the people that I spoke to felt that immediate reconstruction might not be as cosmetically satisfactory as delayed reconstruction.

How did you select the method of breast reconstruction and the plastic surgeon to perform it?

I saw a total of four plastic surgeons because there was a question as to whether I was a good candidate for all the procedures. I wanted to know about all my options so I could make an informed decision. There are a variety of different methods of reconstruction.

I investigated having the TRAM flap, but found that it would be very difficult because I did not have enough abdominal fat. I went to see several plastic surgeons about this. One told me that with as little abdominal fat as I had he would probably have to put implants under the bilateral TRAM flaps to make my breasts large enough. I decided that if I was going to go through major surgery for the TRAM, probably more major than the original mastectomy with a much longer recuperation period, then why put implants under my reconstructed breasts. That would defeat the purpose of natural reconstruction with my own abdominal tissue. In addition to that, I wasn't willing to sacrifice a year of my life: 3 months off work, 3 months feeling lousy, and 6 months of not feeling myself. That was too much. Time is very precious. I feel a sense of urgency to get on with my life and enjoy what I have. My priorities were totally reestablished after facing a cancer operation.

Tissue expansion was another option that I explored. Two plastic surgeons that I consulted suggested that I have tissue expanders placed bilaterally and then later, in a second procedure, after my tissues had been stretched, have the expanders replaced with implants.

Then I went to see another plastic surgeon out of town who reviewed all of the options for me, listened to my expectations, and suggested a different approach. He said that he could use intraoperative expansion and put the implants in to reconstruct my breasts in a single operation, rather than the two-stage reconstruction required for tissue expansion. If I wanted to have nipple-areola reconstruction, I could have that at a later time as a minor outpatient procedure. I elected to have the one-stage intraoperative expansion with implant placement. I felt more confident with that particular surgeon, but also it was an easier, one-step procedure with a shorter recuperation time.

Was your reconstructive surgery painful and how long did it take you to recuperate?

After reconstruction, I had lots of nausea from the narcotics they were giving me. I never pushed the PCA (patient-controlled analgesia) button to get more pain medication; it was already giving me more than I could handle. As soon as I weaned myself from that, I felt much better. Tylenol worked just fine, without the nausea. My level of pain and discomfort, while still significant, was not nearly as bad as with my mastectomies, and I was able to go back to work in 10 days.

How did your breasts look and feel during the first few weeks after surgery?

I have seen so much breast reconstruction that I thought that I would know exactly how I would look and feel when I had it done. But I was wrong. I didn't expect my breasts to be as swollen, tight, and shiny as they became.

The swelling and blueness didn't show up during the 3 days I spent in the hospital. Then my husband and I went to a hotel so that I could be watched to make sure everything was okay before I flew back home. In the hospital I was elevated in this nice hospital bed, sitting almost erect, and there wasn't much swelling. At the hotel I just propped myself up on a couple of pillows; I could barely get out of bed because I was sore and bruised. When I woke up the following morning, my reconstructed breasts were so swollen and tight that I was afraid that they were going to just burst open. (This from someone who is informed . . . who knows what happened to her.) I had dreams that if I sneezed or coughed the seams would open up and the implants would go into orbit. I had this vision of them popping out, so I was afraid to sneeze or cough. Of course, that was totally unfounded. But that's how tight my breasts felt.

They also became totally blue, like two giant ripe blueberries. That wasn't immediate; blue took about a week. They were so swollen and blue. My husband was horrified looking at them. I was blue from my chest above the incisions down to my hips. I spent the weekend looking at those tight, blue, swollen breasts and worrying about them.

Was your plastic surgeon responsive to your concerns?

Yes. He was very responsive and reassuring. In fact, the reason we stayed in the hotel was to see the plastic surgeon before we went home. When I told him how I had imagined the implants popping out, he laughed and said, "You know too much to think that's going to happen. This is fine, a normal postoperative course; your breasts will do just great." Then, of course, I was relieved. And he was right. That all resolved, everything softened, and my breasts have turned out fine.

Did you have any late problems or complications?

I had some sutures coming through the skin when I was on vacation. That was a little bit difficult to handle, but it turned out to be relatively minor. I called my plastic surgeon on the phone, and he told me specifically what to do and that problem was handled very well. Other than that I have had no problems. I have healed as expected, and over time my breasts have softened and become more natural looking.

Was your reconstructive surgery covered by insurance?

Yes, it was, and we have several policies, but the insurance companies are not happy to pay for breast reconstruction. It makes me very angry. When I first called my insurance company (my husband has coverage with a different company), they gave me the run-around. The first person I spoke to said that they would not cover breast reconstruction because it was cosmetic. I said, "I know better—I am a physician. You are not correct. How dare you say this to anybody on the telephone. Of course it's covered. Let me speak to somebody else." Then they referred me to somebody else. And I said, "I am contemplating having reconstructive breast surgery and I want to know what you pay. I want to know what my out-of-pocket expenses will be." And they said, "We can't tell you what we pay. We pay 80% of the usual and customary fee." I said okay, "What is the usual and customary fee?" They said, "We can't tell you that." I said, "What do you mean you can't tell me. I am contemplating very expensive surgery. When I buy a car I want to know what it is going to cost *before* I buy the car. I don't expect to get a bill after I buy the car to find out then how much it is going to cost me. I want to know ahead of time." They refused to tell me. So I called the CEO's office, and I told him who I was and I described the run-around that I had gotten. I asked him how they dared to treat people this way. Didn't they realize that there are many people who might forego breast reconstruction because they fear being saddled with enormous bills. It was terrible to do this to people. The CEO said that he would call me back, and he did 48 hours later to tell me the usual and customary fee they paid for breast reconstruction. It was pitifully poor. Then I called my husband's insurance company to find out what they would pay. They also told me they couldn't tell me, but they did, sooner than my insurance company. And they provided better reimbursement for the surgeon. So my breast reconstruction was covered by two policies that we had, major medical in addition to my husband's policy. But I was incensed at the way it was handled.

Have you had your nipple and areola reconstructed?

Initially I thought, yes. I'm going to do the whole wad. I'm going to do everything. I'm going to do anything that I feel like doing. But I changed my mind. I feel comfortable with my breasts as they are now. It accomplishes what I wanted. I look good in clothes. I don't have to wear prostheses. I don't have to go through any more surgery, and I don't want to. I don't need it; my breasts look very symmetric. They're soft. They look great in a bathing suit, in a nightgown, and in clothes. That is what I wanted.

Has reconstruction affected the way you feel about yourself?

In terms of self-esteem and self-image I can't say that reconstruction has made that big a difference. I value myself enough, with or without my breasts. I did it more for convenience and physical appearance, to feel good about the way I look. I don't feel that my breasts, before or after the surgery, are what makes or breaks me.

Are your reconstructed breasts sensitive? Are they warm?

They're not sensitive. There is pressure sensation, but it's not the same sort of discrimination that you have when you touch the rest of your skin that has normal nerve endings. They are also a little bit cooler than the rest of the body. They don't feel colder to me, but if you touch them, they feel cooler than the rest of my skin.

Are you satisfied with your breast reconstruction? If you had to do it all over, would you choose to have breast reconstruction again?

Without a doubt, yes. It was worth it for me. It was relatively easy compared to the original surgery, and I am pleased with the results. My breasts are symmetric and soft and squeezable. My kids like to snuggle up. I know that when they get cuddly against my chest, they are thinking those are Mom's new breasts and they feel nice and soft. They don't say anything, but I know that they snuggle up against them to observe for themselves. And nobody can tell. If somebody came up and touched my chest, there is no way to know. My breasts feel very natural and normal.

What advice would you like to give to other women considering breast reconstruction?

Become informed. Investigate all of the options so that you can make a choice that meets your personal needs. Identify your goals. Why are you considering breast reconstruction? What do you expect to get out of it? Do you want to look as natural naked as you possibly can or just to look good in clothing? How much time do you want to invest? If you are thinking about a more lengthy procedure, you need to assess what it will cost in terms of time and money. How are you going to pay for it? It is crucial to know what your expectations are. Once these questions are answered, you need to know about all of the different reconstructive procedures before choosing a particular method. You can't just go to somebody and have him tell you this is the surgery for you. There is no such answer. You must have input. First, you must be able to state what your goals are. How do you want to look? How much are you willing to go through to achieve that look? Then, when you feel informed, when you know all of your options, and only then, can you make the best decision for you.

SIMONE: A FRENCH PERSPECTIVE

"You know in my country, the French women, we are not like, how would you say, *prohibited*. You know, not showing yourself. We have a different reaction with our bodies. In France we have the nude beaches and topless beaches. We are more open. We like our bodies and the breasts are for women something special." This charming explanation was given to me by Simone as she described her reasons for wanting breast reconstruction.

Simone is a native of France who has been living in the United

States for over 20 years. She is bilingual and works full-time as a French translator at an export company. Even though she apologized during our interview for her inability to communicate because of her lingering accent, I found her to be articulate and intelligent. A small woman with short blond hair, she has the stunning good looks so characteristic of French women and an almost casual sense of style. At 46 years of age she is married, the mother of three, and the grandmother of four. She prides herself on being health conscious. She eats well, exercises, and loves the outdoors, frequently retreating to the mountains with her husband to hike and contemplate nature. In fact, that is the refuge they sought when her cancer was diagnosed.

Simone's cancer seemed to come out of nowhere. She has no family history and has always been very good about going for physical examinations and mammograms.

Simone describes herself as a strong, even tough, person. She knew she could survive this experience. Fortunately, she didn't have to face it alone. She had her husband. "A wonderful guy . . . he was there with me all the way. The two of us went through it together."

Simone's cancer was treated by mastectomy, followed by 6 months of chemotherapy and then a TRAM flap breast reconstruction combined with a breast lift on her opposite breast. She wanted the TRAM because her new breast would be created out of her own tissue, not an implant. Originally she had worried that she wouldn't have enough abdominal fat to build a breast. But because of her good eating habits during chemotherapy she gained 18 pounds, leaving her with plenty of abdominal fat to fashion a new breast. Simone's story is an uplifting one and her perspective is uniquely French.

How did you discover you had breast cancer?

Two years ago in June I was feeling fatigued, so I went to the doctor for a complete physical; all my results came back fine. No sign of anything. Two months later I went to New Orleans with my husband. I was putting on the sexy lingerie I had bought when I felt a lump on the top of my breast. I knew I had fibrocystic disease, so I thought maybe it was just another cyst popping up. I was drinking a lot of caffeinated beverages. I decided to stop drinking so much coffee and I took vitamin E, but it did not go away. When September came, the lump was no smaller. I had company during that time and did not have much time to myself. So I let it ride, just put myself on the back burner and took care of everybody else. In November I decided "that is not right. I have to do something." I went for a mammogram. When I got the mammogram the doctor sent me to a surgeon who did a biopsy and told me I had breast cancer. He advised me to have the breast removed.

Did the surgeon give you any other options? Did he tell you about lumpectomy and irradiation?

He could tell by the size of the tumor that lumpectomy was not advisable. If he removed the lump, my breast would have been so damaged that even reconstruction would have been difficult. So mastectomy was his recommendation. I trusted this particular surgeon. He was quite special, very caring. I asked him to give me 3 days to think about it.

What was your reaction to the breast cancer diagnosis?

I was not really shocked because of the size of the lump and the way it felt. But I think every woman must ask, "Why me?" "What is it going to do to my life? How is it going to change?" The breasts are for women something very special. I wanted to be around, so I was going to do whatever was necessary to beat this cancer. I was not really bitter. I am quite strong mentally. I come from a strong family. I have been married before and my first marriage was not a good marriage; I learned to be quite tough. I did not think the breast cancer was the end of the world. I thought I am going to do this and I am going to go on with my life with one breast or two breasts. I am going to have a good time. My husband, he is a great guy, and I think he was more concerned about the way I would react.

When I first found out I had cancer, my husband and I took off for the mountains. When I want to think about something, I have to go where it is quiet. I have to go to nature; I relate with the peace and I guess that is closer to God. We went hiking and talked about it and the things we would have to do. I did not know the extent of the cancer and that concerned me more than having the breast removed. We spent the day in the mountains, talking, and came to the conclusion that the surgery was needed and we would make the best of it. Whatever happened we would make it together.

How did you tell your children? How did they react?

I just told them like it was. I do not beat around the bushes. That Sunday I decided to call everybody. I called my children and I told them that I had breast cancer and I needed a mastectomy. They were speechless. Nobody knew what to say. I called friends, the people at work, and my family. I got the same reaction from everyone. "No it is not possible." I said, "You know, it is possible. It happens to one in every nine women and now I am the one of the nine."

How did people at your work react when they knew you had breast cancer?

One lady kept in touch with me. Her father died of cancer so she related to cancer much better than my other coworkers. The other ladies really did not know what to tell me. I received many cards, the preprinted kind, but not really a note. I think that most people do not know what to say to a person who has a serious illness. So I called them and I was the one who approached them. I said, "Look, it is not the end of the world. I am going to make it." And then they began to speak, to open up.

How long did it take you to recover from your mastectomy? Did you experience much pain?

I recuperate quite quickly. I could use my arm right away. My surgeon was totally amazed how much I could do. My husband brought my nice gown and makeup case to the hospital, and the day after surgery I washed my hair and got myself fixed up. I was operated on Wednesday and discharged from the hospital on Sunday. By then I could raise my arm. I really did not have any pain. The drains were probably the most uncomfortable thing I had to endure. I felt good. When the surgeon removed the bandages, my husband and I saw it, and I said, "It is going to be okay. I still have one and I am going to be fine." I was still anxious to find out how far the cancer had gone.

Did you have any positive lymph nodes? Did you require any additional therapy?

I had three involved nodes. My surgeon recommended an oncologist who came to see me at the hospital. I was really impressed by him and he suggested the chemotherapy treatment I should receive; he wanted to start ASAP. He said, "I would like to start right now in the hospital, but I am going to give you enough time to recuperate from surgery." A week later I started chemotherapy.

When did you return to work?

I stayed off work from December to September. I probably could have gone back after the surgery, but I would have been very fatigued when I was taking chemo. I chose to take a leave of absence to recuperate fully, to get my strength back, to go through chemo. I am a strong believer in nourishing yourself correctly. If I would have gone to work, I probably would not have taken care of myself as well as I did. While I was at home, I went to the market and made a point of buying fresh vegetables and a lot of fresh fruit and prepared special meals. My husband said I was becoming a very good chef. I truly believe eating well helped me quite a bit during chemotherapy. I gained weight during chemo. I had a chance to do some reading, and I got involved with modeling for mastectomy patients.

How did you start modeling for mastectomy patients?

I went to be fitted for my prosthesis about a month after surgery. The lady at the lingerie shop was very nice. Mastectomy lingerie is not very sexy, and I made a comment to her that somebody needs to come up with much nicer ideas for lingerie. After all, we are still women. It makes you feel better if you have something pretty to wear instead of those ugly bras, heavy-duty looking things. So she said, "Well I know of a company that makes the prostheses and is currently working on a line of bras." Several days later this lady called and said a person from the company wanted to meet me. I came and she showed me this new bra. She said, "What do you think of my product? I need people to try the new bra with their prosthesis and I need feedback. I would like for you to tell me how you feel about it." I said "Great." They were underwire bras, lace with a nice pocket. Much nicer than the regular mastectomy bra. I tried the bra for a few days, and when I returned it, she asked if I would like to be one of their models? "We need someone like you who is not inhibited and can model the bra for the retailers. We like for them to see it on someone who had a mastectomy." I agreed, I even posed in a photo session.

What was your reaction to having chemotherapy? Did you have any side effects?

Like everyone else, I had heard horror stories about chemotherapy. The oncologist told me exactly what to expect. He said, "I am not going to say that you are not going to lose your hair. Some women do, some women do not. Those are the side effects you may encounter," and he went over them, "but it is very much an individualized type of reaction." The first time I went for chemo his nurse explained what drugs I would be receiving and she stayed with me during the treatment. I went home thinking, "Well, what is this supposed to do to me?" The day went by and I felt fatigue, but they had given me a nausea-type medicine that makes you groggy. That is what I am feeling, more sleepy, nothing happened. No, nothing. No side effect. Second trip, no side effects. So he increased the dosage. We had to do some readjustments, but each time before I would go to chemo, I would always do something special the day before, you know, something to get myself ready and happy. I never took the chemotherapy negatively, I took it positively. I think that has helped me. It was like taking a vitamin, something I had to do to make me feel better. The last treatment was a little bit nauseating, but I did not lose my hair. It only thinned out.

What did you do to cope with your cancer treatment?

Sometimes I had a good cry, and that kind of clears the air. You let it all out. It takes the tension off. I have been here for 26 years in this country, so you know I have experienced down days missing my home, my country. I always find I can have a good cry and feel better.

My husband was a wonderful help. He would look at me and say, "Okay, let's go hiking. I think it is what you need and here we go." We would pack and go. I feel very close to the earth and to nature, so those trips were very calming.

How did you learn about breast reconstruction?

I was not ignorant of breast cancer and reconstruction. I had read about it and I had heard about it. You know, you never think it is going to happen to you, but I was aware of some of the techniques available. Before my mastectomy I asked my surgeon what the scar would look like after he removed my breast? I wanted an indication of how big it would be and where it would be. We talked about that and I said, "Now, what do you know about reconstruction? What type of reconstruction would you recommend?" He said, "That is a personal choice; you will have to make your own choice." He had a book on his shelf that talked about the different reconstructive techniques. He told me to read it. It would give me an indication of what to expect and would help me make a decision. He said, "If you have to have chemotherapy, I would suggest you wait until you finish chemo and fully recover."

Why did you want reconstruction?

I like nice lingerie. I enjoy having a cleavage. With the prosthesis, when you bend down, even with those special bras, it does not feel the same. You never feel complete; it is not attached to you. It does not feel the same in your clothes. I think I had to have it done to feel right, to feel comfortable.

Several years ago I lived in Baton Rouge. After having three children my breasts were sagging. I went to a breast clinic to see about having a breast lift, having the surgeon remove some of the skin and lift the breasts. I always had it in my mind to have my breasts redone. So I was telling my husband when I had the reconstruction, you know, I always wanted a "boob job" and I guess I have it now. You have to be careful about what you wish for because it may come true. I had not planned to have my boob job that way.

How did your husband feel about your reconstruction? Was he supportive?

He knows when I have made up my mind about something I am going to do it. He asked me if I was strong enough to go through it. I said, "Yes I was," and he said, "Okay, you know I will be there. I will be with you every step of the way." We are husband and wife, but we are also best friends. Now he is very complimentary about it. He thinks it is great. Support from your spouse is definitely a plus.

What reconstructive technique did you select? Why?

I was very impressed when I read about the TRAM flap procedure. I personally believe in taking your own tissue. If that was possible, I wanted to do it. But because I was so thin, only 103 pounds, I did not have much of a stomach there. I said, "Maybe it is not going to be possible." If I do not have enough here, we will have to use a back flap. I didn't want a scar on my back. My second choice was to have tissue expansion. I thought I will go with that route. Little did I know then that when I went on chemo, eating the way I was eating, I would gain 18 pounds. I was able to have my TRAM flap after all.

How did you select your plastic surgeon?

My surgeon recommended him, so I made an appointment. My husband and I spoke with him. He discussed the procedure and I was very pleased with his consultation. There is something very honest about him. I trusted him and I had very good vibes about him. I had heard different stories from different women. Some women had suggested that I go elsewhere. One said, "You are going to be one of many and you are not going to have the attention that you should have." I said, "Possibly, but it is a choice that I have to make." I did not feel that way. He is a very busy man, but I had very good care. He always answered my questions.

How long were you in the hospital? Did you experience much pain?

I was in the hospital for 6 days. I heard from other women that it would be extremely painful. But the word "painful" means something different for each person. I did not find it painful. I found it uncomfortable, but not painful.

The most discomfort that I encountered was from my back. When you come back from surgery, you are in a "jackknife" position because you have stitches in your abdomen and cannot really stretch. So they position you where you cannot move very well. You do not want to pull anything. I could not find a position in the bed that was comfortable for my back. My lower back was bothering me, but I did not find my abdomen painful; it pulled when I moved, but the pulling was not a pain to me. When I got up from the bed to sit in the chair, I did it very easily. They kept asking me to grade the level of pain, and I really could not tell them. My breast was not painful at all because the nerves had been cut before, so there was no feeling.

Initially, after the first stage of the breast reconstruction, were you satisfied with your breast appearance?
Were any adjustments needed?

I was amazed. You see the pictures, but the actual marvel of what the surgeon is able to do to shape a breast can only be understood when you see it in person.

I had the other breast lifted at the same time. My breasts matched pretty well, but the new breast needed to be reshaped a bit. It was a little bit larger and not as round as the normal one. Earlier, he had told me that if I needed any adjustments he would reshape my breast when he did the nipple.

Did you have any complications or any problems after your breast reconstruction?

I had the other breast lifted at the same time, so I had drains in the abdomen and in both breasts. But I had no complications.

How long did it take before you could resume your normal activities?

After I got home, it took another week to 10 days before I really could walk correctly. I always felt like I was bending down some because your stomach pulls. Within 3 weeks of the surgery I was feeling pretty good.

It took a good 6 weeks for my full strength to come back. I did not want to force it, so I was cautious. I took my vitamins again, and I went more slowly regarding activities.

Why did you decide to have nipple-areola reconstruction?

When I found out I could use the stomach to build my breast, I decided to go all the way, you know. It is like doing half of the job if you don't go for the nipple. Some of the women that I spoke with told me after the initial reconstructive surgery they would not go back for further surgery. But for me, I felt that as soon as I healed enough I wanted to finish the job. I want my breast complete. It turned out great. I am not totally finished with it because we still have to tattoo the nipple.

What did he use to build your nipple and areola? Did he make any other adjustments at that time?

He took my nipple and areola from the extra tissue left at the end of my abdominal scar (the dog ear) where he cut the flap. When he did the nipple, he trimmed the fat and reshaped the breast. Now it looks great. I am very, very pleased with it.

He also did liposuction around the abdominal scar to flatten it and it turned out great. This was outpatient surgery. I came, had the surgery, and went home.

How do your scars look?

The reconstructed breast itself has a scar all around it. It is a very thin circular scar. Under the breast, coming from the middle of the breast up, you have a thin scar where they attach the fat. For the nipple, on top of the breast at the point where they attach the areola, there is a little circle scar. My scars are beginning to whiten. They are reddish at first, then they turn pink. They are beginning to fade and whiten now.

The nipple itself is a small piece of your tissue sewn on; you really do not see any scar. It seems like it just grew out, but you can see this very thin scar for the areola.

Now, on the abdomen itself, you have a scar, like a smiley face, and that is where he took the flap for the breast.

Are any of these scars visible in your clothing?

If I would wear something very low cut, I am maybe a little more restricted now than I will be later when the scar fades. It has only been 7 months. Within a year the scar will fade much more. Then if I wear something lower cut, I can cover it with a bit of makeup, and it will not be that noticeable. My abdominal scar doesn't show even when I wear a bikini, so it was well done.

Do your breasts match?

Very much. The top of the newer breast may need to be raised a little bit more, but we want to give it a couple more months to let everything settle. Then we may raise that up a bit. If we go that route, my plastic surgeon suggested taking some tissue from under my arm, but it is not an absolute need.

Do your breasts have sensation?

No. I can touch the breasts. I know my hand is there, but there is no actual feeling. If I pinch myself or if I were to stick a needle in my breast, I do not feel any pain.

Are your breasts warm? Are they soft?

The temperature is a bit different. The reconstructed breast is sometimes a little colder than the other one. I think it is due to the circulation of the blood because of the way the breast was reconstructed.

The new breast is firm. When I am walking, it does not have the bounce of the normal breast. You feel it moving, but it does not have the feeling of a real breast. When you touch your normal breast, you feel the mammary glands—it's warm and soft. The new breast feels hard, more like a lump. I must say it takes a little time to get used to that.

Did breast reconstruction meet your expectations? Are you satisfied?

Very much. Extremely satisfied. I never went through the reconstruction expecting my new breast to be like the old breast. You go through reconstruction to make you feel better, to help you adjust to the cancer. I like to be able to wear a regular bra and to have my clothes feel better. My new breast has similarities to my old, but it is not like a real breast. I went through reconstruction knowing that. I think that helped me too.

Did you have any problems or complications with your reconstruction?

No problems whatsoever. I came out of it with flying colors. I would suggest to anyone who wants to go through it to first prepare herself with a good positive attitude. If you are positive, I think you can recover so much better. And you will feel great about yourself.

If you had it to do over, would you have breast reconstruction again? Would you choose the same technique?

Oh, yes. For me it was great. If I had cancer again, I would have reconstruction with no hesitation. I would choose the TRAM again. It is a beautiful operation.

Did your mastectomy or your reconstruction affect the way you feel about yourself? Your feelings of sexuality?

I am French. You can excuse me please. I like pretty lingerie. Before the mastectomy I was always sleeping in the nude. I would start with a gown, but I never finished that way. In the morning I would never wake up with a gown. When I had the mastectomy done, I came back from the hospital and for the first 2 weeks I was wearing a little gown for protection because of the scar and because I had some drainage. My husband looked at me and said, "Are you going to keep on wearing this gown?" and I said, "Well, what do you think?" He said, "Knowing you, you are going to be uncomfortable. I would not think you would want to be wearing a gown." So I took it off and went back to going without a gown. Because of the scar, I had to be more careful, but that did not stop me. It was still me, you know, and I was not ashamed of me. I have read about women who could not look at themselves, and I know someone like this. I never stopped looking. What I saw in the mirror was me with one breast left, but there was still a whole lot of me left to work with.

How do you feel now when you look at yourself in the mirror?

I feel great. I am the type, again, I do not sleep in anything. Many a time when I put on my makeup, I am naked in the bathroom, and I feel comfortable because scar or no scar, it is me and I look good.

LYNN: WHY WAIT?

"I didn't want to see myself without my breasts, and I didn't see any reason to wait. Why wait and heal only to be reopened and have to heal a second time? With immediate breast reconstruction, I never felt the terrible devastation of breast loss after bilateral mastectomies. The hard part was over once I had that surgery and from then on it was an adventure in rebuilding."

It was summer when I interviewed Lynn for the first time. Tanned and fit, she was dressed in a white shirt and shorts with her dark hair pulled back from her face. Married with two daughters, she has an active career as a communications expert at a local high school. Who would ever imagine that breast cancer could strike this beautiful, articulate woman of 47? And yet, true to the statistics, Lynn was diagnosed with breast cancer 5 years ago.

Her diagnosis, while shocking, was not totally unexpected. She had a family history of breast cancer and had herself been plagued with fibrocystic breasts, a long-standing problem. Lynn had been under close surveillance by her surgical oncologist for many years and had had numerous biopsies for suspicious lumps. Just 2 years before her breast cancer diagnosis, after she had three suspicious lumps biopsied at one time, her oncologist suggested that she consider prophylactic mastectomies and reconstruction to prevent the possible development of breast cancer in the future. She had even seen a plastic surgeon about this option, and he also recommended preventive mastectomies. But Lynn was still doubtful; she didn't have cancer and the thought of having her breast tissue removed was not appealing. Reflecting on this early decision now, Lynn admits that "I should have been smarter. My mom has breast cancer and I have a family history." She went to another oncologist for a second opinion. He told her it would be foolish to let them take her breasts off. She should wait until she had cancer, if, indeed, she ever did. That was just the news that she wanted to hear, so she decided to wait and see.

Two years later, shortly after her aunt had been diagnosed with a breast malignancy, Lynn's breast cancer was discovered during yet another biopsy. This time she took immediate action. She had a modified radical mastectomy on the right side and a prophylactic mastectomy on her left breast, a procedure in which the breast tissue is removed and the nipple cored out. Both breasts were reconstructed immediately with tissue expanders.

Lynn's decision to have immediate breast reconstruction was partially explained by her mother's experience with breast loss. "I had seen my mom with her concave figure and staples all across her chest. I watched her battle with a prosthesis. I remember the day that she threw it against the wall. She was so tired of hauling that thing around. She had very big breasts, and after her one breast was removed, she needed a large prosthesis for balance; it weighed 7 or 8 pounds. That's a heavy load to carry. I knew that route was not for me. With immediate reconstruction, I never had to experience breast loss. I never mourned my breasts. My attitude was, 'Now that this is out of the way, let's go.'"

Lynn's initial reaction when she woke after her operation was one of relief. "When I woke up, I lifted the sheet immediately and all I had was two little Steri-Strips on my body. I had expected massive bandages. I had these little mounds and it was like I didn't lose that much. Even knowing that it really wasn't me under there, it was reassuring to have something there."

How long did it take you to recuperate?

I had my mastectomies and reconstruction on a Thursday, and I went home on a Saturday, but it took a good 4 weeks before I felt like doing much. My mom came and stayed for a week and helped out. I went out in public right away; I attended my daughter's graduation a week later. I went to the grocery store. Raising my arms was a little difficult, however, and I didn't want my scars to stretch. So I was careful about lifting and moving. I didn't vacuum. In fact, I still don't vacuum if I can get out of it.

I was off for the summer and I didn't go back to work until late August. I was still having my breasts expanded then. The expansion was not hard once I got over the initial part. In October, when I had my expanders replaced with implants, I stayed off work 2 weeks. I really didn't need that full 2 weeks; 1 week would have been fine. But at that point my priorities were different. I decided that I was going to take all the time I needed to heal. I put myself first probably for the first time in my life.

When I had my nipple reconstructed, it was done the day before Christmas vacation, and I had another 2 weeks to recuperate.

What type of anesthesia did you have for each of your surgical procedures?

The anesthesia was one of the hardest parts of the surgery. I was under general anesthesia for the original surgery when my expanders were inserted. But I also had general anesthesia when my implants were put in and when my nipples were done. It was all done under a general. It's hard for me to come back from anesthesia; it takes about 4 to 6 weeks to get it out of my system. I'm tired and drag around. That's why I took 2 weeks to recuperate each time.

How did you choose your reconstructive technique?
What considerations were most important to you
in making this decision?

I chose tissue expansion with implant placement because that's what my plastic surgeon recommended. He told me about the other operations and about the tummy flap, but because I was so slender, he didn't think I had enough stomach fat to reconstruct both of my breasts. Today there are even more options for the breast reconstruction patient. They can move tissue from other parts of the body with microsurgery. Even so, I really didn't want to go through the pain of a procedure that involved. And I didn't want all of the scars. So tissue expansion seemed to be the best option for me.

Describe the expansion process. What happened when you had
your breasts expanded? Who did it? How long did it take?

Two weeks after my surgery I met with my plastic surgeon and his nurse, and we started the expansion process. My plastic surgeon told her how much fluid to inject into my expanders and over what period of time. From then on his nurse usually took care of me, injecting about 100 ml of fluid into each breast during each session. Expansion proceeded pretty rapidly. It took about 15 minutes each time, and I went every week for the first 7 or 8 weeks and then less frequently. We never cut back on the amount of fluid injected, and we never stopped. But she always gave me the option. She was very responsive to my needs.

Tell me how this nurse helped you? What did she do to make this
process easier for you?

She was one of the greatest supports that I had. She allowed me to have control, to make some decisions about my body, and to decide how fast I wanted to have my breasts expanded. Each time she asked if I felt I could handle it. If I told her something didn't feel right, she never brushed me off or dismissed my concerns. Instead she would say, "Tell me how you feel. Exactly where is the problem?" Not all nurses do that. I've had experiences with other nurses during that process and I've never had that kind of compassion. If I was extremely tight, she allowed me to say whether I wanted to be expanded or not. And a lot of them don't. They say, "You have to get used to the tightness, because the only way to stretch the skin is to expand it immediately." But that's not necessarily true; sometimes your skin doesn't stretch as fast as they think it should. Sometimes you need the time to allow your skin to relax and work itself loose so that it is more comfortable.

Tissue expansion involves some sense of being violated. This is true especially with the original surgery, but even with the expansion you are not in control of making decisions about what's being done to your body. My nurse gave *me* control.

Was your plastic surgeon responsive during the expansion process?

My doctor's schedule was extremely tight, and I couldn't always reach him. But I could always see him when I had a problem. I understand from other people that their doctors don't see them during the expansion process. I saw him every single time. It was important to me that he was still going to check to make sure everything was okay. I needed to be in touch with my doctor during that time.

How did it feel to have your expanders inflated? Was it painful?

I had more feeling on my right side where I had the preventive mastectomy. I always felt the pinprick of the needle being inserted into my expander port. Once it was in, I didn't feel a thing. The other side had no feeling. I could feel some pressure. I was not always comfortable, but I was never in pain.

After the first 4 weeks it felt like I had bricks put in my body. My breasts felt heavier, like I was carrying more weight. That's probably because my expanders were positioned behind my chest muscle and were exerting pressure on it. I just felt my breasts blowing up; I could actually see them as they grew. That was encouraging to me because I didn't want to be flat-chested. As a teenager I was fairly big-breasted. And I think I would have had a hard time being totally flat-chested. But I could see my breasts as they grew, and each time I would go home and think, "They're getting better."

How long did the expansion process take?

Everything went like clockwork. I wore my expanders for about 5 months. It took me 4 months to have my breasts totally expanded and then a month to let my breast skin rest so my breasts would become comfortable.

Was it inconvenient?

No, because it was summertime. Had I been in school it might have been. But my mindset was such that nothing would have seemed an inconvenience. I had tunnel vision with breast reconstruction. Other things went on in my life, but this was a goal; it consumed a large part of my life and my thinking.

Why did you choose to have your nipple-areola reconstructed?

Because I wanted to be complete. I wanted my breasts to look normal and to match. The nipple on my normal breast was preserved after the prophylactactic mastectomy, so I wanted one on the mastectomy side also.

How was your nipple-areola reconstructed and when was it done?

My initial surgery was done in May, my expanders were replaced with permanent implants in October, and my nipple was reconstructed in December. The nipple reconstruction was done at a third procedure to allow my breasts to settle. My nipple was reconstructed from the scar tissue extending under my arm. They sit you up to graft the nipple, and they have to open a fairly decent-size scar to get the skin for the nipple graft. I also had my nipple tattooed as an outpatient procedure.

What type of permanent implants did you have put in and did you have any concerns about implants?

I have textured-surface silicone gel implants. I was upset about these implants for a while during all of the media scares, but I feel pretty comfortable with them now. I haven't had any problems. I have faith in my plastic surgeon to pick the right kind of implants for me. He told me about the possible risks. I was informed. I still think what I have is the best. My medical oncologist isn't worried about the implants, and he would be the first one to tell me to get them out. So I'm not going to have my implants removed. My plastic surgeon would have to tell me it is time to do it before I would consider it.

How do your breasts look? Are you satisfied with the appearance?

My breasts are symmetric and I look terrific in my clothes. I asked to be big and I got bigger than I had planned to be, but I'm very satisfied. Sometimes I have to be careful about buying clothes, because the top doesn't fit the bottom, but that is a minor inconvenience compared to my level of satisfaction.

After the modified radical mastectomy my armpit was hollowed out and it looked funny to me in clothes. Other people probably wouldn't notice if I kept my arm down, but I was self-conscious. To correct this problem my plastic surgeon removed a piece of muscle from my back (the latissismus dorsi muscle) and swung it under my arm, so I now have a fairly normal looking armpit.

My nipples still don't match, but that is because I had my nipple skin preserved on my normal side. At the time I didn't want to lose the nipple on my normal side if I didn't have to. That seemed very important then; it isn't now. Sometimes I wish I had gone ahead and had it taken off so there was a little better match. But that side is more comfortable because I have more skin.

Also, the color of the tattoo on my reconstructed nipple does not match the color of my preserved nipple. I have yellow-toned skin and yellow tones are difficult to replicate. I've heard that they now have tints with more yellow pigment available. After my tattoo fades, I am going to have my nipple-areola tattooed again to try to get a better match. It is hard to do it again. After all of that surgery, Band-Aids are a real turn-off.

How do your reconstructed breasts feel? Are your breasts sensitive? Are they soft? Are they warm?

I have no feeling in about a 3½-inch diameter. I do have feeling around the outside of my breasts, but only in the skin. All of the good, warm sexual sensations are gone. I miss those most of all.

My breasts are cooler than the rest of my body. When it's cold, my breasts get cold. I'm a walker, and I try to counteract that by layering with lightweight clothes. Then my breasts don't get so frigid. On winter nights I use an electric blanket and flannel sheet to keep me warm. The rest of my body isn't cold; I just feel cold when I touch my breasts with my arms, because I have no feeling there.

Is there anything you would change about your reconstruction?

I would like to have the sexual feeling back, and I think someday they probably will know how to do that. If they do it in my lifetime, I'm going to be jealous. But that is the hardest part to me.

Has the mastectomy and reconstruction experience affected your feelings of sexuality and femininity?

Yes. Breasts are important; they are a turn-on. Now that my breasts are no longer sensitive, I don't have that response. As you get older, turn-ons are harder to come by. You are without that and you have to have a pretty good relationship with the person you have sex with, whether it's a husband or another partner. The woman who goes through this has to know that this is a loss.

Your femininity goes with the mastectomy; the reconstruction rebuilds that femininity. I never get in the shower that I don't look at myself and smile. I never feel devastated.

What are your scars like?

I don't scar badly. You would never even notice I had a scar on my right side. The one on my left side from the mastectomy is also faded and barely noticeable. It is a very thin line and the nipple is grafted right over the major part of the scar. I do have a red scar from when he redid my armpit. It will take several years, but I know it will eventually turn white like the rest of my scars have done.

Did you have any problems or complications after your breast reconstruction?

No, none at all.

What coping mechanisms did you rely on to help you get through this experience?

I went through this experience fairly humorously. When I went in, knowing hospitals the way I do, I wrote "prophylactic" on my right breast and "modified radical" on my left, so that they didn't do the wrong side. When I went in to have my implants put in, I communicated further by writing "big" on my breasts. And when I had my nipple tattooed, I also had a little heart tattoo put on my side. I figured it took a lot of heart to get through it all.

Did you join a support group?

Yes, a breast reconstruction support group, and it was important to me. It has been a vital part of the healing process. You talk about this experience with your family, but they can't really relate. They've never had muscle spasms as the muscle adjusted to having a foreign body behind it. They don't know what it's like to lie on your stomach and feel like you are lying on rubber balls. They don't know when you move from side to side that you feel like you've got to push your breasts back into place, which you really don't. But it's a strange feeling because of the lack of sensation in your breast. I can go to my support group and I can talk all I want about my breasts and about reconstruction and nobody says, "Here she goes again." It's a group that wraps around you when you have problems. We share more than just our breasts: the good and the bad. With reconstruction, I knew everything that could go wrong. Women in the group share what has gone wrong with them. Doctors will tell you what might possibly happen, but in my support group I could see firsthand what did happen. Some people belong to the group for a short while and then leave because they don't need it anymore. I still need it, not just as a means to express myself, but because it is pay-back time. The women in the group were wonderful for me; if I can be there for somebody else, then I want to do it. I am one of the lucky people. My reconstruction was aesthetically successful. It looks fantastic. I've not had any major problems. Not everyone is so lucky. One of my good friends who I brought to the group died 2 weeks ago. That was tough to deal with. But that helps me stay in touch with reality. It scares me, but it helps me.

In retrospect, do you feel that you made the right decision when you had a prophylactic mastectomy on your normal side?

Definitely. If I was allowed more hindsight, I would have done it 2 years earlier when my breasts were merely high risk. I would recommend that anyone who is diagnosed with precancerous breasts get them off. What you gain from early prevention far outweighs the loss of a breast. It is just not worth carrying the time bombs around. And that is literally what I did. As my husband said, "Somebody has to hit you with a 2 by 4 to get your attention." Second opinions are great. But if they are different, go for a third or a fourth and then weigh all of your information. I'm sorry I stopped at two.

Was reconstruction worth the time, pain, and money?
Would you do it again and would you choose the
same reconstructive approach?

I would do it again in a heartbeat. And if something were to go wrong with my implants tomorrow, I would probably have tissue expanders and implants again. I know that 20 or 30 years down the road I may have different options, but I really don't want any other major surgery unless it's absolutely necessary. Tissue expansion and implant placement are not major surgery. I also know that the flap procedure is available to me if my implants should fail or if something should happen and I cannot have implants anymore.

Aesthetically, tissue transfer is not as pretty a result as you get with expanders and implants. With the TRAM there are more scars. Not only do you have the scar across your stomach, but you end up with two scars across your breast, rather than the one. The scarring bothers me.

Has your mom had breast reconstruction?

My mom decided to have reconstruction after she saw me go through it; she had my plastic surgeon do her reconstruction. She was 72. She also had her second breast removed and had prophylactic mastectomy and reconstruction. She's had more problems with her reconstruction than I had. She had an infection and had to have her implant removed. She ended up having a latissimus dorsi back flap transferred to give her better skin cover for her implant. She is having some problems with her other breast right now and is scheduled to see her plastic surgeon.

Is she happy she did it?

Yes, because she doesn't worry anymore about developing cancer on the other side. But she isn't as comfortable as I am. I feel somewhat guilty knowing that she did it because I did, even though I didn't pressure her. In fact, I tried to discourage her because I worried about surgery at her age. I wanted her to do the reconstruction for her self-image, but I didn't want her to go through any pain or discomfort. She came through it better than I did to begin with. But her aesthetic result has not been as successful as mine. She has one breast that is hard and she will probably have to have that implant replaced.

How did your family react to your mastectomies and reconstruction?

They were with me all the way; they were as involved in it as I was. We engaged in a lot of humor to keep us all going. My youngest daughter is the funny bone in the family and she kept it light. She called the state department to get me a handicapped parking sticker as a double amputee. They didn't give me one. But that was her type of humor. Even now, she jokes, "Those are the biggest things I have ever seen, Mother; what do you do with them?" My husband chose to stay with me in the hospital and take care of everything, even though my aunt was director of nursing there and offered to stay. But I was more comfortable with him. It was a bonding time for us.

Are your daughters concerned about the threat of breast cancer? How has this experience affected them?

It has brought us much closer together. It has also made us aware of what's in their future. They have to be careful. My oldest daughter is very open and talks freely about her body. She is very large-breasted, and she is a tiny person. She is aware that her breasts could be time bombs and that cancer could come earlier for her than it did for me. It seems to be hitting younger people all the time. My gynecologist has recommended that she come in every 3 months to have her breasts checked. My younger daughter is 19 and is very hard to work with. She is self-conscious about her body; no one sees her body. We found her a wonderful female gynecologist. Even so, my daughter said it was the most horrifying experience she's ever been through. She has even said things to me in jest, yet not really joking, "Thanks, Mom, look what you have given me to look forward to." I know that it hangs in her mind.

Do your daughters do breast self-examination?

Yes. My oldest one does BSE. She told me she could not find any lumps. When I ask my other daughter, she'll say, "Mother I'll take care of that." She really won't open up about it. I worry about her more. She probably is the one that checks the most because she is more frightened by it. I don't know if she knows what to look for. We have a friend who is 25 and was diagnosed with breast cancer in December. That brought it home, but my younger daughter still doesn't talk to me about it. I know that this experience has heightened both of my daughters' awareness of the threat of breast cancer. They talk about it with their friends. Their friends are all aware that I've had it, and when they come over to visit, they never meet my eyes when they are talking to me. Their eyes are right on breast level. They ask me a hundred questions about how it feels. What does it feel like inside? How does it feel to touch? I'll say, "Why don't you touch my breasts and see?" I don't ever push. They always want to.

How have your friends reacted to your breast cancer and breast reconstruction?

It took my friends a long time to ask me if my breasts look right. I said, "They are beautiful; you ought to see them." My support group made it easy to do show and tell. I touched other women's reconstructed breasts before mine were ever finished. I knew what they felt like, I knew what they looked like. That was really important to me to know beforehand what it was going to feel like.

When my mom had her breast reconstruction, her friends thought she was ridiculous and vain. After all, she was 72. Since then three of her friends have had mastectomies, and now they want to touch and feel and see her breasts because they are considering reconstruction. These women are all in their late sixties or early seventies, but they see how great it's been for her.

Did your plastic surgeon meet your needs? Could he have been more responsive?

When you are dealing with somebody on a very busy time schedule, you have to come prepared with questions written down or so well implanted in your head that you don't walk out and say, "Oh, I wanted to ask him this." My plastic surgeon hung the moon as far as I am concerned. He is probably the most caring man I've ever been around. He was responsive, but I wish he would slow down a little. He is in and out. He moves like a butterfly. Although all my needs were met, I would like him to sit down in a chair when he comes into my room. I would like him to talk to me after he has examined my breasts. I did learn to express these feelings to him. I would say, "I didn't get my money's worth yet; sit down, I want to talk." I didn't want small talk; I know his time is valuable, but I want to be able to express my concerns, to let him know when my breasts are uncomfortable.

It has been a bit more difficult for my mother to communicate with him. I would send her there with a list. Sometimes I went with her because I'm more assertive than she is and I would say, "Here's your list of questions; make sure he listens to them before you leave." Or I would come in with her. Some people are intimidated by doctors. And you can't be. You are paying their bills. You have a right to decide what's going to be done with your body. You have a right to tell your doctors how you are feeling about things and expect them to respond to that.

What advice would you like to give to other women about breast reconstruction?

Most people think reconstruction is just going to be more surgery. But it is different. It is uplifting, upbeat; it's the healing process. You're back looking like you did. Don't let the threat of cancer stop you from doing it. I think people are so afraid once they have cancer that they worry that reconstruction is just an extension of their illness and it's not; it heals you. Cancer is terrifying; it is horrifying and I will live with that every day. Wondering what's going to happen next. But reconstruction is nonthreatening. It is a rebuilding process. Although I was a whole person without my breasts, reconstruction restored me physically to the person I was.

LIBBY: I WOULD NOT BE DISFIGURED!

"I just wanted boobs! I couldn't walk around with a 36C breast on one side and a flat chest on the other. It was inconceivable to me to do that. I had augmentation years ago and it turned out very nice. I am a nurse, a professional, and there was no question in my mind that I would have breast reconstruction so I would not be disfigured." This explanation was given to me by Libby for why she opted for immediate breast reconstruction with tissue expansion and a latissimus dorsi (back flap) reconstruction after her breast cancer was discovered.

Libby is married and has a 16-year-old daughter. She has light brown, curly hair and wears glasses, which lend an air of seriousness to her demeanor. Her carriage is very erect, which I would later learn is partly from her effort to counteract her shoulder falling forward as a result of her transferred back muscle. She had been in nursing for over 20 years; yet she found that she had as many misconceptions about breast cancer as people far less familiar with medicine. She was fortunate, however, in having access at her own hospital to the best possible care from people who knew her and took a personal interest. Even so, she took the time to investigate the different reconstructive options before making a final choice.

Libby is an intelligent woman with a sense of self-confidence and self-assurance. She describes herself as an "involved person who always wants to know more." She is 5 feet 8 inches tall and laughingly admits that "she sees herself as a tall, slender person and probably always will even if she really turns out to be a tall, dumpy person." When she found out she had breast cancer, she was not going to let this disease rob her of her positive body image. She drew on all of the resources she had available, chose the best plastic surgeon to perform her breast reconstruction, and now, 2 years later, is ready to share her knowledge about what she learned in her experience with breast cancer and breast reconstruction.

How did you discover your breast cancer?

I have a history of fibrocystic breasts. For years my breasts would get sore at the end of my monthly cycle. I used to think one day I would

have a prophylactic mastectomy and implant inserted so I would never have to worry about getting cancer, but I never did. Even so, I
was always careful about checking my breasts. But you get lax with
BSE because of so many lumps and tough spots. A year ago, as I was
lying in bed, my hand fell across my chest and my ring finger fell on a
spot right below my rib in the middle of my chest, not in a spot that I
perceived as being breast tissue, but high on my chest. I felt a lump
there; I sat up, put a finger on both sides of it, and could palpate the
edges. I went downstairs and had my husband feel it. I said, "That's a
lump; it could be cancer." I called an oncology surgeon the next morning. He examined me that day and told me I had a 50/50 chance that
the lump was cancerous. In my mind I knew when I felt it that it
probably was.

Did your surgeon give you a choice between lumpectomy and irradiation and mastectomy and reconstruction? Which did you choose and why?

The surgeon was blunt; he said we're going to have to make some
decisions. We need to do a biopsy to see what this is. After the biopsy, if it is cancer, we will need to decide what to do. We can do a
lumpectomy; I will make an incision right over the lump and remove
it. This will require follow-up radiation therapy. Or you can have a
modified radical mastectomy with immediate reconstruction. I will
send you to see one of the plastic surgeons I work with. I must tell
you that right now the survival statistics are equal for these different
therapies.

It was all moving very quickly. I had a mammogram done, but my
lump was so high that it was hard to get enough breast tissue to get a
picture of it. By the time we did the biopsy I had to know what I
wanted to do and what I wanted to do as follow-up because it would
make a difference as to how he would cut my chest. I had an appointment with the plastic surgeon and he thought he could do reconstruction at the same time. Then it was a decision as to whether to do
lumpectomy or mastectomy with immediate reconstruction. I called
another oncologic surgeon and asked her opinion. She said that she
was seeing people who had lumpectomy with irradiation come back
with cancer in the same breast. She felt that I was just too young, in my
early forties, to have a time bomb in my chest. She had seen reconstruction and it was good; she recommended that I get rid of it. That
really fit with my surgical background. If it offends you, get rid of it. If

I'm going to have a part of my body that's attacking me, then I want it gone. What she said sounded sensible. So I decided to have the mastectomy with immediate breast reconstruction.

How did you react to the possibility of having breast cancer?

I was under a lot of stress. Another girl in my office had discovered a lump and had already had a mastectomy. Then a third lady in our office developed breast cancer. So out of 35 women in one department three of us had breast cancer. My boss's sister, my age, died 2 weeks earlier from breast cancer. It was as if someone sprinkled breast cancer dust all over and we were caught in the spray.

Why did you decide to have breast reconstruction?

I did not want to be a victim. I wanted to be in control of this whole process to the best of my ability. By getting the reconstruction I was more in control of my own sense of self. The plastic surgeon I went to gave me a book of pictures of patients who had breast reconstruction. I looked at the pictures and thought there's really little difference between their breasts no matter how they were reconstructed—whether a TRAM, a latissimus dorsi flap, or an implant. I would be foolish not to do this. I had augmentation years ago by another plastic surgeon, so I was already familiar with breast surgery. It turned out really nice. I just wanted boobs. I would not be disfigured. There was no question in my mind. And if I could do it immediately, as opposed to having a second surgery, then why not?

Did your plastic surgeon explain all of the reconstruction options? What type of reconstructive approach did you chose?

My breast was too big for an implant just under the muscle unless I had a breast alteration on the other side. My friends said, "Oh you can have a tummy tuck and do this all at the same time." But I was too thin for the TRAM, so that was not an option. I don't think I would have opted for that anyhow. My best option was a latissimus dorsi flap with tissue expansion. My plastic surgeon thought he could get good balance with a flap.

Are you happy you had immediate reconstruction?

Yes, it made this experience a whole lot easier to deal with. I came back similar to, although not exactly the same as the way I left. I didn't have to deal with the idea of having cancer and disfigurement and the potential of chemotherapy and my hair falling out. I mean, "Why don't you just cut off my arms, too, or give me a scar around my face?"

Did you experience much pain from your mastectomy and immediate reconstruction?

There was remarkably little pain. I was tight. They didn't want me to lift my arm higher than elbow or shoulder height. I was afraid that I would have a lot of pain. So I had them hook up a PCA pump after my surgery. That's a pump that is attached to a jug of morphine; every time you hit the pump, you get a little dose, just enough to keep you comfortable as opposed to getting a shot in your hip, which gives you zonk time for 20 minutes to 2 hours until it wears off and you are uncomfortable for another hour until it is time to get your medication. I'm also very sensitive to narcotics and a little bit goes a long way for me. I only used the PCA pump three times after surgery and then I switched to Tylenol.

I also did not have difficulty moving around. It isn't like the TRAM flap where your abdominal muscles are cut and you can't get in and out of bed easily. I could do anything. I had drainage tubes coming from my donor sites and I think I had two coming from my side; one was from the breast tissue somewhere up in the reconstructive site. I could get in and out of the tub with no problem to take a bath, but I couldn't take a shower.

What was your reaction to your breast reconstruction when you woke after your surgery?

I looked down to see what I looked like, and I was pleased with the immediate picture of this little stretchy thing holding my gauze in place. I was round on both sides. I had a new baby boob and it was nice looking; I flashed everybody. I didn't have time to incorporate it as part of me yet. It was something new they had built on me. I showed everybody; I really think women need to see this. People don't know what this looks like; if they could see it, they wouldn't be so frightened of it.

How did your breasts look and feel after your reconstruction? Did you have any surprises?

When they tunnel under your armpit to drape this tissue into your chest, it leaves a roll of tissue under your arm that resembles a rolled-up washcloth. When I put my arm straight down, it hung forward so it would miss the bulging tissue under my arm. My shoulder fell forward and I didn't like that. I asked the resident why my shoulder was forward. He said it was because the latissimus dorsi muscle had been moved; when it's in its normal position, it pulls your shoulder back. I was constantly having to remind myself to pull my shoulder back. Now I just remember to try and use other muscles to pull my shoulder back.

Also the roll of tissue under my arm was an annoyance. Fortunately, that tissue atrophies and weeks later I realized I wasn't going to have to live with this huge lump under my armpit. It goes away. Now my arm lays flat at my side the way I would want it to.

I didn't expect a roll of back tissue under my armpit, I didn't expect my shoulder to fall forward, and I didn't expect the suture line on my side to be as tight as it is. It felt like somebody had taken a sewing machine and sewn a seam right into my chest wall. It did not move at all. There was no give. And it wasn't until I asked one of the plastic surgeons that he told me that it would become looser as I exercised. I didn't know those things. If I had, I think it would have been easier for me. Also nobody ever told me when I should start exercising. I was told not to exercise because of all that drainage. Just don't move your arm. I probably did a whole lot more than I should have.

When were you able to resume your normal activities? Did you experience any problems after surgery?

I stayed home from work for 2 weeks. Most people probably stay longer, but I was having problems with drainage and was having to drive 10 miles to the hospital to be drained; it seemed stupid to make this drive when I could just mosey over across the street and be working. So I came back to work. I was a little tired at first and worked half days for the first week.

I drained a lot after my surgery. I went home on a Monday, and I still had all these tubes and the little Jackson Pratt drains in me that I had to keep measuring and draining. I wondered when the drainage would stop. They took the drainage tubes out on a Wednesday or Friday and it still didn't stop. I had to come in three times a week to be drained; they drained 60, 80, sometimes 100 ml.

Describe the technique that was used for your reconstruction.

They took a big slab of muscle and piece of skin tissue from my back and then tunneled it up under my armpit and laid it across my chest.

Then they connected the skin that was left from the mastectomy to this back skin and placed a tissue expander underneath the transferred muscle and skin.

Did they expand the tissue? If so, when did the expansion process begin?

Approximately 2 months after my surgery they started adding saline solution through the port in the expander. I needed tissue expansion because I didn't have enough skin to accommodate a breast that would match my remaining breast. After the surgery, my right reconstructed breast was 34B as compared to my left breast, which was a 36C.

Was the expansion process uncomfortable? Did you have any pain?

I had a sensory nerve removed with my tissue and the whole breast was numb. But when they put the needle in during my first expansion, it really hurt. I'm a fairly stoic individual, but when the nurse pulled that needle out, I thought I would die. I started crying; I was white. They were all concerned about me. I said I can't do this and with that I left. Evidently, they stuck a needle into a nerve. Then they started using Novocaine with the injection; I didn't have another bit of trouble.

What was your primary goal in breast reconstruction? Did you achieve it?

Symmetry. My breasts are perfectly balanced. I wanted to look like I did. And I do. I scar terribly, so I knew I was going to have bad scars. And I do. But I wanted to look good in a bathing suit. I have a pool in my backyard, and people come over. I can't be sitting there in bathing suits that are odd looking because I've had surgery. I wanted to be able to wear whatever I wanted to wear, and I also wanted to jiggle. And I do. So it worked out just fine.

Where are your scars placed and what do they look like?

My scar starts about 4 inches under my armpit and then it curves down about 2 inches above my waist. I'm a very tall lady. But it's about 10 inches long and it's curved toward the front as opposed to the back. It's totally hidden by my bathing suit. It's also hidden by any backless dress. I also have a scar on my breast that's like a keyhole with two ends; it's an elliptic piece with two straight lines on either end.

Can you wear the same clothes now or have you changed the way you dress?

I've not had to change anything. That was the nice thing about this whole thing. I didn't have to do anything different. I've always been tall and thin. I weigh around 140 pounds now at 5 feet 8 inches, and this is the most I've ever weighed in my life. I got the best bang for the buck actually. I just can't tell you how good it felt not to bother with a prosthesis and all that. I didn't have to sew a pocket in my bra. I didn't worry about facing the embarrassment when you jump in the pool and the damn prosthesis floats to the surface because you didn't get your little pocket in perfectly. I didn't have to sew elastic pieces onto my bra to prevent my bra sliding up over my suture lines when I raised my arm. I have enough to deal with without having to worry about how to get dressed in the morning, is everything hooked properly, is it going to shift or move, am I going to end up with a boob under my armpit. I don't want to have to deal with those kinds of issues.

Is your reconstruction complete? Are any adjustments still needed?

I'm not done. I haven't had the final implant yet. I still have the expander. I haven't had time because of my job. I only stayed out 2 weeks when I had the big surgery; this time I want to stay out 2 weeks for the small surgery to get a real rest. My plastic surgeon said that when you have larger breasts you probably ought to do this slowly and take your time.

Do you have any concerns about breast implants?

I had implants before, so I have an idea of what to expect. I didn't form a capsule the last time and so I said why should I this time. My prior surgeon gave me the name of the implant that was used last time. I thought, well, I'll just have him special order it because it worked the last time. I wasn't terribly worried, knowing how the media is. They want all the hype so you'll buy their magazines. I thought I would wait for the dust to settle before I could find out more. I really trust that my doctors will not willingly expose me to something dangerous. So I thought I would just wait and see what the current knowledge is when I go to have this expander taken out and have the final implant put in.*

*Since this interview was conducted, Libby has had her expander removed and replaced with a postoperatively adjustable expander implant during an outpatient procedure. This implant has a small valve in the underarm region to permit future adjustments and to provide long-term control over her breast size.

Why are you having the nipple-areola reconstruction? When will it be reconstructed?

I told my husband that maybe I won't get a nipple put on. He says, "You can't go to bed without straightening the sheets. Do you really think in the long run you're going to be satisfied with one breast without a nipple?" So I'm going to have that done and just be finished. Get total closure to the whole thing. I also want it for symmetry. I've got a good-size nipple on one side and it leaves an impression; the other side is just smooth. My nipple will be done when my permanent implant is put in.

How long did it take to incorporate your new breast into your body image?

It took a couple of months. I was so pleased to be symmetric and to be comfortable. But it wasn't incorporated until I started wearing my own bras again. Then I felt back to normal.

Was your plastic surgeon responsive to your needs? How could he have helped you more?

One of the drawbacks to being at the university center is that many times the people that you are dealing with are teaching around the country. That was true of my particular surgeon. He did the surgery on a Friday night and I didn't see him again. I was taken care of by an extremely nice resident. Since that time I have seen him, but just briefly.

I guess if I had needed him more, I probably could have gotten to him. But I was able to get to the resident, and he was everything that you would want. He was focused on me and would answer any question no matter how ridiculous it seemed; he was just so good that I didn't feel the need to go any further. I felt very much supported by him.

The master surgeon, the designer, gave me the benefit of his design, but the follow-up I got from the resident. I didn't feel lacking.

What questions do women need to have answered when they are considering reconstruction?

You get information in small portions. People need to see the whole picture, even if it's just bullet points so you know what to expect. They need to explain what they mean when they say they are going to *overexpand* you. Who knows what that means. When my new side got to be equal to my old side, I thought I was done. Then I found out that they were going to put 300 cc more in this sucker. It turned out to be like a watermelon on one side of me. It was huge and it was heavy. I didn't understand that there were other considerations, like having your breasts sag the same. They told me not to wear a bra for a month to let this tissue hang so it would have the same sag as the normal side. After a month of not wearing a bra I had equal droop and equal projection; then I said, now can we take some out? It all made sense, but it would have been better if they had explained it all to me initially.

MARCY: YOU CAN'T TELL THE DIFFERENCE

"It's amazing! If you didn't know that I had breast cancer and reconstruction, you could never tell. Just look at these pictures; aren't they great? My husband is so proud; he shows them to everyone." Slim and pretty, Marcy's face is framed by bobbed dark hair. This former teacher is married with two small children. She blushes as she pulls several photographs out of her purse and hands them to me. Her delight in her restored appearance is infectious. "These were taken of me wearing the same bathing suit before my mastectomy and after my reconstruction and you just can't tell the difference. If anything, I look better now."

Marcy's breast cancer was discovered on her first mammogram, right before her fortieth birthday. Fortunately, it was in its earliest stages, making her prognosis excellent. Nevertheless, decisions about which treatment approach was best for her were not always easy, even though her husband, a cancer specialist, helped her to sort through her options and find the best care possible. She is well informed and the type of woman who wants to know all the facts. Because of her husband's profession, she looks to physicians for expertise and sound advice and does not come to the doctor-patient relationship with the trepidation that many others exhibit. Even so, Marcy frequently found herself puzzled and needing more information and direction in selecting the best treatment for her breast cancer and the right reconstructive technique. Her decision-making process was further complicated by the FDA's moratorium on silicone gel implants right after her mastectomy. She and her husband had already decided that silicone gel–filled breast implants would give her the best breast reconstruction and would also provide the augmentation to make her breasts appear balanced. They had done their research, were not concerned about the media stories about implants, and wanted to go ahead and have the silicone gel–filled implants despite the moratorium. Marcy offered to sign a release, but her plastic surgeon said he had to abide by the FDA moratorium. As one of the women in the "urgent need" category subsequently identified by the FDA, she was stymied by the intervention. Now she would have to rethink her decisions.

How did you decide between lumpectomy and mastectomy?

That was frustrating. I kept asking my cancer surgeon what he would recommend. I said, "If it were your wife, what would you do?" All he could say was, "I can't tell you what to do."

I realize it is hard, especially for male doctors, because they feel that breast cancer is a uniquely female problem and they don't know what to make of it. But patients come to doctors for their expertise. I hope that doctors haven't become afraid to recommend a course of action for their patients or to say that mastectomy can cure. I wanted some direction and I persisted in asking him what he would do. He said, "I can't tell you what to do." I protested, "I *want* you to tell me what is the best thing to do. That's why I am here; you are the expert. You should know." We kept going around in circles; it was frustrating. He said, "You have to do what you feel is right. You have to make that decision." But I was coming to him for an answer, and he wasn't willing to give me one. He said, "You can have a mastectomy or a lumpectomy, or at this point you can choose to do nothing. We can watch it; it is so early."

I said, "Does mastectomy guarantee me better results then a lumpectomy?" He replied noncommittally, "It's an option many people have chosen and they have done well after a 5-year follow-up, but in 10 years, I don't know. We don't have long-term results; we don't have 15- to 20-year studies on lumpectomy. We do on mastectomy." I saw another cancer surgeon for another opinion and he said the same thing.

It was frustrating not to be able to have my doctor tell me what was the best course of action. There is so much controversy surrounding breast cancer, so many different options. I wanted him to say, "This is the way to go." But I guess maybe they really don't know.

Are you happy with your choice of mastectomy over lumpectomy?

Yes. I am very happy with my decision. I would do the same thing tomorrow. Knowing that I could have the reconstruction made my decision for mastectomy that much easier. It took away any anxiety. The only anxiety that I experienced throughout the whole ordeal was when I had to wait those 2 days in the hospital before I got the final path report back. My cancer is so early that it would have been 4 to 5 years before I would have felt it on self-exam.

I would recommend what I did to anyone. After the mastectomy they were able to study the whole breast, and they discovered that the cancer was multifocal. Had I had the lumpectomy they would not have gotten every little area of cancer. For me, the procedure I had was the right one. Of course, I didn't know that 100% until after it had been done. But on hindsight it was. Even before that I knew in my heart that a mastectomy was the best choice for me. I could not put more value on saving a breast than on saving my life. Long-term survival is important; I want to watch my children grow.

Why did you seek breast reconstruction?

It is comparable to someone losing a limb and wearing an artificial leg, losing an eye and wanting a glass eye. Your breast is a part of you. It doesn't define who you are sexually, but you want it back. You want to be whole.

Sexual feelings between my husband and me were fine following the mastectomy and prior to reconstruction. I didn't have reconstruction to feel sexy, just to feel complete, to be *normal*, not necessarily bigger or better than before. I wanted to dress normally . . . to not be concerned with what I could wear and what I couldn't. I felt I was young, just 40, and I wanted to look normal for me, for my husband, and for my children.

How did you learn about breast reconstruction?

One of my husband's scrub nurses gave him your book to give to me. It turns out she had a double mastectomy and reconstruction. My husband was astounded. He said, "I operate with you every day. I never noticed anything different and you never mentioned it." She said, "Well, I don't talk about it, but this book was a tremendous help to me. I thought it would be a big help to your wife."

She talked to me about her experience. She had some complications but still had a positive experience. Her plastic surgeon and the whole team continued to work with her till everything was okay. Now she is finished and she looks wonderful. She is very happy and has since married.

I came home that weekend and read the book from cover to cover and said, "Thank goodness, everything is going to be fine." That next week I went in to have my mastectomy and never once gave it a second thought or felt that I was making a mistake.

How did you select your plastic surgeon?

He was recommended by people we knew in the community and by my husband's surgical colleagues. When my husband found out I had breast cancer, he got on the phone and called everyone he knew and asked, "Where should we go? Who is the best?" They said we had the best right here. It made it easy. He called people at Mayo Clinic, people here, friends at Stanford, and he kept hearing the same thing. My surgeon also recommended him, and we had friends of relatives who knew people who went to this plastic surgeon for reconstruction. We kept hearing his name so often that it gave us a feeling of confidence and security. We never thought to look elsewhere.

Have you been happy with your plastic surgeon? Was he responsive to your needs?

He was just wonderful. He went over the different reconstructive options with me, talked about immediate vs. delayed reconstruction, answered my questions, and was very reassuring. He was confident in his ability to reconstruct my breast, and he took away any fear or doubt that I had. His staff was also wonderful, especially the nurses. When I have problems, I call. It has been a terrific experience.

Why did you decide not to have immediate reconstruction?

My surgeon and plastic surgeon were at two different hospitals, and I felt comfortable with the surgeon at the local hospital; it was where my husband practiced. We were well known there. I wasn't sure what operation I would choose for reconstruction, but I knew I wanted to go ahead with the mastectomy. I decided to get that out of the way and then take time to read the book, talk to other people, and decide what type of reconstruction I wanted. The plastic surgeon also gave me names of former patients and suggested that I call them and talk to them.

Did your plastic surgeon and general surgeon coordinate your care even though they were at different hospitals?

Yes. They spoke before my cancer surgery, and my plastic surgeon told my cancer surgeon what type of incision would be best for the reconstruction and how much skin to leave.

What type of reconstructive operation did you choose?

I considered all of the options and decided on tissue expansion with simple reconstruction with an expander implant. During my recovery from the mastectomy I met a woman who had the abdominal flap. She was unhappy with it. She had her reconstructive surgery a number of years ago, and I am sure it was not the state-of-the art operation it is today. Even so, she said that she still can't sit up straight in bed; she can't bend over and pick up a basket of laundry. She has never felt right; she has a very uncomfortable feeling in her midchest area where she thinks the flap was turned. She said that if she had it to do over she would not have such an elaborate operation. It was a huge surgery with a very long recovery period. I didn't want anything that dramatic. Also, I wasn't rebuilding a huge breast. I didn't need a lot of tissue. I am not that large physically, so I didn't feel they would have a whole lot to work with anyway. So I eliminated the possibility of an abdominal flap.

We talked about the latissimus dorsi back flap. Implants are often used along with that flap. I rejected that option because I figured why subject myself to a major flap procedure with additional scars on my back. I decided I might as well just go with the simple implant.

My husband and I came back to see the plastic surgeon with our decision and said, "What do you think of this; would an implant be good?" He said he thought it would work in my situation.

Why did you decide that implant reconstruction was the right choice for you?

I wanted reconstruction; I wanted the breast back, but I didn't want to go through a horrendous process to get it. I wanted the simplest, easiest operation. I wanted a nice cosmetic effect with the least amount of trauma and disruption in my life. My children are small, 7 and 11; I wanted as little time away from them as possible.

Did you have any surgery on your opposite breast?

Yes, I had an augmentation with a textured saline implant. We decided to do a small implant on the other side to give that breast the same type of lift and look; plus, since I was going to have implants, I thought it would be a nice bonus if I could go a little bit bigger than I was. My plastic surgeon thought he could do that without any trouble. So he put an expander on the left at the mastectomy site and a saline implant on the right side for augmentation.

Augmentation was not what I initially requested, however. Originally I wanted to have a prophylactic mastectomy with an implant on the other side. But my surgeon said that the type of cancer I have is not normally bilateral and they discouraged it. Even so, I knew by just having breast cancer in one breast you have a higher risk of getting it in the other breast, and why would I want that? Why not just do both? But all the doctors said that I was being a little too reactionary because of my type of cancer and the fact that I had no family history. I was not in a high-risk group. I thought, well, if it happened once why would it not happen again. They told me yearly mammograms would be able to catch it soon enough. They said that the pocket for the implant would be already made and it would be a very easy procedure. So I didn't have a prophylactic mastectomy and implant. Instead, I just had an augmentation with an implant. I still think that the prophylactic mastectomy would have given me more peace of mind.

Describe your hospitalization.

I went in the hospital at 6:00 A.M. and had the procedure done at 8:00 A.M.; I went home at 9:00 the next morning.

Did you have much pain after reconstruction? How did it compare to the pain you experienced after your mastectomy?

The mastectomy was a breeze. I was in the hospital for three nights, and when I went home I felt almost no pain. I was back doing almost everything I wanted to do within 10 days. I had no complications. It went great. I wanted to start reconstruction as soon as possible. We waited 3 months because my plastic surgeon felt that would allow enough time for my tissues to heal.

I had a lot of pain after reconstruction. That was surprising. None of the patients I spoke with mentioned that reconstruction was very painful. When I came for the preoperative workup, I was asked if I generally have a lot of pain. I said no; generally I have a very high tolerance for pain. With the mastectomy, I was pain-free after the first day and then and I took Tylenol. So they didn't order any special pain medicine for me, and I agreed with that decision. But I was wrong. I can remember waking up in recovery and not being able to move, not being able to take a breath. I was afraid to breathe. I think I was hyperventilating. The nurse kept telling me to calm down. If anyone touched me, I just gasped. I felt a tremendous burning sensation in my chest. I would try to take a breath and it would hurt. Both sides hurt. When the nurse asked if I would like something for pain. I said, "Yes!" She said, "They have nothing ordered for you. They didn't think you would need it." That was my fault. It was very painful and I don't know why.

I talked to people who didn't think it was that painful. When I spoke with people later, they admitted that it might have hurt at first, but they really didn't remember anymore, and since I didn't seem to think it would hurt, they hadn't wanted to tell me any different. I thought, oh thanks!

They gave me Darvocet when I went home and that took care of the pain, but it would wear off. It took about 4 days before I felt better. I could move around, but trying to sit up or turn over in bed was painful.

Did you experience much swelling with the reconstruction and augmentation?

Yes, after my surgery, I was huge and swollen. At first I was petrified. "Oh, my God, I've gone overboard. What am I going to do. This is terrible." My husband says, "This is great." I was like, oh, "This is too much." But then, the swelling started going down and my reaction was, "No, stop—it's going too low—it's not going to be big enough." I went from one extreme to another, but then it leveled out and was fine. It is a nice size, although every time I get expanded I am off balance again because they overexpand and overstretch the skin. They do this so that when the permanent implant is in, the breast will fall naturally and appear more normal.

Did you have much bruising after your reconstruction?

The breasts themselves were not black and blue. But on my side and across the front of my chest there was a little bruising; it healed fairly quickly.

How long before you could return to normal activity?

After 7 days I started feeling better and I wanted to drive; they said I could try it if I felt up to it. We have a Ford Explorer and the steering wheel was hard to turn with no power steering, but I wanted to drive. I wanted to get back on the road, pick up my children. I knew when I left my driveway it was a mistake. We have a curve in the driveway, and I could barely make the turn. I couldn't turn the wheel. As long as I was going straight I was fine; a turn really hurt. I continued on and then got back home; I didn't drive for another week. I think I set myself back a few days. After the second week I could do just about anything. I don't do aerobics or jog; I am not big into physical activity right now, so I wasn't anxious to get back to something strenuous. For me, normal activity was just regular housework, driving, walking, and riding my bicycle.

Do you have any restrictions now?

No. We went to Florida 3 months after my surgery, and I tried to swim; that was difficult because it was hard to stretch. But everything else I can do fine.

What type of implants did you choose? How did you make that choice?

When I had my mastectomy and we made our reconstruction decision, I wanted to have the silicone gel implants. I didn't have any objections to those; I had never heard any horrible stories involving implants. I knew there was a risk of contracture; they could get hard and might need to be replaced. But I felt that any time you deal with a foreign object in the body there is a chance of a problem. Every person's body is going to react differently. I didn't worry about silicone gel implants.

Did your plastic surgeon get your informed consent before implant surgery? Did he explain potential problems and complications?

My plastic surgeon explained all the different types of implants. We asked him what he preferred, what he had used most often, and how his patients had done with them. Then we spoke to patients who had this implant surgery. They were all very happy with the results. I didn't talk to a single woman who was unhappy with her silicone gel implants. They were all very pleased, not only with how they looked but how they felt, every aspect. So I was fully intending to have silicone gel–filled implants, one for augmentation and one for reconstruction after the tissue expander was removed.

Were you able to have the silicone gel–filled implants you desired?

No. While I was healing, getting ready to begin the reconstruction, the FDA controversy erupted. When I came back to have my surgery, I asked if I could still have the silicone gel implants if I signed a waiver or release. My plastic surgeon said no; he was going along with the moratorium and he would use a textured-surface saline-filled implant instead.

Were you unhappy when you couldn't have the silicone gel implant?

I don't know if I would describe it as unhappiness. I just felt that my choices had been limited. I felt that I didn't have a decision. I wanted to go ahead with the reconstruction. I wouldn't consider a flap procedure as an alternative; that would have been out of the question. When the silicone gel implants were ruled out, a saline implant was all I could have. My plastic surgeon felt this would be fine for me. If I couldn't have had the saline implant, I would have been very unhappy.

Did all of the media attention on implants cause you concern?

No, not really. I know many women came forward with stories that their breast implants caused this and that problem. But I didn't necessarily believe all that I heard. All of those problems just can't suddenly surface. Sometimes, when things happen, people need to find a scapegoat, somewhere to place the blame. For many of these women, it was simple to just blame implants for all of their problems. I read the information that was available to me.

Obviously there is a risk when you have an implant, any kind of implant; you don't know how your body is going to react to the foreign material. But you face risks with any operation. I felt that if I had a complication I would get it fixed. I would do it again; I would keep trying. But I wasn't going to panic just because of television or newspaper reports. That's just hype. Tomorrow it will be another danger. I talked to so many people who were totally pleased with their silicone gel implants, and we asked the plastic surgeon if his patients had serious problems or were upset with their implants. We trusted him; he is an expert. You have to have faith in your doctors, particularly when you have cancer. I trust him. People come to see him from all over the United States; surely he knows what he is talking about. I certainly would believe him more than I would believe any sensational talk show. Where's the science in that?

My plastic surgeon said that in his experience most patients had been pleased with their implants. He didn't whitewash the issue or try to sell me. He told me that some patients have problems and explained what they were. I could accept that. Everyone reacts differently to implants, to medications. Some people have problems with penicillin. Anyway, I trust his judgment. I don't think that a doctor of his reputation would recommend something for me that he felt was bad. He is not a plastic surgeon out in the private sector doing this for big bucks. He is at a university hospital, a teaching hospital. I do not think he would do anything that was harmful to me or that he felt was injurious. There has to be a level of trust between a patient and her doctor. The news programs did a real disservice to women by attacking that bond and making women fearful.

As a cancer specialist, did your husband have concerns about silicone gel–filled implants?

No, he really didn't. He did investigate them. He called people he knew at the FDA. They felt that in some women there possibly could have been leakage with resulting problems, but they said that there are going to be certain risks and possible complications with any device. We were both willing to accept that. My husband knows about cancer and about implants and he wasn't worried. We both agreed; he understood that I did not want to go through a big operation.

Are you concerned that your breast implants will interfere with mammograms?

No, I asked the doctors and the radiologist; they said that as long as you go to a technician who is experienced in doing mammograms with implants there is no reason to worry.

What type of implant did your plastic surgeon decide to use and how did it differ from the silicone gel–filled implant?

It had the same textured silicone cover but was filled with saltwater instead of silicone gel. I wanted to know if there was a large difference between the two. They explained to me the main difference was how the implants felt; the silicone gel–filled implant feels more natural. I was not primarily concerned with feel; however, my concern was how my breasts were going to look. My plastic surgeon said that the saline implant would not look significantly different from the silicone gel implant. So I said fine. Now, I have a saline implant on the right side where my breast was augmented and an expander implant on my left side for my reconstruction.

How does the saline implant feel?

It feels normal, not to the touch, but when I walk or move. I don't feel like I have an implant. Now, if I touch or palpate it, it feels like a little water balloon, especially on the underside of my breast. It has more "give." If I push on it, it pops right back out like a balloon. On the top or sides my breast feels like it did before. Underneath I can feel a difference.

How does the expander implant feel? How does it differ from the saline implant?

It feels fine. The main difference between my expander and my saline implant is the valve. The expander implant has a small fill valve that is positioned under my arm. I can feel it as a small bump in my underarm area, but it is not a problem. The saline was injected through this valve, and if I need any size adjustments later, these can be made through this valve without my having to undergo another operation. This expander just stays permanently in place, and I am happy with it. It is really a good solution for me because I can have control over my breast size with minimal discomfort.

Have you had any problems?

No problems on the right side with the augmentation. The only problem I had was on the left side with the expander. My incision opened a little bit; it wasn't a serious problem, but we had to delay the tissue expansion for several weeks.

Did your surgeon know why that happened?

After the first expansion, I still had Steri-Strips covering the incision; we didn't take them off and reapply them. When the tissue stretched, my plastic surgeon thinks the expansion process might have caused a tape burn, causing my incision to open. After a few weeks it healed, and then we left all the Steri-Strips off. I have never had another problem.

What happens when you have your tissues expanded? Describe the process.

Oh, it is very easy. They have a device inside of you, and they plug the syringe into this device that hooks up like an IV. Saltwater is injected to expand it. You just lie on the exam table, and they give you whatever quantity they have determined is needed to expand your breast that day. You can feel it gradually dripping in. One time they were going to put a little more in, but it was feeling tight and a little sore, so I asked to stop for the day. I had a busy weekend coming up. It was nice to have that control.

Is tissue expansion painful?

It is a full feeling . . . not painful, just tight every time it is expanded. Then after a few days it gives and then feels normal until the next expansion. I guess the tissues stretch so that they will be ready for the permanent implant. Sometimes I take Tylenol right after it's done, but that is all I have ever needed.

How often was your expander implant inflated? How long did the expansion process take?

My skin was expanded about every 3 weeks. I went to the office and it took about 20 minutes. I had three sessions; then further expansion was delayed because the incision opened up. I started in January and the expansion process was completed by May, so the total process took approximately 4 months.

Why are you going to have nipple-areola reconstruction?

I want my breast to be complete. When we were in Florida, I wore a regular bathing suit. The only time there was a noticeable difference between my breasts was when I came out of the water and was cold, and you could see that I had a nipple on one side and not on the other. I have seen it done on other women and it looks beautiful. Someone described it as "the icing on the cake." If you are going to go this far, why stop? Why not take it through to completion? People who see the pictures think my breast reconstruction is marvelous. I tell them I am a *work in progress*. I am not finished yet. They are very impressed. A lot of women I have talked to who have seen the bathing suit pictures say now we know that if it happens to us we will not be so afraid because we can see what can happen afterwards.

Aesthetically, are you pleased with your breast appearance?

Yes. Here are some pictures of me wearing the same bathing suit before the mastectomy and after the reconstruction. My husband took these to the hospital and showed them to the nurses on the floor who had taken care of me. I was so embarrassed. The results are marvelous. People think I am finished, I am done. They think, my gosh, you look great. My husband is very proud. I am also. My husband feels that if I do not do another thing, I look great. But I'm not finished yet. I want the nipple done.

Does the reconstructed breast have any feeling or sensation? How does it compare to the opposite breast that was augmented?

Sensation is normal in the right breast that had no mastectomy and a simple implant. There is feeling in the left reconstructed breast, but it's blunted. When I push on my left breast, I can feel the pressure but not much sensation.

Is there any sexual feeling or sensitivity?

To be perfectly honest I have avoided sexual contact on the left side; I don't feel right yet. My husband has no problems with it. But I don't feel finished yet. The shape of the breast still needs some adjustment; it is fuller on the top and below. There is no nipple. I still feel we are working on it.

Was your husband supportive? How did he react to the idea of your having breast reconstruction?

He was wonderful. Being a cancer surgeon himself, he understood what we had to face. My husband deals with cancer every day and he has to tell someone they have cancer. The idea of disfigurement never entered into it. The total focus was on the cure.

The minute we found the cancer it was, "We can take care of it," and "If you want, you can have reconstruction." "This isn't the end of the world." He was finding out as much information as he could and as quickly as he could so that we could make the decisions we needed to make.

He supported me all the way and went through the whole learning process with me. I remember one funny incident when my husband and I were looking over the pictures of some patients that the plastic surgeon's nurse was showing us. My husband asked where were the women who had the mastectomies and were re-done? It turned out that was just what we were looking at, but you couldn't tell. It was very reassuring.

It was a learning experience for both of us. Right before I was to have reconstructive surgery one of my plastic surgeon's patients who also had a simple implant reconstruction came to see my husband for a medical problem. As he was taking her history he asked her what other surgeries she had had? When she said that she had a mastectomy and reconstruction, he asked her who her surgeon was and if she was happy. She said she thought he was wonderful. My husband told her that I had just had a mastectomy and was about to have breast reconstruction and she just said, "Well, let me show you!" She was so proud and thrilled with her result. He immediately had her call me on the phone, and she talked to me from his office for 20 minutes, telling me how wonderful everything was, what a positive experience she had, and how terrific my plastic surgeon was. She offered to meet with me and show me how she looked. My husband came home and said, "She looked incredible. She looked wonderful and you would never have known." He said, "I'm a doctor looking and I would never have known. She looked that good."

How have your children reacted to this experience?

My children have been understanding. My daughter had been through open heart surgery, which was far more serious than what I had to undergo. In fact, when she came to see me in the hospital she said, "Mommy, you only have two tubes. This is no big deal." When she was in the hospital, she had tubes everywhere. We have two girls and we were very open with them from the beginning. We said, "Mommy is going to have her breast removed to take away the cancer and disease so I can be healthy and live a long life." We told them that I was going to have reconstruction and explained what that meant; we were going to rebuild the breast. It won't look exactly the same, but it will look very close. They handled it very well. They did not seem afraid or worried. They know their daddy is a doctor and operates on people every day, and so they had confidence that the doctor would make me better and it would be fine. My older daughter's concern was, "Will my friends be able to tell? Will you look different?" Really, I never did look different, and right after the mastectomy surgery I bounced back very, very quickly. The children couldn't tell. They looked when I came home; we took the bandages off and they looked. The only thing my older daughter keeps asking me about the reconstruction is, "Why did you make your breast so big?" I said, honey, I didn't make it that big. I was a 34B. I wanted a slight enhancement and that is what we decided to do. So now I am a little larger, a 36C.

What about this experience would you like to share with other women?

I would like to tell women not to risk their lives to save a breast. I was never very big-breasted. That was never the focus of my feelings of self-worth or femininity. Maybe if it had been I would have felt differently. Not all women feel that way. In fact, I talked to a woman doctor who had breast cancer; her husband also was a doctor and he said mastectomy was the way to go. She said she couldn't or wouldn't have a mastectomy. She couldn't do it; it would be very difficult. I said, "But Susan, when you are faced with the statistics?" She said, "I know but I don't think I could deal with it emotionally." Even her husband admitted that her breasts had always been very important to her and that is why she couldn't face breast loss. I never had that feeling. Anyway, with what can be accomplished with reconstruction today, I would not take the risk of keeping my breast; I would not want to live day in and day out worrying if the cancer is still there? Is it coming back? I would not want to make cancer an everyday part of my life. I would want to take the form of treatment that would be the most definitive and proceed with my life.

If you had to do it over, would you have reconstruction again? Would you have the same kind of reconstructive approach?

I would do exactly the same thing. It was the right approach for me and I am very happy with what I did.

Did knowledge about reconstruction make it easier for you to cope with your cancer surgery?

Knowing that it could be fixed made all the difference. Knowing that, my attitude was let's get on with it—take care of it, get rid of it, and move ahead as opposed to, "Oh no, this is terrible." I went to my mastectomy almost jubilant; I wanted to get this breast off and rebuilt again. So I coped pretty well because I knew I could have reconstruction. I could do something.

It's the feeling of powerlessness that gets you. Around Christmas we were having company and a string of Christmas lights went off on the tree. When that happened, I just lost it. I decompensated; I panicked. My sister was astounded. She laughed at me and said, "You had cancer, had a mastectomy, and you never said anything. Now you are getting upset about your Christmas tree?" Well, this was important because I couldn't fix it. I had people coming and I couldn't get the lights on. But my breast I could fix. I could take care of it. That made all the difference. I was in control.

How have your friends reacted to your breast reconstruction?

They didn't realize how easily breast reconstruction could be accomplished. They never expected me to continue to look so normal throughout the whole procedure, even with the expansion. My friends have just been amazed. They think breast reconstruction is marvelous. Knowing about my experience and about the possibility of breast reconstruction has done wonders for their peace of mind. Now they know that should it happen to them it is not the end of the world.

DENISE: A JOYOUS ADVENTURE IN REBUILDING!

Talking with Denise is like visiting with an old friend, no need for small talk—just an immediate connection. She is effusive and friendly and virtually embraces you with the warmth and generosity of her personality. Her soft, gentle voice seems in keeping with her loving, yet unassuming manner.

Denise is a slender brunette of 58 years; she has been married for 24 years and works full-time as manager of a cosmetics and fragrance department at one of the exclusive stores in the city. Despite her cosmetics career, she wears little makeup, and her long hair is simply pulled back from her face and tied at her neck. Her tailored dress reveals an excellent trim figure.

Denise has a history of severe problems with fibrocystic breasts and has been under close physician surveillance since she was 19 years old. Breast self-examination has always been difficult because, as she explains, "I had so many lumps that I really didn't know what I was checking." Thirteen years ago, during one of Denise's periodic breast examinations, her doctor discovered a suspicious breast lump. He was "98% sure that it was nothing" but sent her to a surgeon for a biopsy. The results of the biopsy proved otherwise. She had breast cancer. It was the type of cancer that usually occurs as a mirror image; most likely it would show up on the other side. She required a mastectomy on one side, and her other breast would need to be carefully watched in the future. "Unfortunately," she admits, "I didn't know enough at that time to tell the surgeon to just go ahead and do the other side." Denise was emotionally unprepared for this diagnosis and was traumatized by the possibility of breast loss. Her doctor convinced her, however, that she had no choice. Several days later she had a modified radical mastectomy, and because she desired breast reconstruction, she had her surgeon leave skin flaps to allow for this eventuality.

Once recovered from her mastectomy, Denise approached her doctors about the possibility of reconstruction. Neither of them recommended it. And so over the next 13 years Denise continued to have periodic biopsies and mammograms for suspicious lumps. During this time she did not forsake her desire for breast restoration and never stopped urging her doctors to allow her to pursue this option. As Denise explained, "Although I had learned to live with my mastectomy, I still didn't feel right. Something was missing. I love being a woman. I love being feminine. That had been taken away from me, and I wanted it back."

Then Denise's surgeon suffered a stroke and she was referred to another surgeon, an expert in breast cancer and breast surgery. She once again broached the topic of breast reconstruction; only this time she got a different answer. This surgeon considered her a strong candidate for breast reconstruction and also recommended a prophylactic mastectomy and reconstruction on her opposite side. Denise was ecstatic; this was the news that she had been anticipating for 13 years. Not only could she get her breast rebuilt, but she could get the worrisome precancerous tissue removed from her other breast and have it reconstructed at the same time.

Denise's husband was not enthusiastic about breast reconstruction. He worried about her health and possible risks from the surgery. He had to be convinced that reconstruction was safe and that the prophylactic mastectomy might even save her from future breast cancer. Then, with her husband fully supportive, Denise embarked on what she describes as "a joyous adventure in rebuilding." She had a prophylactic mastectomy on her right breast, and then both breasts were reconstructed with temporary tissue expanders, which were later replaced with permanent implants. Denise still glows with enthusiasm as she recounts how this experience has virtually transformed her life.

What was your response when your surgeon recommended that you could have breast reconstruction after years of waiting?

I yearned for breast reconstruction for over 13 years. When I had my original mastectomy, I went in with the idea that one day I would be able to have reconstruction. So when they operated on me, they left the flaps. My surgeon's attitude about reconstruction was a letdown. The week after my mastectomy he said that I was doing great and healing wonderfully. So I came back in another week and I asked, "What about my reconstruction?" He was evasive. He asked if I had a plastic surgeon. I said "No, I was hoping he would refer someone." He said he wanted me to wait until I healed. A couple of months later I went back and asked him how long would it be before I could have my reconstruction done. He told me he wasn't recommending it for me because of the kind of malignancy that I had. I accepted his decision, but I would always look and see those flaps and think, "Well, maybe one day." Even though I was getting older, I always had it in the back of my mind. When my new surgeon said I could have it, it was like a dream fulfilled. I was ecstatic.

Why did your husband object to breast reconstruction? How did you convince him?

I have a wonderful husband. He was worried about me. He said, "Denise, I do not want to see you go through surgery again. Breasts are nothing but a bunch of trouble anyway. I do not want you to have reconstruction." But I wouldn't let go of it. I said, "Bill, this is really important to me. I want you to be a part of it and I want you to be happy with it." He didn't even want to come with me to talk to the surgeon until I told him that the surgeon had said that the prophylactic mastectomy might even save my life. Then he agreed to go with me to see the surgeon and later to see the plastic surgeon.

What happened during your consultation with the plastic surgeon? Did he answer your questions? Did he calm your husband's fears?

We consulted with the plastic surgeon several months after we talked to my general surgeon. I was anxious to get going. Both Bill and I liked the plastic surgeon immediately and that helped to raise Bill's comfort level. At the beginning of our consultation the plastic surgeon asked me a lot of questions and Bill and he talked. He told me about the different reconstructive options, and then he took me in and examined me. He took pictures of me. I thought, "What is this all about? Why is he taking pictures of me?" Now I know it was for his records, but at first, I thought, "Oh, my word, what is he doing?"

I was nervous that day, hoping that the decision was going to be in my favor. I was hoping that the plastic surgeon would say, "Denise you are a candidate, and yes we will remove the tissue from your remaining breast and we will be able to do the implant." When he was still examining me, I told him that I wanted to go ahead and have this done. He said, "Okay, but I want to see you one more time before the surgery so we can go over any questions and talk about what is going to happen." Then he sent me out to talk to his secretary, and we scheduled another consultation and a date for surgery.

Before we left his office he gave me a book on breast cancer and breast reconstruction and told my husband and me to read it and then come back with questions for our next meeting. Bill read the book before I did and he underlined everything. He wrote out questions. He said, "Really, Denise, I want you to read this. Do you understand what you are getting yourself into?" After he met the plastic surgeon he felt much better, but he still was not sure that he wanted me to go through this.

Bill came with me to my second consultation. He talked to my plastic surgeon again and asked his questions. Was I going to be able to lift? Was I going to be able to exercise? Were my breasts going to look normal? The plastic surgeon answered everything. He also told Bill that the prophylactic mastectomy might prevent me from getting cancer in my other breast. After Bill heard that he felt much more comfortable. He said, "Okay, go ahead. I want you to have the surgery because I want you to do what you want to do." But I kept reiterating, "Bill, I want you to be happy, too." Finally, to convince him, I agreed to consult with some other doctors who were familiar with my history to see what they said. These doctors also consulted other cancer specialists, and by the time we were through we had opinions from seven doctors. My surgeon said it is very hard to get three doctors to agree on anything, but all of these doctors unanimously agreed that I really needed to have it done. I said, "Bill, That's seven doctors that have given their opinions; what else do you want?" He said, "Fine."

How did you decide what reconstructive technique you wanted to have done? Did your plastic surgeon recommend a particular technique? Did he explain what it involved?

My plastic surgeon discussed all of the different techniques, and I read the book he gave me so I knew something about what was possible. I also had several friends that had reconstruction, two with the TRAM flap and one with implants. They were all delighted with what they had done, but it took my friends with TRAM flaps a good 6 months before they could stand up straight and were active again. I wanted to get back to work right away: I am too active to be incapacitated for that long.

My plastic surgeon recommended implants combined with tissue expansion. He did not want me to have to go through the TRAM flap because the recuperation time was longer. He also felt that implants would work best for me because I was slender and needed both breasts rebuilt. He explained where he would cut me and that after he put the expanders in I would be coming back for 4 to 6 months to enlarge the

expanders and stretch my skin. When I had been expanded sufficiently, he would replace the expanders with permanent implants. Several
months later, in another operation, he would reconstruct the nipple.

**Was it hard to go back for reconstruction? After all it was more
surgery.**

It wasn't hard for me; I was looking forward to it. I had this inner
strength. My ladies at work said, "I can't believe how positive and
upbeat you are." But I said, "You do not know what a wonderful thing
this is for me." After meeting my plastic surgeon and all the people in
the office I felt so confident.

The morning of surgery I was a nervous wreck. It was awful. Every
2 minutes I had to run to the bathroom. I had the worst case of diarrhea. I think my surgery was scheduled for 7:30 A.M. and they
started it at 8 o'clock because I could not get off the john. It was like
there was nothing else left in me.

What was your reaction when your expanders had been put in?

When I woke up and looked down, I had this new, lacy bra on. This
bra was so feminine, so wonderful. The things you have to wear with
a prosthesis are so ugly. I was always pulling that prosthesis down
because it would ride up and I would have one up and one down. I
looked at some pictures of me, and you could actually tell that one was
setting up higher than the other one. I was thrilled with this beautiful
bra filled with my own breasts.

**How long did it take you to recover from the first stage of your
breast reconstruction? Did you experience much pain?**

That was unbelievable. When they first removed my tissue and put
the expanders in, they had a pain pump next to my bed. They told me
to push that button when I wanted the pain medicine. I only pushed it
one time. I don't know if the positive thinking made me oblivious to
the pain or if I was just fortunate. When the implants were put in, they
had the pain pump there, but I didn't need it.

When I was to be released, my plastic surgeon gave me a prescrip-
tion for antibiotics and one for pain. I said, "Oh I don't think I am
going to need anything for pain." My husband said, "If she hasn't had
any pain yet, is she going to have it now?" My plastic surgeon said not

likely. I am not the martyr. If I have pain, I am going to let everybody know about it or I am going to do something about it. But with reconstruction I have not had one ounce of pain.

Did you experience much bruising or swelling?

When I first went in for my expanders, my whole back was bruised. After I thought about it, the bruising made sense because I am sure they had to pull the skin around my chest to be able to put those expanders in because I was flat. That skin was attached to my chest wall for over 12 years. I am sure that the initial shock of just stretching it out caused the bruising, but that went away after a week.

How long did it take before you could return to work and to normal activity?

I probably could have gone back to work in 2 weeks because I felt good and I was ready to go. But I had some vacation time coming to me. Because I drive a stick shift car and my husband is very protective of me, I was out for 4 weeks. I felt pretty normal and was back doing things within 2 weeks. When I went back to work, I had no problem lifting stock or moving around.

How did your recuperation compare to your recovery from your mastectomy?

With my mastectomy, I was out for 5 weeks and it took me a good year before I really felt up to par. I have a high energy level, but I was not myself for that first year. I was always exhausted. I'm sure a lot of it was mental fatigue that was dragging me down. I think I was upset by the mastectomy and worried about the cancer recurring. Now the fear is gone. I go to bed at night and I say, "Thank you, dear God, for taking such good care of me."

Are you happy with your decision to have the prophylactic mastectomy?

Yes. I only wish I knew about the option earlier, at the time of my mastectomy. It would have saved me years of worrying about my breast. That was probably the most traumatic time in my life. You think it is over. You want to be positive, but you hear so many horror stories. It was a constant worry. I went every 3 months to be checked and there were always recurring lumps. My hands would start perspiring, and I would hold my breath until those results came back. I remember when my plastic surgeon examined me the first time. He commented on how many lumps I had. It would have been great if they had been able to remove my breast tissue when I had my first mastectomy and then have done the implants immediately. I think I would have healed mentally and physically so much faster. This time, to wake up with the tissue removed and to hear that it was benign and I don't have to worry about this ever again was wonderful. I am just glad that the breast tissue is finally gone.

What was involved with tissue expansion? How long did it take you to get your breast tissue fully stretched?

I had my expanders put in at the end of January and for the first 2 months I came back once every other week to be expanded. It took about 30 minutes each time. The expanders were sitting high up on my chest and I worried that my breasts would not look normal. But my plastic surgeon explained that they would look more natural when the implants were in. They would be more centered and not as much to the side. He was right; they look just fine now.

Did you experience any problems or complications during tissue expansion?

I had a leaky expander. I got up one morning and my breast was almost flat. The saltwater had leaked out. I thought, "Oh, my gosh, what is wrong, what has happened?" The nurses explained that sometimes there are faulty expanders. It's rare, but it happens. Then I had to come every week for them to pump me back up.

How did they fix the leak? Did they need to take the leaky expander out and replace it?

Fortunately, it was a slow leak. My expanders did not need to be removed, but I did have to come back every week to have my breast pumped up until I got my permanent implants. One time I did go for 2 weeks without expansion because my plastic surgeon said, "Let's just wait and see; if you really go flat, come back." I went down quite a bit. I wore loose clothing so nobody could really tell.

When did you have your permanent implants put in? What type were used?

After 3 months my plastic surgeon was ready to put in the permanent implants, but I had a busy schedule at work so I delayed it for an additional 2 months. I had saline implants inserted and I am happy with them.

How do your breasts feel? Are they natural? Are they soft? Are they sensitive?

They are very natural and soft. They are not at all sensitive. I can feel my hands when I place them on my breasts, but it is pressure, not sensation. When I was first reconstructed, my breasts felt hot to me, but now they feel pretty normal.

I sleep on my stomach. When the expanders were first put in, I had difficulty sleeping. I slept on my back until they put the permanent implants in. Since then I am back on my stomach and I am much more comfortable.

Why did you decide you wanted to have your nipple and areola reconstructed?

Whenever I decide to do something, I don't do it halfway. I go all the way. I think the nipple and the areola are an important part of the entire breast and I wanted my breasts to be complete.

Are you satisfied with the results of your breast reconstruction? Has it met your goals?

My breasts look better than I thought they would. I never dreamed that they would look so normal. It's just wonderful. At night, God forgive me, when I take off my bra I find myself just standing there and looking at myself and thinking, "Is this really me?" He did a beautiful job. It was not important for me to be bigger than I was. I just wanted to be put back together. If all my plastic surgeon could do was to make me a size A, I would have been happy. As it is, I am a little bigger than I was. Now all I still have to do is have my nipple reconstruction and then I will be finished.

Has reconstructive surgery had an impact on the way you feel about yourself? Has it affected the way you act?

Reconstruction has changed my life. I have always been a positive person, but this has been the most inspirational and exciting experience. I can't tell you how happy I am. I feel younger than 58 now that I am whole again. I have more confidence in myself and in the way I present myself. Most people don't realize that I am a little timid because I work at being more outgoing for my job. Now, however, I have this wonderful air of confidence. I just feel good about myself. I feel comfortable about what I am saying, and I think I am saying it better because I am all put back together again. It's amazing what that can do for your image. When I walk, I feel taller. I do not know what it is, but it's great.

Has reconstruction affected the way you dress?

Now I can wear what I want and I feel more comfortable with my body. After my mastectomy I made up my mind that I wasn't going to let it get me down, but deep down inside I never felt whole. I had some fine, feminine clothes, and I just stopped wearing them. I changed my style of dress because if I wore something more feminine, my prosthesis always seemed to slip up, and if I leaned over, you could see that one side was flat. Now I get up in the morning and put on my bra; I do not have to worry about putting that prosthesis in. I think every woman likes pretty lingerie, although I am still wearing the bras that they gave me from the hospital because they are so lacy and feminine. It's just so wonderful to get up. I haven't had a bathing suit on in 12 years. I will put one on now. I always worried before, even if I was not conscious of it. I was always tugging and pulling.

Are you happy with the technique that you chose or is there another one you would have preferred?

I am thrilled with the technique I selected. I look very natural. It was not painful and I love the way I look.

If you had it to do over again, would you have breast reconstruction?

In a minute. My only regret is that I couldn't have done it 13 years earlier. Breast reconstruction is the most fabulous thing I have done in my whole life.

Has reconstruction had an impact on your relationship with your husband?

I am more relaxed now, more open. After the mastectomy, even though my husband never made me feel uncomfortable, I was reluctant to let him see me unclothed. When I undressed, I would go in my dressing room and slip my nightgown on. I would never turn toward him when I put on my bra. He never had a problem with it, but it bothered me. That was my stigma. Mentally I always had it in the back of my mind that I was not whole, not a total woman because a part of me was missing. Even though I was not that big and it was not important for me to show my breasts off, deep down inside I knew something was gone. I guess you really never get over it, although no one else ever knew it but me.

Has breast reconstruction altered the way you relate to your husband sexually?

After my mastectomy my husband never had a problem with intimacy and the sexual part of our relationship, but I did. Sometimes I would make excuses, like I am tired or whatever. But now it's fine. It has changed me. I am more loving. I have a husband who is very endearing. He loves to give me a hug when I come home from work. He is really a sweet person. Now I am the one who is there with arms open. I just feel so good. I feel like everything's going in my favor.

How does your husband feel about your reconstruction now that you have had it done?

Wonderful! He is so glad I did it. As a matter of fact, after they started to expand my breast, my husband really got involved and he said, "I want a size D." I said, "Excuse me—a size D? I don't think I am ready for that." Anyway he is so proud. He thinks I look great. Even though he said it didn't bother him, I know that he is happy now that he can look at me and say, "Oh, gosh, she really looks great." His secretaries at work told me that I was blessed with the most wonderful husband. And he is. He is so proud of how well I have done and he is so happy that I am over this. But he was a nervous wreck. Bill suffered more than I did.

Were you pleased with your plastic surgeon? Was he responsive to your needs?

I told him that if ever he needs a public relations director I am going to apply for the job. He answered every question in great detail. I was very satisfied. So was my husband.

How did you pay for your reconstruction?

My husband researches everything; he told me that we have to cross our T's and dot our I's to make sure we get full insurance coverage. He said that we needed a letter of approval. So we got my plastic surgeon to send a letter explaining why I needed this operation. Then my insurance company paid every single penny.

What advice would you like to share with other women faced with decisions about breast cancer and breast reconstruction?

A woman should never lose sight of the fact that she has rights. If she believes in and wants reconstruction, she really needs to pursue it. Yes, you want your family, your husband, your friends to share in this wonderful experience and you want them to be part of it. But if they are negative, then you have to turn their doubts into positives. If you believe in it, you are the one that needs to pursue it. I could have easily been swayed by my husband because he felt that adamant about my not having reconstructive surgery. You are responsible for your own body. You have to go out there and you have to make it happen if that is how you feel.

FAITH: I COULDN'T FACE BREAST LOSS

"Please be sure to tell your readers that not only people with beautiful bodies are vain. We with the run-of-the-mill-type bodies also want to have the best image of ourselves that we can. . . ."

Thus began the letter that I received from Faith several weeks after our interview at her plastic surgeon's office. Faith is a pretty young woman with short dark hair and glasses. She was only 28 when her breast cancer was discovered. She courageously investigated her treatment options. As a young, single woman, Faith was unwilling to face breast loss. Unfortunately, living in a small town, she had few people to consult about reconstructive options. There was only one general surgeon in town and no plastic surgeons. The only women she knew who had had mastectomies were considerably older than she was. Therefore she took it upon herself to write to a Cancer Helpline in a neighboring state and request information on breast cancer and breast reconstruction. The information she received proved a godsend, and she studied everything she read until she found the procedure that she felt was right for her. She used the same research methods to locate a medical center, surgeon, and plastic surgeon to do an immediate breast reconstruction. Faith braved this trauma alone, traveling to the hospital by herself.

She cried through most of our discussion, taking off her glasses to wipe her eyes periodically. This experience was still very fresh and her emotions overwhelming. As she explained, "The doctors and nurses really need to stress that a person is going to be very emotional after any surgery, especially this one. I'd like to see a person assigned to the breast cancer team whose function is to provide emotional support. Because you already have a permanent breast shape in place, people tend to believe you are 'all well.' You are not. You still have to cope with surgery, with having a mastectomy, and with having cancer."

Faith chose the most complex and extensive method of breast reconstruction, an immediate TRAM free flap, a microsurgical operation in which her abdominal tissue and muscle were transferred to her breast and the nerves and blood vessels were reconnected under an operating microscope. She was in surgery for approximately 10 hours, and even though she would have liked to have had better information about her operation, she is delighted with the technique that she selected.

How did you discover your breast cancer?

I found a lump on January 1. Three days later I went to see my family doctor. He felt two lumps and I had a mammogram, but nothing showed up. My doctor said, "It's just fibrocystic disease. It's common in big-busted women. Nothing to worry about." He referred me to a surgeon who also thought they were just cysts. But I wasn't satisfied. My gut told me something was wrong, and I wanted them out. The surgeon tried to discourage me. He said, "You're 28. You'll have a scar." I told him I didn't care; let's get these lumps out and see what they are. So he removed them and he was right. What we had felt were cysts. But when he lifted the cysts, he found extensive intraductal carcinoma.

How did you get your information about breast cancer and breast reconstruction?

I saw a breast cancer documentary on TV. It was presented by a hospital in North Carolina. They had an 800 number; I called it and they sent me a packet of literature on breast cancer and breast reconstruction. This information was wonderful because it gave me something to read to base my decisions on. I'm a research person. I have to know all the options before I make the decision. I had to make a quick one and they got me the information in 3 days. By the time I got my second opinion I knew what I wanted done.

Why did you decide to have a mastectomy to treat your cancer?

The doctor in my town suggested a lumpectomy and irradiation, but I went to a neighboring city for a second opinion. That doctor said I needed a mastectomy for the type of cancer I had. I took the pathology slides to this second surgeon, and he had a complete pathology report done on them. I was devious, however; I took the old report out and said, "Here are the slides; tell me what this is." They had another pathologist look at them, and his diagnosis came back word for word as my other pathology report. He told me to have a total mastectomy and get it over with. He said, "If you were my wife, there would be no way I would let you have a lumpectomy. This type of cancer cannot be felt because it is so deep within the tissue." So I said, "Okay, but I want a TRAM flap breast reconstruction done at the same time."

How did you select the TRAM free flap breast reconstruction? Why did you choose to have microsurgery?

I knew that's what I wanted done because I had read about it in the material I received from the American Cancer Society; it contained a pamphlet on reconstruction with about a 3-inch paragraph, no pictures or anything, describing the TRAM flap reconstruction technique. I wasn't really sure about the difference between the regular TRAM flap and the free TRAM flap, but I knew that I liked the idea of using my stomach tissue. I have severe allergies, and I was afraid of the implant technique. With my luck, I'd be allergic to them. Anyway, I have plenty of extra abdominal tissue and this seemed to be the right approach for me.

Why did you want immediate breast reconstruction? What did you do when your surgeon was unwilling to perform an immediate TRAM flap?

I could not face leaving the hospital without a breast. This surgeon I went to for the second opinion told me to have the mastectomy done and to come back in 3 to 6 months and have the TRAM flap. I said, "No, I want to go home with something. I cannot handle just having a skin flap with an expander underneath to stretch the skin. I want to have a breast when I leave the hospital." He told me that they had never done an immediate TRAM breast reconstruction.

I said it's being done somewhere; I am going to find out where. I called the American Cancer Society and got the name of a good plastic surgeon and cancer surgeon in a nearby city at a major medical center. Then I called my doctor back home and said I want a referral; this was about 4:00 P.M. on a Friday afternoon. He called me back at 4:15 and said be in there Monday morning at 9:00. So I went in and on March 5, 2 months after I found my lump, I had a 10-hour operation.

Did your plastic surgeon explain the different reconstructive options to you? Did you know that you were having a free TRAM flap and not a pedicle TRAM flap?

I came in with my mind made up. This was my choice. They saw how hardheaded I was. I came in and told them that I wanted a TRAM flap. I even had my booklet with me with information about TRAM reconstruction. I think they assumed I knew everything about it. They just agreed to do it. I qualified with my weight; I had a stomach for them to use. I heard them refer to it as a free flap, but I didn't really understand that it was a more complicated form of TRAM flap operation. Nobody explained the difference to me, but I think I fooled them; they thought I was much better informed than I really was.

Did you require blood transfusions?

Yes, I had to have 3 units of blood donated. At first I couldn't think of someone we could trust to give blood and so I had to give my own. They kept telling me, "We'll never get the three out of you in this short period of time." So I called my pastor, and within 3 hours there were 10 people from my church volunteering to give blood for me; it was great! And they all called and came to see me; I saved the cards and counted them. I think I have 900 cards. People just pulled together.

How long did the operation take?

It took about 10 hours total. The only thing I remember in recovery is the nurse leaning over me and asking, "Can you tell me what they did?" I got so indignant with her because I thought she should have known what they did to me. Then she said, "Send her to her room she's okay." So I'm sure I had to talk to them before I got to my room.

Describe your hospital stay. Did you experience much pain?

I was in the hospital 6 days. My surgery was on a Tuesday and I was much better and functioning on my own by Sunday. I came out of surgery with three drain tubes and a catheter; at one time I had nine items going into three needles for IVs. Also I had a morphine pump.

The incisions themselves did not hurt because they were so deep and the nerves had been cut. Most of the pain was through the stomach where they had done the "tummy tuck" to take the tissue. My stomach was very tight. I would try to sit up and I couldn't. I guess my pain resembled the pain of childbirth. A person never realizes how the simplest movements use the stomach muscles. A sneeze will just about kill you. Reaching is impossible. Laying down you don't even think about. I also had trouble from my back. I had hurt it years ago, and it really ached from having to sit and lie in the same position. I had difficulty finding a comfortable position and I had to sleep on my back, propped up with pillows. I'd never have made it without my aunt staying with me during the days and my mother staying at night. After all, the nurses can't be by your side at all times.

I think the main contributor to my pain was the length of surgery. Ten hours is a very long time. I had two major surgeries in one. I remember feeling as if I had been beaten. Every muscle hurt. To help get rid of the aches I did what the doctor advised, I exercised. That meant I shuffled back and forth down the hospital corridor.

I also had trouble with my veins and the IVs. Because I had so many needles in, my veins started rupturing. I was taken back to surgery and had a jugular vein IV inserted. Believe it or not this made me feel much better. It gave me back the use of my one good arm. Until this was done, I couldn't even reach and get my own water or get into bed by myself. I decided that the next time I have major surgery I will have the jugular IV installed during surgery. The larger needle and blood supply in my jugular vein let them draw blood samples directly out of the IV instead of being stuck again when they needed to see if I needed another transfusion. Also, all other medications could be placed directly into the IV.

Did you require any special monitoring because you had microsurgery?

When you have microsurgery, they need to see if the blood vessels have been connected and that there is blood flow through the tissue. The way they check is to literally take a syringe with needles and stick it into the breast tissue, into the flap. If it bleeds, then they know that the blood circulation is good; if it doesn't bleed in an area, they know that the blood vessels have not healed properly and that they may need to do something else. They also touch the reconstructed breast to check it's temperature. If there's a cold spot, they'll know that the blood is not flowing through that area correctly. The first time they checked me I was just about terrified. They were sticking needles in me. I said, "What are you doing?" I didn't understand what they were talking about. They were saying, "Oh, good, it's bleeding." As far as I knew, things aren't supposed to bleed. Later they told me that was the way they checked to see if the blood vessels were connected properly. Once they explained it, I was okay, but they really need to warn a person before they do that.

Did you have to adjust to any other surprises during your hospital stay?

In a medical center you have to adjust to these young doctors always coming to see you in groups of five or six. I think that's one thing people need to get used to. Even though you have one doctor, he comes attached with five behind him. They were not all students; these were people who already are doctors, but they are studying that particular field and training specifically with someone. It was intimidating at first, but eventually you lose all inhibitions. They just come in and give orders. "Unsnap the top of your gown." You're just sitting there, and the feeling is, "Excuse me, who are you?"

How long did you recuperate before returning to work?

After my 6 days in the hospital I was at home for 4 weeks before I returned to work. My job requires a lot of lifting. I'm on my feet and it is also hot where I work. You can't cool off. So I stayed home for 4 weeks to make sure everything was fine.

Did you have any problems or complications?

I had an infection; it was the kind you get when you cut yourself and the surrounding area swells. It occurred because the knots from some of the stitches were not dissolving; the stitches dissolved, but the knots didn't. The infection spread. Because I live some distance from the medical center, I went to my family doctor and he gave me an antibiotic for it. The next week when I saw my plastic surgeon for a checkup, the incisions were already looking better. My plastic surgeon told me to continue on that medicine because the infection was healing just fine. It was just a skin infection. There was never any chance of losing the flap, even though that's the first thing that went through my mind. "I can't lose this. I don't have anything else to replace it with, so let's get this infection out of here!"

How long did it take until you were standing straight again and feeling like yourself?

Everybody kept saying that I was going to walk bent over at first, and they were right. But I thought I would be bent over by choice, not because I couldn't stand up. You should be told that. The muscle is gone. You have to stretch it out in order to be upright again.

At first I was miserable every time I stood up. But I made myself do it. Each time I would try to stand up just a little bit straighter. I noticed by the end of the day as I got tired I also got more slumped over. It was very hard to stand erect. We live on a farm, so I would go out and take walks to try to get my energy back. Within 3 weeks I was standing up straight. It's taken about 5 months to really feel like myself again.

Did you have nipple-areola reconstruction? Did you have any other adjustments made during that operation?

I came back for the nipple reconstruction 3 months after my initial surgery. My plastic surgeon reconstructed the nipple and areola from the little patches of skin (dog ears) that he left where he made my initial abdominal incision. I felt better before we did the nipple reconstruction than after. The scars were healing. I had some bad scar tissue from the infection. During the nipple reconstruction he cut the skin all over again and took out tissue; so now I have new scars. The nipple looked gross when I first had to start changing the bandages. I was just like, yuck, I shouldn't have had this done. We should have left it the way it was. But now that some time has passed the nipple reconstruction looks better, and the more I see myself in the mirror, the more I like it.

He also did liposuction to smooth my stomach and hip area. That was the worst. I never knew liposuction could hurt so much. My whole hip area was black and blue where they had just rounded and trimmed it off. That hurt worse than any of the other surgery.

Are you satisfied with your breast appearance? Is it what you expected?

Now that my breast has been shaped and trimmed and my nipple has been reconstructed, it looks pretty normal. As time passes my breast appears more natural. It's not perfect, but I am pleased. My breasts still don't match; they are not exactly the same shape. My new breast is too full in some aspects. My plastic surgeon is not happy with the shape, but I don't want to be put back to sleep again unless it's absolutely necessary to reduce the fullness. When I have a bra on, you can't tell. When I put on a swimsuit for the first time I was like, "Yuck, I can tell it." I could notice that the shapes were not the same. But I'm not in a swimsuit that much, so I don't mind. The surgeon had to cut so low to get part of the breast tissue out that even when I have my bra on you can see the lower part of the scar. I keep thinking I need to pull my bra down.

What do your scars look like? Where are they placed?

I have a circular scar all the way around the right breast area and underneath the arm. I'm also cut from behind one hip all the way across the abdomen to behind the other one. When you see this scar in the mirror, it's like somebody railroad-tracked you; it looks just like a pair of braces, only it's scar tissue. But my scars are doing better. Every week they seem to fade a little bit more. I'm sure that in a couple years, they will be fine. I have seen pictures of women who had this technique, and I could barely see any scarring. You could tell that their breasts didn't look exactly the same, but who could tell which was the reconstructed breast. I'd have to look on the back of the photographs to see which one was the reconstructed one and which one was the natural breast. Hopefully one day people will look at mine and comment, "I can't tell which one it was. They don't look the same, but. . . ."

How does your reconstructed breast feel? Is it sensitive?

The new breast is more solid feeling and looks a little different from my other breast. I wish it felt a little more like my normal breast. It also has some sensitivity, and as time goes by it is getting more sensitive.

If you had it to do over again, would you have reconstruction again? Was it worth the pain and trouble?

Yes. The results are so important and lasting that the memory of pain fades. I look natural in my clothes. My breast feels natural; it jiggles when I walk. When I had the surgery, it didn't move at all at first, and my plastic surgeon kept telling me when it's healed it'll start jiggling like your other one does. The first time it jiggled, I was so excited! I was like, "It's attached, it works!" My mother said, "What is wrong with you?" and I said, "Watch it, watch it. It jiggles!" It's been worth it, most definitely. I feel more confident because I feel like it is natural. I'm not going to be allergic to it; I'm not going to reject it. I'm not going to have to go back in 2 years to have an implant taken out and another one put in because that one sprang a leak. It's done.

Are you pleased with the technique that you chose?

Wonderfully. I am very happy. I'm very pleased because now I consider mine finished, whereas some women are still having to go through the process of having the skin stretched and the implant inserted and they're just not finished. Mine's finished.

Do you think your age had some impact on your desire for immediate reconstruction?

Most definitely. Most people my age are healthy and vibrant. If you've got something wrong or you've got a prosthesis, it makes you a lot more self-conscious. Psychologically I couldn't have handled going home from the hospital with nothing there. I probably would have gone bananas if I had gone home with the scar and a hole.

Have you altered the way you dress because of reconstruction?

I went to very big baggy shirts at first because before I had the second operation my reconstructed breast was a whole lot larger than the other breast. I was very self-conscious about that and so I would buy larger blouses.

How do people react when they learn that you have had breast cancer and breast reconstruction?

I work with the public in our business and it's a small town. Everybody knew that I was having surgery. They would come in and they wouldn't look at my face. Instead, they'd be looking down below the chin level going, "How are you feeling?" You just want to cover up. I wanted to say, "Stop staring. I've got a face; look at me."

The only women who've had mastectomies that I have talked to about my breast reconstruction are older women who are in their sixties and seventies. They're still wearing their prostheses. They are all curious. They want to know if I liked it. They will say, "I may go back and get it done."

What can people do to be supportive of someone who has had a mastectomy or breast reconstruction?

I live in a small community, but there are an amazing number of older women here who have had breast cancer, and they were calling to talk. I found it a little disheartening that I was the youngest person. I still don't know anyone my age who has had breast cancer, but my friends were great. They still talked to me and did not treat me as if I had something contagious. They would say, "Let's go to the races. Come on you're not going to lay around, you lazy little thing." They were constantly pushing. I think I had more visitors in the hospital than the rest of the floor put together. My room was just full of stuff. A friend of mine knows I collect antique perfume bottles; he brought me one. They brought food, candy, even jewelry. They all knew I was allergic to flowers, so everyone was sending green plants. They called. I had a friend who lives in Chicago now and he called every day. They didn't treat me like I had already died. They teased me, and accused me of being lazy and just laying in bed. They acted like they always acted around me and that was wonderful.

Do you feel you were fully informed about the details of your breast reconstruction? Was there more information you could have had? Are there questions you think a woman should ask?

Personally I wish I had been supplied with all the gory details, not just simple before and after pictures. I would like to see the information written out in simplified medical terms so you can understand what is going on, so that you can anticipate what will happen, and so you will know how your appearance will change. They should tell you that it is going to take three or four surgeries to get your breasts to look right. I was told there would be more than one operation, but it seems like every time I come here there is going to be another one. You should know that you are going to have a year of bad scarring, so when you wake up you will know what to expect. I was able to handle it. I know some women who would be horrified to wake up and see all the stitches and scars. Their response would be, "What did they do to me!" A lot of times, unless you know what you want or are good at asking questions, the doctors won't tell you everything. It simplifies things for them; they just go ahead and do their little procedure and you wake up and that's it. I would like to see the information written out, so if you knew you were going to have the TRAM flap they would explain in detail what they would do. I didn't really understand fully until after I had the surgery what it meant to have the TRAM done with microscopes and to have the blood vessels sewn together. I wish I had known beforehand; I still would have had the procedure done. It was the perfect operation for me. Still . . . I needed more information. After all, these are life-changing decisions.

PAM: I DANCED MY WAY THROUGH IT

We spoke of ballroom dancing and of the frilly, low-cut gowns that she wore as she whirled around the dance floor. It seemed an unusual topic for an interview about breast cancer and breast reconstruction, but for Pam, ballroom dancing was a goal to focus on to help her cope during breast cancer treatment.

Pam is a registered nurse with a master's degree in critical care. She has a soft voice and a gentle manner, which is reinforced by her physical appearance. On the day we were visiting her curly, light brown hair was loosely tied back with a ribbon and she wore a flowered dress that revealed a trim, graceful figure. She was only 30 years old when her breast cancer was discovered 5 years ago. Single, with no family history of breast cancer, Pam was shocked and devastated by the news. Because of her youth and passion for dancing, she was unwilling to face life with only one breast. She had a mastectomy followed by 6 months of chemotherapy for one positive lymph node. Then, in July, a month after she had finished her chemotherapy, she had a tissue expander placed to reconstruct her breast and an implant placed to augment her other breast. Her expander was replaced with a permanent implant in November, and her nipple-areola was reconstructed a few months after that. Pam performed in dance competitions throughout this whole experience. She kept a positive attitude and focused on the reconstruction that was to make her whole again. Her story is an inspiring one.

How did you react when you discovered you had breast cancer?

I was devastated. My whole family was traumatized at my diagnosis. I have five brothers and sisters and nobody has ever been sick. It's been difficult for everybody, particularly me, because I don't see myself as a sick person. I've always seen myself as a strong caregiver.

How did you learn about the option of breast reconstruction?

I knew about reconstruction because my surgeon told me about it when he discussed my options for breast cancer treatment. He gave me a choice between total mastectomy with reconstruction or lumpectomy with irradiation. Because of the location of my cancer he felt that a lumpectomy would not produce an acceptable cosmetic result and that a mastectomy and reconstruction would probably be a better choice for me.

Why did you decide to have breast reconstruction?

I knew that whatever I had to go through I just couldn't face it or face life afterward with just one breast. I was only 30 years old at the time, too young to be without a breast, particularly when something could be done about it. I was also involved in a meaningful relationship and didn't feel that I could be comfortable with this man unless I could make myself as close to normal as possible.

My love for ballroom dancing also motivated me. I couldn't imagine having to wear my beautiful, semi-low-cut ballgowns with only one breast. I couldn't have done it without having breast reconstruction.

How did you select your plastic surgeon? Did you consult with him before your mastectomy?

I didn't have a chance to talk to my plastic surgeon before I had the mastectomy, even though I had his name. My girlfriend told me about him, and several other people mentioned that he was considered an authority on breast reconstruction. My general surgeon also recommended him.

When I was on the operating room table before my mastectomy I was nervous and upset. I had been crying my eyes out. Before I was put to sleep I made a feeble attempt at humor to try to lighten up the situation. I said, "You guys make a pretty scar, 'cause my plastic surgeon [and I named the plastic surgeon that I had heard about] is going to fix it once you finish." Somebody must have heard me say that and told him because the day after surgery the plastic surgeon walked into my room. I'd never seen him before. He was such a gentlemen; he came to introduce himself and see who I was. He told me to come see him when I recovered from my surgery and we could talk. I said okay, and I decided right then and there that he was going to be the one that worked on me. I wasn't going to look anywhere else.

How long did it take you to recuperate from your mastectomy? When could you resume dancing?

My recovery was pretty quick and relatively painless. I figured the best way for me to recover from this surgery was to just keep a goal in mind. When I had my mastectomy, I had a dance competition coming up 3 weeks later. I had already paid money to enter, and I was determined to perform in that competition. I love ballroom dancing; that's the extra thing that I do, my special hobby. So we modified my dresses, stuffed one side of them, and I performed in that competition with my drains still in. I won first place in all events except one, where I took second place.

It was a wonderful experience. As the weekend passed, everybody around the room found out about my surgery and they cheered every time I stepped on the floor. It was encouraging. I almost didn't make it through the last dance. I just about gave out. But I had a goal—to win that dance competition—and it kept me going.

What type of reconstructive approach did you select and why? Did your plastic surgeon discuss all of the options with you?

My plastic surgeon presented all the options; then he told me his recommendation. He thought the expander would work better for me. I didn't have an abundance of abdominal tissue to pull up for a flap, and I didn't want a latissimus dorsi muscle flap because I didn't want a scar on my back. So this was the best bet for me, even though it would require three procedures. Personally I wanted to go with tissue expansion rather than have major surgery. He also felt that he could get a pretty good match, and he was right.

Did you have any surgery on your remaining breast?

Yes, I had my other breast augmented with a small implant for a better match.

Did you have any worries about breast reconstruction before you had it?

Just if my breasts would match. I had read enough and I had spoken to my plastic surgeon enough to realize that people have this done every day. I also knew a girl who had breast reconstruction, and she never regretted her decision. That helped me.

Were you concerned about having implants?

Yes. I asked what was in the implants. My plastic surgeon explained the different kinds to me, and he told me about possible complications. He said that he had not found implants to be a problem in most of his patients, but he wanted me to know what the potential risks were. I was satisfied with what he had to say.

Was it difficult to face more surgery after your mastectomy?

Yes, I was really anxious. I had been dealing with not having a breast for 6 months. All through chemotherapy I was impatient for my missing breast to be fixed. At times I wished that it could have been done when I had my mastectomy; I didn't want to go back in and have a second operation. But I don't regret it now. When I got discouraged, it helped to talk to my boyfriend and to my girlfriend who had the latissimus flap reconstruction. She did well with hers, and she showed me her reconstructed breast. That helped. Now I show mine to other women who want to know about it. The girls at work were so curious I took them in the back room and showed them, and gosh, they think it looks really good! You can hardly tell the difference; it looks so natural. Of course, none of them had ever seen a reconstructed breast before. They didn't know what was possible. When you see what can be done, it takes away some of the fear.

How long did it take you to recover from the first operation when your expander was placed? Did you experience much pain?

When they put in the expander, they also put an implant in the other side for symmetry, so I was really uncomfortable with that first surgery because they did both sides. I was hurting so bad they kept me overnight in the hospital. It was hard to breathe for the first 2 days. It felt like there was a big pressure on my chest and it was pretty uncomfortable. I was much better as soon as they gave me a shot of Demerol. It was hard to lay on my side, and I don't sleep well on my back, so that was a little trouble. But I hugged a pillow most of the time and that helped. After a week's time it was as if I hadn't had it done.

How often did you go to have your expander inflated?

I went in every 2 to 3 weeks and they put more saltwater in it. Each session lasted about 5 or 10 minutes.

How long did it take for your tissues to be fully expanded and your breast reconstruction to be completed?

I had my initial expander placed in July, and in November we replaced it with a permanent implant. Then I had my nipple-areola reconstructed several months later.

Was it painful having your tissue expander inflated?

No, not at all. I could feel tightness at times. I still feel some tightness, especially if I don't massage the implant behind my chest muscle. It usually feels tight when I get up in the morning. Once I move around a bit it's a lot better. But it's hard to tell if the tightness is from the implant or from the mastectomy.

Was tissue expansion inconvenient? Did it interfere with your ballroom dancing or with other activities?

No, I just kept on going. I did a competition with the big, fully stretched expander in right before I came in and had it replaced. It looked funny. One side was really big and tight, and the other one was not. Most people probably didn't notice, although I was a little self-conscious. But since there wasn't anything I could do about it, I just went with it.

Why did you have nipple-areola reconstruction? How was it done?

To finish the job. He took some of the nipple from my remaining breast and grafted it on my reconstructed breast. He also tattooed my nipple and my areola. This was all done in a third operation.

Have you had any problems or complications associated with your reconstruction?

No, none at all.

Are you happy with your breast appearance? Are your breasts soft, warm, and sensitive?

My breasts look slightly different and they feel different sometimes, but I'm satisfied with them. They feel pretty normal. One of them gets colder than the other one and one is a little firmer than the other, but the difference is barely noticeable. The tatooed nipple-areola doesn't match my normal side any longer because it's faded and needs to be redone.

Did your plastic surgeon create any new scars during your breast reconstruction?

No. He reopened the mastectomy scar. Now it's just a faint line and he has tattooed over that.

Was breast reconstruction what you expected?

I don't know if I knew what to expect. It takes a while for you to assimilate your new breast, to realize that it is part of you. Now, when I look at the reconstructed breast, I think, this is just me; this is what I look like. In the beginning, however, I looked at it and thought this weird thing is not really me; this is something stuck on my chest. But it's second nature; it becomes a part of you. Then you don't think of it as foreign any more; you really don't.

Have you altered your dress habits because of reconstruction?

I changed the way I dressed before I had the reconstruction done. I wore T-shirts all the time. I would never take them off. I never got one of those prostheses because I knew I was going to have reconstruction. I just made my own form and wore it in my bra. I kept my bra on all the time.

What has been the psychological impact of breast reconstruction?

Your body image is different. For me, it is better than not having anything. It may be different from what I had, but it's as close to what I had as I can realistically expect. Now my life is as close to normal as possible; that makes me happy. That's fine with me.

Were you happy with your plastic surgeon? Was he responsive to your needs?

I have the highest regard for him. He is a gentleman and inspires confidence in his surgical skills. His manner is gentle and caring and he is truly concerned about his patients. He takes time with you and explains everything and answers every question. If you are going to have something like this done, you have to trust your surgeon. I did. I trusted him from the beginning. I trusted his judgment. I knew I was going to have my breast reconstructed and I figured he knew the best way to do it.

Do you think your decision was any easier because you are a medical professional?

No, because I didn't know anything about breast cancer or breast reconstruction. I was coming in off the street just like anyone else. I understood more of what the plastic surgeon was explaining to me, but as far as knowing anything about reconstruction or which way to go, I didn't know anything until I read a little bit and talked to him about it.

If you had the decision to make again, would you choose breast reconstruction? Was it worth the time, pain, and money?

Oh, definitely. It was worth the minimal discomfort that I went through. It's been 5 years, and I have lived a normal life.

How did you pay for your breast reconstruction?

My insurance covered 80% and I paid the rest. The insurance companies now look at reconstruction as a part of the process of recovery
from a mastectomy and that's how it should be. Breast reconstruction
is not considered cosmetic anymore. If you lose an arm or a leg, they
give you a prosthesis to replace it, and the insurance company pays for
it. So what's the difference; just because a breast doesn't have an obvious function I don't see what difference that makes. So what if you
can't pick something up with it. It is still an important body part,
especially for your mental health.

If you had it to do over, would you consider having your reconstruction at the time of your mastectomy as an immediate procedure?

I might. At the time I didn't know anything about immediate reconstruction, and with the chemotherapy I may not have been able to
have it. Still it would have been nice to know about that option.
When you're young, immediate reconstruction has an important effect on how you deal with the cancer itself and how you feel about
yourself. A woman needs to have all the facts available to her so she
can make an informed choice before her mastectomy. She needs to be
given the option of going ahead and having the mastectomy and
reconstruction done at the same time. I really feel like this option for
immediate reconstruction has opened a lot of avenues for women they
didn't have before.

How can a man be supportive of a woman when she is coping with breast cancer or reconstruction?

The boyfriend that I had at the time was very positive. He told me that
everything was going to be okay. He never let me feel any less
desirable, even though I wore T-shirts and I never let him see me.
After all, why did I have to? I was getting my breast fixed in 6 months;
we could wait out the 6 months. It seemed to be fine with him too;
when somebody loves you, he doesn't care about that kind of thing.
My boyfriend was really supportive throughout this whole experience.
He helped me get through the chemotherapy. When I was depressed
and didn't want to go through another operative procedure, he reassured me. He said, "It is going to get better; you've got to have it done.
It is going to be all right. You can get through this." Men have to be
positive, but they also have to let the woman take the lead. If she

wants to talk it out, then they need to be there for her. But if she doesn't want to talk about it, then she shouldn't be forced to.

I broke up with that boyfriend, and now I have a relationship with somebody else. We got together after I had all the surgery done. He knows all about it and it has not been a problem for us.

What advice would you like to give to other women about breast cancer and breast reconstruction?

Control is important in coping with cancer and it's difficult to come by. You don't have much say in the mastectomy decision. It has to be done. Even though you can choose lumpectomy vs. mastectomy, you still have to accept what your surgeon recommends for you. You need to play a role in what is happening to you. To do that effectively, to exercise some control, you must be informed. If it means reading a book before you make a decision, then do it. Ask the questions, read the books and articles, learn what you can so you don't feel powerless. Then decide what is best for you.

For me, reconstruction provided some control over my life. It was a way of making my life as normal as possible. I know it's not for every woman. But if it makes a difference in the way a woman sees herself, she should investigate it. If it's important to her, if it will make her life more bearable, then it's the right thing to do. Nobody wants to feel like she is not a whole person. There is no need to be afraid of a little discomfort if it is going to make the rest of your life a lot happier. It's just not that bad. If they can do a little surgery on me and give me back the part that I was missing, then I say, "Go for it."

MAGGIE: A WOMAN'S SEXUALITY

"Flamboyant" was the word she proudly used to describe herself, and I had to smile at the accuracy of her self-assessment. An imposing woman of 5 feet 8 inches, Maggie has an air of self-assurance that dominates her conversation. She is also somewhat of a flashy dresser, which only serves to complement her personality. The day of our interview she was dressed in a bright red blouse draped in comfortable folds over her ample bosom. Her waist was cinched by a gold belt, several gold chains encircled her neck, and her long fingers tapered into finely manicured nails, lacquered in bright red to match her lipstick. She wore black slacks and black high heels and her black hair was carefully coiffured in a short, bouffant style. Her gold bracelets clinked as she talked to me about the importance of breasts and sex appeal to women of all ages and why she, as a widow in her early sixties, felt it was particularly important to have breast reconstruction.

Maggie's striking appearance is consistent with her open and appealingly honest personality. She likes herself and the image she portrays; she was determined not to let breast cancer diminish her body image or make her uncomfortable interacting with others. Her cancer was discovered when she was widowed after 34 years of a happy marriage; one married daughter lived in a nearby town. Even though she was involved in a busy career in retail lingerie, she did not want to spend the rest of her life without a partner. She liked socializing and also frankly admitted that she liked her breasts just as they were. She had always worn clothing that was "sexy" and she "didn't want to change her image now." Of particular importance was her desire to be able to feel free to engage in an intimate relationship without inhibition. Therefore, when she was diagnosed as having breast cancer, she was determined not to delay breast restoration any longer than necessary.

Living in a small town, she did not have an experienced reconstructive surgeon available to consult, so she undertook her own research to find out all she could about the different types of reconstructive operations and the best surgeons to perform them. She decided to have a TRAM breast reconstruction. Although this was one of the more complicated procedures, she selected it because she did not want an artificial substance in her body. As Maggie explained, "I'm an original and I want everything about me to be real." Even though immediate breast reconstruction was not an option for her, she was determined that the delay would be as brief as possible to curtail the period of breast loss. Her deadline was to have her breast reconstruction completed and be totally recovered 1 year after her mastectomy. She set about this goal with style, humor, and determination. Now, 3 years later, this gutsy lady has remarried and is enjoying life more than ever. Sometimes Maggie even forgets that her new reconstructed breast is not her original one.

How did you discover your breast cancer?

I found a lump while I was examining my breasts in the shower. I had fibrocystic breasts, so I had lumps before, but this one felt different. It seemed to be attached to the skin; with the others the overlying skin was more movable. I decided to follow up with my gynecologist. He referred me to a surgeon in my community who sent me for a mammogram and suggested a biopsy. When I came out of the anesthesia after the biopsy, my daughter was there and she told me they had found a malignancy.

What was your reaction to your cancer diagnosis?

I wanted to know how bad my cancer was and what was going to happen to me. When my doctor told me that I was going to need a mastectomy, I told him that I couldn't have one. I was alone. I was unmarried. My breast was a very important part of my body. I felt that I needed my breast if I was to get on with my life. I just couldn't have a mastectomy, but he said that I must. That's when I started my research. I needed to find out quickly what my options were.

What type of research did you conduct to investigate your options?

I got on the phone and started calling people. I had heard of a lady in my town, a friend of a friend, who had a mastectomy and breast reconstruction; I called her. I contacted everybody I could think of. I even called people in other states. Somebody would know of somebody and I would call. This was all new to me. I am the kind of person who wants to know what lies ahead of her and what is the best direction to go. In 3 days I did quite a bit of research, and I learned about cancer treatment and breast reconstruction.

Why was reconstruction so important to you?

My mother's oldest sister had breast cancer. She had her mastectomy many years ago and she never had reconstruction. To me it was a horrible sight. I felt that I would have to change my image if I lost my breast. I am a flamboyant dresser. I have always liked low, revealing clothes. I am that kind of person, that's just me; I have been that way from the age of 16. I didn't want to lose my breast. I liked me. Even though I was not involved intimately with a man at that time, I did not feel that I could ever be comfortable with the opposite sex if I had only one breast.

How did you learn about reconstruction? What type of reconstructive technique did you select?

I heard about reconstruction through my phone calls to women with cancer. I would call these people and ask them questions. "Did you have reconstruction?" "Where did you have it?" "What was it like?"

"Who did your surgery?" "Were you satisfied?" I never spoke to anybody who had anything but implants, but I knew flaps were being done because I had read about these techniques in some books. I decided early on that I didn't want implants. I am not that kind of person. I've never wanted false teeth. I've never wanted anything artificial if it was possible to have the other. I would settle for implants before I would do without, but I wanted the best, and I felt that my own tissue was best. I also wanted immediate reconstruction so I wouldn't have to go without my breast.

Were you able to have immediate reconstruction?

No. As it turned out my cancer surgeon did not feel comfortable with my having a TRAM flap or with the idea of immediate reconstruction. At that time the tummy flap was pretty new, and there was no local plastic surgeon who could have performed it. My cancer surgeon's focus was on saving my life and getting all of the cancer removed. He felt that I shouldn't delay treatment but should go ahead and get my cancer taken care of immediately. Even though I desperately wanted my breast, I decided that I was putting the cart before the horse. I wanted my doctor at home to do my mastectomy because he had a very good name. I also felt that he would take a more personal interest in getting all the cancer. Since there really wasn't anyone in town who could have done the reconstructive surgery, immediate reconstruction was out of the question. So I had my mastectomy and then I was ready for reconstruction. And despite my cancer surgeon's warning that no plastic surgeon would touch me for 6 months, I was determined to get my breast back sooner.

How long did it take you to recover from your mastectomy? What was your emotional reaction to the surgery? Did you experience much pain?

The pain wasn't too bad. I had my surgery on Tuesday and checked out of the hospital on Friday morning. The mental anguish was much worse than the pain. I didn't let anyone but my mother see me without a breast. I had the surgery at 9 o'clock in the morning and that afternoon I sent my mother out to get an artificial breast to put in my gown. I still insisted on wearing my low nightgown, and I lay there very straight so that nobody could tell that the prosthesis was pinned in my very sexy nightgown. I wondered if I could go on with my life. After all, I had lost something very important to me, something that made me a whole person. I couldn't concentrate on the pain; breast reconstruction occupied my thoughts. I'm impatient that way. If I have anything facing me, good or bad, I am anxious to get on with it.

How did you find the plastic surgeon to perform your TRAM breast reconstruction?

I had heard about him from several of the women I talked to. He had a good name, and he was at a major medical center. I decided to consult with him. If I didn't like him, I could always go to someone else in the city. I live in a small town, and I just felt that a major medical center was the best place to go. I went to see the plastic surgeon just 3 weeks after my mastectomy. As it turned out, he suited me just fine, so I didn't need to consult with anyone else.

What was your consultation like? Why did you decide to select this plastic surgeon to perform your breast reconstruction?

I came all dressed up and in my high heels. I was afraid that because of what I had heard about a 6-month delay, he wouldn't operate on me right away. My goal was to have everything complete, behind me, and out of my mind as much as possible within a year. When I was filling out my medical history, I would not write down the month that I had my mastectomy. I just wrote the year. I made up my mind before I went into the plastic surgeon's office that I had to stay in control. I wanted to tell him what I wanted and what I could stand; I wanted it my way. If he had not listened to me, I would have gone elsewhere.

At the beginning of our consultation he asked me why I had come to him for reconstruction. I said, "Because I heard you are the best and I won't have anything but the best. I don't want implants. I want a TRAM flap." I just told him exactly what I wanted. Later, when he saw me undressed, he said, "When did you have this done?" I said, "It doesn't matter when I had it done; I want this reconstruction done during your first opening. I want it now." He grinned. He is a quiet, laid-back person, so it was easy for me to stay in control, which I liked. I loved him from day one. A woman in this state of mind doesn't need sympathy, but she needs someone who is calm and gentle. I felt his caring from the time that he started talking to me. He smiled and said, "We'll have to see when I have the next opening." I said, "You're going to do me?" and he said, "Yes, but this type of surgery is not for everybody." He did not paint a very pretty picture.

***What did he tell you about the TRAM flap? Did he describe the
risks and benefits? Did you understand that this was a major
operative procedure?***

He said that the TRAM flap was painful. You have to be in good
health and it can be time consuming, possibly 6 hours of surgery with a
long time for full recovery. He also said that several steps or different
operations are usually needed to get the breast and abdomen to look
just right. He explained that it would probably take close to 9 months
to a year to complete it, the nipple and everything. I would need to
have blood transfusions. I said I would give my own blood because I
didn't want anybody else's blood. He thought that was a good idea. He
told me that it was a hard surgery. He said I would have to be off work
for quite a while. He told me about all the possible complications. He
explained them in great detail so that I would understand what I was
getting myself into. Of course, I didn't listen, not really, because I
know me and he didn't. If he would do his job, then I could do mine.
My plastic surgeon gave me a book to read when I left his office. Even
with all of this information, I did not realize what I was facing; only
experience can teach you that. As far as I was concerned, I felt I could
tolerate anything for a few days in order to have peace of mind and to
feel whole again.

***Did your plastic surgeon take pictures of you during your
consultation?***

My plastic surgeon took pictures of me from my first visit through my
final operation; he took some before and then some each time I had
another surgery. It is uncomfortable for any woman to be totally undressed in front of a stranger, no matter if it's your doctor, and have
him taking pictures of you. I'd joke about it because I was uncomfortable. I'd say, "Why are you making all these pictures? Am I going to
be in *Playboy?*"

***Was your plastic surgeon reluctant to perform your reconstruction
just 3 weeks after your mastectomy? Did you have to make any
special preparations to meet that deadline?***

He said, "You know it's been just 3 weeks since you had this other
surgery." I said, "I know but I am very healthy despite the breast
cancer. I am also very headstrong and determined to do this." So he
agreed to operate on me in 3 weeks; that made 6 weeks to the day since
my mastectomy. But he let me know that I was pushing it. I would

have to follow his directions to get ready or else my breast reconstruction would have to be delayed. I was happy with that. I said, "You tell
me what to do and I will do it. I will be ready." Normally he asks a
person to do sit-ups to improve blood circulation to the abdominal
tissue. I would still have to do these exercises, but I would have less
time. He also said, "You have to give 3 pints of blood in the next 3
weeks—that's going to be tough." He gave me iron tablets. He told
me to eat all the raisins I could, the rarest meat, livers—the blood-
building foods. I did exactly what he said and more. I did my sit-ups; I
ate raisins at work all day. Every week when I went to give blood they
would say I was on the borderline and probably wouldn't make it the
next week. But I did. I was able to give my 3 pints, and in 6 weeks to the
day I checked into the hospital to have reconstruction.

How long did it take you to recuperate from your reconstructive surgery? Did you experience much pain?

The reconstructive surgery lasted 4½ hours. Afterward, when they
rolled me to my room, they bumped my bed. I knew then I was in bad
shape. I hurt all over from my breast to my lower abdomen. The pain
was concentrated more in my abdomen than it was in my breast, but it
was all connected. When they transfer the muscle to the breast, they
open a tunnel from the abdominal area to the breast area, so there is a
large area that needs to heal.

I had four or five drain tubes coming out of my abdomen and
breast, a catheter, a morphine pump for pain, and oxygen. The next
morning when two nurses came to get me up, the pain was almost
unbearable. One of the nurses, unfortunately, wasn't well trained in
how to get a person back into the bed. She let me fall back, which was
the worst thing. I had stitches and it hurt terribly. I know the morphine helped, but by the third day it was making me deathly ill and I
told the nurse to take the pain pump out. I felt I could tolerate the pain
better than I could tolerate the nausea. I told them I would ask for a
shot if the pain got too bad.

Knowing that they had taken part of a muscle and transferred it, I
had this horror of not being able to straighten up, like an old woman.
So my next step was to get on my feet to see how far I could straighten
up. I was looking forward to that although I knew it was going to be
like death itself. I surprised myself when I did get up to go to the
bathroom on the third day. I was still quite bent over, but I knew if I
kept on I would be able to straighten up pretty soon because I wasn't as
bad off as I expected. I am very tall, 5 foot 8 inches. A little person

wouldn't have as far to stretch as I did. It was very important to me to be erect again, so I really worked on it. By the fifth day I was in the hall walking, taking tiny steps. I had to hold to the rail, but I was straight.

I was in the hospital 8 or 9 days. When I left the hospital, I stayed with my mother for a week and a half. During that time I was not always able to dress because I was so sore that I could hardly stand for anything to touch me. Even so, I exercised. I found a flat place in my mom's yard, and five or six times a day, with just my night clothes and my tennis shoes on, I would walk one way and then another and then I would go lie down. Then I would walk again. Three weeks after my surgery my daughter asked me to go to a shopping center with her. I called a hospital equipment store, rented a wheelchair, and went shopping in a wheelchair. I was totally exhausted when I got home. I could hardly stand any bumps, but I did it. I still had on the stretch halter top they had given me in the hospital to wear over the bandage. I wore my clothes and jacket over that.

It took 2 to 3 months before I felt like myself again. As far as the pain was concerned, the first step of the reconstruction was the most painful. The rest was a breeze.

What was done during this first step of your breast reconstruction?

I was cut from one side of my abdomen to the other, all the way in front. The abdominal skin was then grafted from the navel to the hairline to move up to my breast with the accompanying abdominal muscle (the rectus abdominis muscle) and fat to give me enough skin and tissue to build a breast. It is my understanding that this flap of abdominal muscle and tissue was threaded up through a tunnel into the left side; that's where my mastectomy was. Then my plastic surgeon shaped a breast from it. He also had to make a new navel. I have a very pretty navel, almost as good as Mother gave me.

Was your breast what you expected after the first stage of reconstruction?

I had been told what to expect, but it's always a surprise when you see yourself after surgery. It was difficult to face the scars. I didn't expect my stomach to feel so hard; it was also numb and that lack of sensation was quite disturbing to me. It resembled the numbness you experience after you have Novocaine at the dentist; you know you are touching something, but it has no feeling. My breast was also numb, but I was expecting that. Even so, it still felt strange and it looked funny without a nipple.

I had more swelling than I had anticipated. Immediately after my operation the area under my breast where my flap was tunneled was swollen as big as another breast. I worried if it would ever go down. That was my first question to my plastic surgeon. He assured me that the swelling would go down, and if it didn't, he would take care of it during the next step of surgery. That eased my mind because I had all the confidence in the world in this doctor. I knew that after a few more operations he could make me look the way I wanted to. I was anxious to get on with it. I kept asking when he planned to do the next step.

What other procedures or steps were required to complete your breast reconstruction?

I had some hardening almost under the arm; that's where my lymph nodes had been stripped. You could feel stitches. It felt like scar tissue. It was a hard knot and it pooched out. In the second step he took care of that; he reopened the incision, removed that tissue, and it was fine. It bothered me that he had to make another little scar on my breast to remedy that situation. When I looked at it I thought, "Oh Lord, another scar."

He also suctioned the swollen area under my breast that I was so concerned about. By this time it had shrunk to the size of a lemon, so there wasn't much contouring to do. In the lower abdomen on each side where he started and finished the incision, I had little areas of skin that seemed to hang over. He called them "dog ears." He told me not to worry about these dog ears because he planned to use them to get tissue grafts for my nipple-areola reconstruction. Fortunately, one side leveled out and we didn't disturb it; he got his graft from the other side.

Why did you decide that you wanted nipple-areola reconstruction?

To make the reconstructed breast look like the other breast. It would not have been complete otherwise. I knew I had gone through the worst and I would never settle for an unfinished job.

Did he tattoo your reconstructed nipple-areola, and if so, was it a good match with your opposite nipple-areola?

Yes, I had a tattoo and, no, the match is not good. I hurried too much for the first tattoo. I was so determined to get it all done. They told me that they felt they were doing the tattoo too soon. It might not take because the tissue had not healed enough. It didn't. I had to have it done over, but the match still isn't good. My plastic surgeon is not happy with the coloring on the tattoo and neither am I. It's too dark. I have a lot of yellow tones in my skin and that is one of the hardest colors to match. It is much too dark, but my plastic surgeon said that he can take care of that.

Did you have any complications, any problems?

No. It just took some time to recuperate, but I really didn't have any trouble.

What were your primary goals in having reconstruction?

To be like I was. I never thought that I had the prettiest breasts in the world, but once I had lost one, I wanted a replacement just like the old one. Until you lose something, you never appreciate it; you take it for granted. I didn't really want any miracles. I didn't expect to mess with nature. Nature does a great deal for most people. But once I had lost my breast, then I felt I owed it to myself to find a way to restore what cancer took away.

Are you satisfied with the appearance of your breast? Is it soft, natural? Does it have feeling?

Yes. I cannot tell now that it has not been there forever. I also cannot tell any difference in feeling. I was told by my plastic surgeon that I would not have any feeling in this breast, no sensation. But I am one of the fortunate ones; I do have feeling now, but no sexual feeling. The nipple has no feeling, but all around the breast and at different places on the breast I know when I'm touched. When they did the tattooing, they had to numb me. They were quite surprised because I had feeling.

Where are your scars located and how do they look?

The scarring is disturbing. I have a scar completely around the breast on the left side and an inch long V-shaped scar extending onto my breast from my underarm. I also have a scar that extends across my entire lower abdomen. But now my scars are fading into hairline scars that are more acceptable.

If you had the choice to make over again, would you choose to have breast reconstruction? Would you select the same technique? Was it worth the pain, the time away from work, the expense?

Yes. I think the direction I went was best for me. I don't know anything that I could have done to make it turn out any better. I have been totally pleased. I feel complete. I feel attractive again. I feel comfortable undressing in front of a man. I look good in my clothes again. I can go on with my life.

How does breast cancer and breast reconstruction affect a woman's relationship with a man? Is it difficult when you are single and dating? What are the worries?

Divorced, widowed, or single women have mastectomies and reconstruction just the same as married women who have companions and support. At the time of my mastectomy I was not involved in a sexual relationship, and it would have been impossible for me to consider one with only one breast. Even though I had reconstruction, I wondered how I could explain what had happened to me. I wondered if a man would feel that I was complete, sensuous. Then I decided that any man that doesn't accept me as I am isn't worth my time. This sounded good, but I still had to give myself a pep talk every time I went out on a date. When I met a guy, I would think about how I would tell him. When you are dating, this is a worry. Most men like to love a woman and a woman likes to be loved; a breast is an important part of that. Even if you don't have a sexual relationship with a man, the first thing most men do after they get pretty well acquainted with you is fondle your breasts. I didn't tell anybody about my breast, however, unless our relationship developed and I saw that I was going to undress. Then before I reached that point, I would prepare him for what I had to say. I would begin by telling him that I had breast cancer and had a mastectomy and breast reconstruction. Sometimes I wouldn't go any further. It was surprising how the men related; I don't think it made a difference to anyone I became involved with. And men don't hide their feelings well. Usually they were shocked to hear about it at first, and then they would say, "Well, if it weren't for the scars, you couldn't tell you've had anything done." I said, "That's right, and in time it will be less visible."

When you met your present husband, what was his reaction to your breast reconstruction?

I met him through a friend, and we had several phone conversations prior to our face-to-face meeting. Of course, I didn't tell him anything about my surgery at that time. I really didn't even like the guy the first meeting. He continued to call me though. Several weeks later I was coming to the city where he lived, so I called him and told him that I was going to be there. He insisted on taking me to dinner. At dinner we talked and found out we had mutual interests and that we both liked to travel. When he asked if I wanted to go to Nashville with him that weekend, I surprised myself by saying yes.

I like to dance and sing and I was looking forward to a good time in Nashville. It didn't worry me that I had this reconstructed breast and would have to tell him about it. That wasn't on my mind until the time came. That's the way that I handled it with everybody I met. So I didn't think the breast would make or break my relationship.

That night we checked into a motel and made dinner arrangements at a nice steak place. I thought, "Well, I like this guy and I'm probably going to wind up in the bed with him." Before we went out to dinner, I pointed over to the other bed and told him to sit down because I had a story to tell him. He sat down and I said, "I had cancer a year ago and I had to have a breast removed." I was always a little "hyper" about telling someone even though I never thought I was. As I was telling my story, I looked over and big tears started rolling down his face. He reached over embraced me and kissed me. I asked him, "What are you crying for?" Here's this big old 300-pound man crying and I'm the one who's had the surgery. He said, "You're just the most remarkable person that I have ever seen in my life." You know, I had several male friends that I dated after having my breast reconstruction who said the same thing to me. They said, "You're marvelous. I admire you, and there is nothing to be ashamed of." I always told them that I wasn't ashamed of it; I just felt that I should tell them in case they questioned the scars. I think that men accept this better than women accept it themselves.

How has your daughter reacted to your breast cancer and breast reconstruction? Has she been supportive? Is she more aware of the dangers of breast cancer herself?

She accepted my cancer well, but she was worried about my health and about my mental state. When she saw that I wasn't going to die, she was very glad that I decided to have breast reconstruction. She knew that it would take that to make me happy. So she was all for it.

I have been told by my doctors that she should have regular checkups and should start earlier than most women because of the hereditary link. So I encourage her, and I remind her to examine herself. She is aware of her risk and has already started having mammograms.

***What advice would you like to give to other women considering
breast reconstruction?***

A woman at any age owes it to herself to consider breast reconstruction. It does wonders for you mentally. It helps you to bypass self-pity
and move on to life.

CARLYE: I WANTED TO KNOW AS MUCH AS I COULD

She was strikingly attractive with her hunter green suit and upswept
red hair. A green and maroon scarf was tied stylishly around her neck,
and she smiled easily as she introduced herself as Carlye, my next appointment.

Carlye's cancer was discovered during her very first mammogram,
when she was only 39. At the time the doctor thought it was probably
nothing to worry about but, as a precaution, sent her to a surgeon for a
biopsy. She didn't bother telling her husband because she was so sure
that nothing was wrong. The surgeon also was reassuring, and even
though he talked about breast cancer and treatment options, he told
her that he was positive that she was too young for breast cancer.
These reassurances from two different doctors made the discovery of
her breast cancer all the more shocking and distressing to Carlye and
her husband. She thinks that if they had been less optimistic initially,
she might have been better prepared for the news that she received.
This was also a complicated and somewhat harried time for Carlye,
her husband, and their three young children. He was in the process of
being transferred out of town. She held down a full-time job as a public relations representative for an advertising agency and also had full
responsibility for their children since her husband was out of town for
long periods of time. The burden of her breast cancer treatment seemed
particularly heavy.

The biopsy confirmed breast cancer, and the recommendation for
her type of cancer, lobular carcinoma, was a mastectomy. She decided
that she needed a second opinion. She was not especially happy with
the first surgeon. It was at this point that she became her own consumer advocate and started researching the topic, interviewing surgeons, and taking control of her health care decisions. In this process
she interviewed three general surgeons and two plastic surgeons; consulted with numerous other physicians, cancer information services,
and support groups; read medical books and articles; and educated
herself until she was sure that she knew what she wanted to do and

that she had chosen the best doctors to provide the treatment that she needed.

Carlye's treatment consisted of a modified radical mastectomy on her left breast and a preventive (prophylactic) mastectomy on her right breast. Breast reconstruction was an integral part of her treatment. According to Carlye, "There was never any question whether I would have breast reconstruction. I was just going to have it done because I wanted it. I never thought otherwise." Although she originally considered having a TRAM flap because she desired abdominal contouring as well as breast restoration, on further investigation she elected for a simpler procedure. She had bilateral reconstruction with tissue expansion and implant placement along with liposuction of her abdomen. This seemed the ideal solution for her and involved less surgery. The amount of abdominal tissue for reconstructing two breasts with a TRAM might be inadequate. This way she could have larger breasts and still have a smaller stomach. It has now been 5 years since she had her reconstruction, and Carlye is delighted with her choices and with the fact that she did not "take the first answer that she was given."

Why did you seek breast reconstruction?

It wasn't a question. I was just going to have it done because I wanted to. I never thought otherwise.

How did you choose the plastic surgeon to perform your breast reconstruction and the particular technique that you wanted? Did you consult with more than one plastic surgeon?

I was never a person who takes the first answer. I went to three surgeons before I decided on someone to perform my mastectomy. I also did some shopping for my breast reconstruction, consulting with two different plastic surgeons before I made my choice.

After my mastectomy I started checking around to see who was the best plastic surgeon in the field. I asked everybody I could find and read anything I could. I saw the first plastic surgeon because he was well respected. He does the flap procedure; that's his thing. He let me talk to a lady in his office who had the stomach flap reconstruction. She let me see her breast reconstruction and her breast looked great; it matched the other side. It was amazing. I thought if this woman can look this good; that's not so bad at all. The plastic surgeon told me about all of the other methods of breast reconstruction, but I thought it would be great having my stomach bulges removed. Also I had always been extremely flat-chested, a 32A. I really wanted to be a little bit larger. This plastic surgeon told me that if I selected the TRAM flap, I could only use this flap once. If I was considering having both sides done, he would need to know that now, so he could plan the flap accordingly. I decided I would rather have both sides done and get it over with so I wouldn't constantly worry about getting cancer in my other breast.

I then went to the second plastic surgeon, and he recommended tissue expansion with implants. If I was concerned about my stomach, he said he could do liposuction. I wasn't sure about that. So I dragged my husband along to speak with these plastic surgeons.

I went back and forth between the two doctors three times. I talked to other women who had different procedures done. I talked to anybody who would talk to me. I went to my breast cancer support group and talked to everybody there. I talked to a Reach To Recovery volunteer and a nurse in the hospital. I called the American Cancer Society and asked to talk to somebody. They sent someone who was my age and who had the flap procedure. I saw hers; it looked great. I saw a lot of different people's reconstructed breasts. I got a medical book on breast reconstruction and spent hours reading it and looking at the pictures. One of my friends asked me how I could look at that gory stuff, but I wanted to know as much as I could before I had anything done.

Now the question was which procedure I wanted to have. I made my decision after attending a conference where both of these plastic surgeons were lecturers. At this seminar I watched videotapes of the different reconstructive operations. Finally, I decided that I wanted to try tissue expansion with implants. I wanted to be bigger busted and I felt that tissue expansion would provide more flexibility in determining my breast size since I was having both sides done. The TRAM was always an option if the implants didn't work out or if they were rejected. Even so, I wanted to try implants first.

The plastic surgeon I selected was the one who had suggested tissue expansion to me. He is supposed to be one of the best; he was considered one of the innovators in breast reconstruction. I felt confident with what he had to offer. The pictures he showed me didn't show the best results. Every patient that I saw actually looked better than those pictures. I didn't feel like I got a rosy picture that everything was going to be absolutely perfect, but I still thought he had the best to offer.

Are you happy with your choice? Did you experience any problems communicating with your plastic surgeon? Was he responsive to your needs?

Some of his other patients told me that he was kind of quiet. I said, "Okay, I can talk a lot." I always came prepared for my appointments with a list of questions for him. Then he would sit down and talk to me. I wanted his undivided attention and I got it.

How did you decide how large you wanted your breasts to be?

I used my temporary prostheses to estimate the best size. When I bought my prostheses, I tried on small, medium, and large ones. Because I had the option, I decided to experiment to determine what I wanted. I had worn an A bra cup previously, but wanted to be larger. I decided to try a C cup. I didn't want to get accustomed to prostheses that were too large, because then I would be disappointed if the reconstructed breasts weren't that large. So I wore the C cup and it felt good. Then I waited a year before I had reconstruction.

How did your recovery from the reconstruction compare to recovery after your mastectomies? Did you experience much pain?

The drains were uncomfortable and I was happy when they came out. It was also difficult having both sides done. I couldn't use my arms to pull myself up, but I could use my stomach. My doctor told me to take it easy and I did. My mom came to help with the children, and I was ready for her to go back home after 2 weeks. The neighbors were great; everybody brought in dinner. After 2 weeks I could get up and move around. I was a little stiff when I started exercising my arms, but it wasn't a bad pain. I went back to work 6 weeks after my surgery.

Recovery from the first stage of my reconstruction, when my expanders were put in, was easier than the recuperation after the mastectomy. When I had the expanders placed, I also had my nose done to help me breathe better. I decided to get something extra out of this experience, to have everything done at one time. I expected some discomfort after the reconstruction, but I never really felt much pain. I just considered it part of the normal procedure. I didn't feel that bad. It was not unbearable. I was off work for another 6 weeks.

Did you have any problems or complications after your reconstruction?

No, none at all.

After the tissue expanders were placed, how long did it take you to get your breasts expanded? Was expansion painful?

It was done in 6 weeks; I came once a week. I was petrified the first time I came, but they used this tiny IV bag and this little, bitty needle. It was nothing. I went about five times to have my expanders inflated. Once the IV bag was in, I felt a little prick and then pressure under my arm. After the first few times I adjusted. Immediately after each expansion my chest was tight, but it would get better within a day or two. It didn't bother me.

When did you have the permanent breast implants put in?

I had my expanders inserted in July and I waited until early November to have the permanent implants put in. That timing was better for my work schedule. I also decided to get rid of the stomach during this operation. That morning when I went in I was a basket case. I was pleased with how the expanders looked, and I wanted to be sure that the permanent implants didn't make me look any smaller. The plastic surgeon and I talked about size before the operation. He asked if I wanted to be the size I was or bigger. I said maybe a little bit bigger, and I am plenty big now. I am probably a double D.

Did you have any pain after the implants were placed?

No more than I had expected. I didn't feel bad.

Why did you have nipple reconstruction? Where was the tissue graft taken?

I just wanted it. That was part of the complete process. I said no to the groin area because I did not want a hairy nipple. I have too much hair there. He decided to take the graft material from underneath my arm.

Was your nipple-areola tattooed? Does it match the nipple-areola that was preserved on the breast that had the prophylactic mastectomy?

I was perfectly happy with everything except the coloring of the nipple. I had this real dark nipple, and I cried. Every time my plastic surgeon changed the dressing on it, I would say, "It's too dark. It's like a headlight." He kept telling me it would fade, but I would still cry over it. That was the only time I cried about the reconstruction. He told me to put salt on it. So every night I sat with a salt press on it, and I would look at it and say to myself, "I can deal with this." But it really upset me. I was impatient. I had my natural nipple on one side and I was trying to compare it to that. It was hard. The color is fading now. It takes a while. Besides the color, the nipple itself looks great; it matches the other side perfectly.

Have you had any problems with the implants?

No. They have been just fine.

Did you have any concerns about having implants?

When I was considering implants, I asked if they could cause cancer. My plastic surgeon said there had been no reported cases of cancer and no evidence to link implants with cancer. I have not experienced any problems with them.

Are you satisfied with your breast appearance?

I am a perfectionist, a nitpicker. I look very good, but I probably would have placed the nipple higher. I think it's a bit low, but the placement may have been influenced by the location of my mastectomy scar. My breasts are still a tiny bit imperfect. But if I have a bra or my clothes on, you could never tell it. I turned out better than I thought possible. I feel free to show my reconstruction to any of my friends who ask to see it, even the friends that haven't had a mastectomy. They can't believe how good it looks. I don't think the pictures in the books do it justice.

Do your breasts have sensation?

I don't have any feeling from the top up or in the bottom halves of my breasts. It's strange. I have some remaining feeling in my nipple; it hurt when they tattooed the corner of my nipple. I must still have some underlying nerves there because I could feel it and they had to deaden that area. My nipples still have a sense of touch, but the sexual sensation is gone. I had hoped that by saving the one nipple I could also retain that, but it is gone. I had read that I could lose it, but I assumed that I wouldn't. That was a big disappointment.

How do your scars look?

I have no new scars. My plastic surgeon reopened my mastectomy scar when he placed the expander and then the implants. I was fortunate because my mastectomy scar was in a good place. The plastic surgeon marked where he wanted my scar before surgery. It runs horizontally across my chest as opposed to being oriented across my upper chest area. I much prefer having my scar go sideways. I can wear a sundress. I can wear anything I want; the scar does not show. I love that; it is just great. I don't know why all surgeons don't do it this way.

Have you adjusted to your reconstructed breasts? Do they feel a part of you?

I feel completely together, but I still don't feel like they're totally mine. I am more protective of my breasts now. Having been so small before, these big lumps are an adjustment; they don't mash down totally and I feel pressure if I lay on my stomach. Now I sleep with a pillow under me. Maybe large-breasted women have this problem. I don't know. I could lie flat on my stomach before; now that position is uncomfortable for me.

Are your breasts soft and natural?

They are very soft. My husband says they feel great. He also loves the way they look.

Has reconstruction had an affect on your self-image, your feelings of femininity? Has it affected the way you dress?

I feel more feminine; that is a plus. I look better. I feel and look good in my clothes. I look great in a swimsuit. After I had my expanders put in, I bought absolutely gorgeous lingerie because I felt comfortable. Before, when I was a 32A, nothing fit very well; my gowns would always just hang on me. I never had anything form fitting because it never looked right. Now I put on a sexy nightgown, and it fits at the top and doesn't hang loose. I don't feel that I am a different kind of person. I didn't go out and suddenly buy everything that was low cut. I wear most of my same clothes, except for a few blouses that are too tight now, but it was a pleasure to have to replace them.

How have your children coped with your breast cancer and breast reconstruction ? How did you tell them about your breast cancer, the mastectomy, and the reconstruction?

When I first found out that I had cancer, my husband and I didn't tell the kids right away. Before my mastectomies we sat them down and talked to them. We tried to be real positive. I thought we had done a good job; the kids seemed to take it very well. They even visited me in the hospital and saw that I was fine. It wasn't until later at the teachers' conference that we realized that they didn't really understand. My son had told his teacher that I had AIDS. They knew I had something bad. I guess they just missed the cancer part. I said, "Gee it's bad, but it's not that bad." We have tried to explain to them that my cancer was found early and the chance of my recovery is good.

Do you have concerns about your daughter's or other relatives' risk of developing breast cancer?

I have concerns; my daughter needs to be monitored more closely than the normal person. She asked, "Will I get it?" I said it's something that needs to be watched. There is always a possibility that she could. She just needs to be aware of her risk, so if cancer develops, she can find it early like I did mine. My mother is concerned. She goes routinely for breast exams, like she should.

Since my cancer was diagnosed, I have an aunt who has developed breast cancer. It spread into her entire breast. It's an extremely severe case, so extreme that they can't even perform a mastectomy because they couldn't close the wound. I couldn't believe that she would let it go. I mean she knew she had a lump for 6 or 7 years and didn't do anything about it. I guess she's from a generation that wasn't aware or informed. They can't accept it and don't want to know about it. Since then I have met many people through Reach To Recovery and my support group who don't want to know about anything. They just want their surgery or reconstruction done.

How have your friends reacted to your breast cancer and breast reconstruction?

It's amazing how many people my age are being diagnosed with breast cancer. It's pretty scary. After I had my mastectomies, everyone in my office had mammograms; they were in shock. One other woman found she had breast cancer; she was one of those people who doesn't want to know. She just wanted to have her surgery and get it over with. She didn't want reconstruction, whereas I couldn't wait to have it done. Later she changed her mind and had a latissimus dorsi flap breast reconstruction. She was thrilled.

How can a man be supportive to a woman undergoing breast cancer treatment or breast reconstruction?

My husband was there for me as much as he could be. He always came with me for my doctor's appointments, and he would discuss the problems with me. He wanted to know what was happening. It was also good because he would remember what I missed. He took notes and was a great backup.

After my mastectomy he was transferred and was commuting back and forth each weekend. It would have been easier if he had been in town during the week and could have helped with the kids and the house. That part was hard for me, having to do it all day and night with no relief. But it was the best we could do considering the circumstances, and he really wanted to be there. Knowing that he cared helped a lot.

He also supported my decision for reconstruction. He said, "You don't have to have reconstruction; it doesn't matter to me." He never pushed me to have this done. Reconstruction was my idea, not his, but he was willing to go along with it. He thinks I look great with my breast reconstruction. So does my mother. She says I look better than I did before, and I do. My husband has always been a boob man anyway; now he has everything he ever wanted.

Were they supportive of you at work? Did you feel that they were sympathetic to your needs after your mastectomies and after your breast reconstruction?

They were okay after my mastectomy and my first reconstructive surgery. Then, after my second reconstruction surgery, when the implants were put in, it was different.

Two weeks after I had been back they called me in and said, "We know you've been out sick, but you need to improve your attendance." I was devastated and totally shocked. I said, "I don't need this." I didn't think that sort of thing happened; I thought people were more knowledgeable and understanding. I had enough to deal with. My husband was transferred right after my mastectomy. He commuted back and forth every week. He could not be with me physically from Monday through Friday. I had to do everything myself, and I was recuperating. I had to be out for anything that came up with the children. There was no one else to do it. Plus I had to be out for doctors' appointments. After you have cancer, you go steady with your doctors for awhile. You have to go back and see this doctor and that doctor. You don't just say, "Okay it's over now." I expected them to understand and I cried and cried when they didn't.

Did you talk to anyone about this reprimand about your attendance record?

They did that to me Friday afternoon; you're not supposed to ever do a conference on a Friday afternoon. All weekend I cried hysterically, and I cried at work for months in the privacy of my office. Just thinking about it I sniff. On Monday I got the nerve and went in and said I didn't appreciate that treatment. The warning still stood. I now think that my manager was responsible; he is from the old school. His wife stays home. I think that he never felt that I needed the reconstruction. He probably felt that the additional time I was off work for reconstruction was unnecessary. I don't care what he thinks. It was the right thing for me to do. But their reaction was hard to deal with. People need to be sensitized to this issue. Reconstruction is an important part of treating a woman's cancer; your sense of well-being is crucial to your recovery and rehabilitation.

If you had it to do over again, would you have reconstruction? Was it worth the time, the pain, and the trouble? Are you happy you did it?

Oh, yes. It was never an option that I wouldn't do it, and I would do it again. It was a positive light at the end of the tunnel. I am glad that the cancer surgeon I chose sent me to a plastic surgeon before I had my mastectomy because that provided me with something hopeful to look forward to. The first doctor I saw avoided the issue of reconstruction. He said, "We'll talk about it later." I didn't want to talk about it later. This was something good, not something bad. I didn't want to put it off; that is why I looked until I found a cancer surgeon who understood my feelings.

MARILYN: A POSITIVE ATTITUDE MADE THE DIFFERENCE

"Hang nails hurt me, so I don't know why I didn't have any pain with this whole experience. It's probably because I had a positive attitude from the beginning and that helps more than anything else, especially with recovery." This optimistic attitude and her decision to "just get on with it" characterize Marilyn's approach to life. A large, full-figured woman, Marilyn found herself coping with the dual traumas of divorce and breast cancer at the age of 46. As a busy professional and the mother of three sons, she could ill afford to succumb to depression; too many people were depending on her. Instead, she decided to "take one step at a time." Her divorce she admits, while not a particularly happy event, actually may have helped to divert her attention from her cancer. As she explained, "I usually do well in a crisis, and then I fall apart after it's all over. This time I haven't fallen apart too badly. I guess I just had too much to deal with—there wasn't time."

Marilyn's cancer was detected after she noticed a burning sensation in her right breast and went to the doctor to check it out. She did not feel a lump in her breast and was astonished when her gynecologist's examination revealed a golf ball—sized lump, which necessitated a modified radical mastectomy, chemotherapy, and finally, "because I never considered going without," breast reconstruction. Her breast was reconstructed with a latissimus dorsi (back muscle) flap with tissue expansion and implant placement, and her opposite breast, which was quite large, was reduced to provide the best symmetry.

As a nurse from a family of medical professionals, Marilyn knew where to get the best care, and she relied on these experts to guide her through this experience. "My thought was, you do what you have to do, and I will make the best of it."

Why did you decide to have breast reconstruction?

It was something that I never questioned. I just wanted to have it. As I wore the prosthesis I knew even more that I wanted it. I have big breasts and the prosthesis just made me more aware of my loss. Each time you change clothes that thing is there and you have to take it off. I didn't like being flat-chested on one side. I was self-conscious wearing nightgowns around the children with one side flat; I didn't feel whole. I couldn't wear a bathing suit. The prosthesis was so large that when I bent over it would fall away from my body. Reconstruction has been wonderful.

How did you select your plastic surgeon?

My friend had gone to this plastic surgeon and recommended him. I just called him and made an appointment. My brother is a physician; he checked my plastic surgeon out and said I had the best surgeon for breast reconstruction. I was confident with my choice.

What breast reconstruction technique did you select?

My plastic surgeon caught me off guard when he said he wanted to do the latissimus dorsi back flap. My friend had tissue expanders and implants for her reconstruction, and I just assumed that was what he would do for me.

I did ask him why he felt this procedure was right for me, and he said it was because I needed the fullness. I took his word; I figured he had done this and had good results. He was the one that knew, not me. I certainly would not second guess him.

What were your goals for reconstruction? Did you have any surgery on your remaining breast?

I wanted to be back to normal and I accomplished that. But the really great thing that happened was that he reduced the other breast. He took one look at me and said, "Marilyn, I can't put back what was there." I said, "Great! What can we do with this other one?" He said that he could reduce it. For me that has been even better than the actual breast reconstruction. I was tired of having big "boobs," but it never occurred to me to have breast reduction because I thought you lost sensation, and I didn't want that. But I haven't lost any sensation with the reduction. None whatsoever.

Was it easy to communicate with your plastic surgeon? Was he responsive to your needs? Could he have served you better?

I'm crazy about him; he is wonderful. He is a very warm person. If I had questions, he would answer them. If I demanded more time, he gave it. But I had to work at the relationship and the communication.

During my first visit in July when he told me he wanted to do the latissimus dorsi flap, I was shocked and I didn't ask the questions that I meant to ask. I was also flustered by the pictures he took of me. My former husband is a lawyer, and so I had seen pictures of patients before and after surgery. I knew why my plastic surgeon needed to take them. Even so, being overweight, I was horrified at having pictures made of me. I also wasn't sure I wanted to go through that much surgery, and he hadn't spent that much time explaining the operation to me. So, although I had my doubts, I didn't say anything.

During that office visit in July my surgery was scheduled for November. As I left I said, "Will I see you again?" He said, "No, I'll see you the day of surgery." That puzzled me. I wondered how he could see me once and then operate on me 4 months later. I wasn't sure that I wanted to come back to him. And, as it turned out, my operation in November had to be postponed. That was the best thing that could have happened because it gave me a chance to establish a better line of communication and make sure that he was the right surgeon for me. I called him and made another appointment. I told him that before I let him operate on me I wanted to see him again because I had questions. So I went back with a page of questions, and I just went down my list and he answered them all for me. Of course, I already knew the answers because I had done research and carefully read what I could find. I just wanted him to say, "Yes, this is what we need to do and why we need to do it." And he did that. I'm mechanical; I like to know how things work. I wanted to know about the flap and the way it was twisted in the tunnel. My plastic surgeon did not take the time to do that, but he did give me a book to read that explained those details. It might have helped if he would have spent a little more time explaining how the flap was done.

I did one really neat thing to communicate my expectations to my plastic surgeon. Two or three days before I had my reconstruction done my son and my daughter-in-law and I went through *Playboy* and *Penthouse* magazines and I selected some pictures of breasts that looked like I wanted to look. I took these pictures to my plastic surgeon and said, "Now I know you can't make me look just like this, but I'd love to come close." That was really great; it was good for him to have that visualization. By looking at those pictures he understood what I meant when I said that I wanted to be "small." "Small" to somebody else might mean something else.

What did your breast reconstruction involve and how long did it take?

He reduced my normal breast and then did the latissimus dorsi flap and inserted the tissue expander during the same operation. Then I came back two times for tissue expansion. I had a total of 300 ml of saline solution injected into my expander. I had the reconstruction done in December, and I had the permanent implants placed in March.

How did your recuperation from reconstruction compare to your recovery after mastectomy?

With the reconstruction, I was in the hospital from Thursday until Sunday. It was similar to the mastectomy, only not as bad. I was out of work the same amount of time, 1 day short of 3 weeks. After reconstruction I could move and lift my arm, whereas I couldn't do that after mastectomy. There was no pain. When he put in the permanent implants, it was done on a Thursday and I went home on a Friday morning. I went home with a drain. Monday I had a friend take me to his office to get the drain out, and Tuesday I went back to work.

Did you have much drainage after the latissimus dorsi flap? How long did your drainage tubes stay in?

Nothing that the tubes didn't take care of. I had two drains to begin with and they took one out right away. They were both out by the time I went home after the first stage of my reconstruction.

Did you have any complications, any problems?

Part of my breast turned a little red. My plastic surgeon thought it might be an infection, but it was never sore and there was never any discomfort. It just had a little fever in it. He gave me some antibiotics and the redness disappeared after about 4 or 5 weeks.

When did you begin your tissue expansion? Was it uncomfortable or inconvenient? How long did it take?

I had my first expansion 1 week after my surgery and it was fine. I didn't have any problem with it. The second one was more difficult. I was really wrung out by the time it was over. The needle wasn't long enough, so the nurse had to press down on my breast to inject the saltwater into the expander. It didn't hurt, but it took a long time to drip in. When I went back the third time, I said I didn't want to be expanded any bigger than I was. My plastic surgeon looked and said that was fine.

Describe the scars from your reconstruction. What do they look like? Where are they placed?

My scars are gross, but that is not the surgeon's fault. That is the way my body reacts to being cut open. I've had gallbladder surgery and an appendectomy. I had the appendectomy when I was young, so you really can't see it. But my gallbladder scar is just horrible. It's ¼ to ½ inch wide and very long. The scars from the reconstruction and from the mastectomy are the same way.

I have a scar down my back from the reconstruction; it's perpendicular to the floor, straight up and down, and it's terrible. I mean it's very red and angry and wide. It doesn't show in my clothing, and I can wear a bathing suit. I couldn't wear a bikini, but then I wouldn't want to wear a bikini anyway. On my breast I have a triangular scar from the back flap; it is also wide and red. I know it will fade with time because my gallbladder scar has faded. These scars don't bother me. They don't hurt, although sometimes they itch. But that's normal and I just put lotion on them.

Was reconstruction what you expected? Any surprises?

I expected the reconstruction to be similar to the mastectomy and it was, but better. It was great to wake up and feel my upper chest and find something there . . . instead of a hole. It is not identical to my original breast, but it is the nearest thing to it.

How is it different?

The reconstructed breast may be a little bit harder than the other breast. The tissue expander sort of fell under my arm a little by the time I had the implant put in, so my plastic surgeon was careful to secure the permanent implant in place. My reconstructed breast also hangs a tad differently, but if you saw me without any clothes on, you would be amazed. I think you would have to feel it. Down at the crease there is a sharper curve. I'm sure that's where the implant sinks down. But it's great.

Are you going to have your nipple-areola reconstructed?

I have not had my nipple done. I have not decided if I am going to do that. I'm tired of being operated on.

Are you limited in activity from your reconstruction?

No, not at all. In fact, I've taken up golf. My 15-year-old son is teaching me. I have never played before, and my swing isn't bad.

How did you pay for your reconstruction?

My insurance company has been wonderful. I have insurance through the hospital and it has paid almost everything. My divorce agreement provided that my husband would pay for the rest of it. Not one penny has come out of my pocket.

Was your family supportive?

My family was very supportive. My boys did not hover over me, but they did anything I asked them to do. My attitude with them was very straightforward: I have cancer, I have to have a mastectomy, and then I'm going to have reconstruction. They never questioned me. Of course, they were upset about the cancer, but I think they are proud of me because of my attitude. I just said this is the way we are going to do it and I did . . . one, two, three.

If you had it to do over again, would you have reconstruction?

Absolutely. I don't even think about having had cancer anymore. Before reconstruction every time you dress you have to put the prosthesis in and get it fixed just right. It's just bothersome; this way it's almost like nothing ever happened.

What advice about breast cancer and breast reconstruction would you like to share with other women?

A positive attitude helps you to cope in the most trying situations. You can't choose the circumstances; you can't change the fact that you have cancer. It's best to take action, find the best people to help you, learn as much as you can, then do it and get on with your life.

SARA: NO LONGER A VICTIM

I could feel her tension when we shook hands at the beginning of the interview. Sara sat down tentatively on the edge of the chair, and she remained there throughout our discussion with her arms crossed and her fingers tightly clenched. As her story unfolded, she cried silently, wiping away the tears.

Sara is pale and fragile with the youthful good looks of a cover girl model; no one would suspect that she is a married woman of 40 with three young children. Five years ago Sara was diagnosed with breast cancer. She chose mastectomy as treatment for her malignancy because she worried about the possibility of cancer recurrence after lumpectomy. Recovery after her mastectomy was particularly devastating for her, and she is still shaken by the trauma that she has endured. She did not want to face her deformity or deal with this experience. Sara describes herself as "squeamish and emotional." Surgery, with its accompanying blood, scars, stitches, and drains, was terrible for her. The only good news she had was that her cancer had been discovered early and chemotherapy would not be necessary. But even that report was reversed as her pathologist and oncologist, on analyzing her mastectomy specimen, discovered several other malignant sites. These were microscopic, but they felt that she should have chemotherapy to "cover her bases."

Chemotherapy was another terrible trial to endure. Her anger at this point was hard to control. She found herself screaming at her oncologist and saying how unfair it was. It was at that point in her treatment, she admits, that she began advocating for herself and took back control of her life. When Sara finished her course of chemotherapy, she set about investigating the option of breast reconstruction.

Although Sara did not want additional surgery, she felt that she needed reconstruction so that she could get on with her life. She hated the way her chest looked, and she couldn't bear the thought of her young daughter seeing her in that condition. She did not, however, want a major reconstructive procedure. Flap surgery was out of the question for her. She had seen someone with a TRAM flap and she could not understand how anyone would choose to undergo that operation "in the name of a breast." She had no desire for additional scars. She wanted the simplest operation possible with the least chance for complications. She knew she was thin and that her skin was tight and stretched, but she wanted an implant reconstruction and wanted a plastic surgeon who could meet her needs.

Her efforts to find a plastic surgeon were not trouble-free. The first plastic surgeon she consulted assured her that he could reconstruct her breast with a tissue expander and an implant. She was scheduled for surgery with him when he called her in and informed her that he had changed his mind; he felt that her skin couldn't stretch enough to build a breast symmetric with her remaining breast. Her only choice would be a TRAM flap or she would be very disappointed because her breast reconstruction would be a failure. She was shocked and angered by this news, feeling that her confidence had been betrayed and that he should have told her initially if he couldn't perform the operation that she had requested. She decided if she couldn't have an implant reconstruction she wouldn't have anything.

She next consulted two other plastic surgeons who both felt that they could successfully reconstruct her breast using tissue expansion and an implant. She chose the surgeon whose approach seemed most logical to her and whose standards of perfection were as high as hers. She wasn't willing to accept a mound on her chest; it wasn't enough to just look good in her clothes, she wanted to look good naked. Now, after several procedures, Sara is delighted with what she had done. Her plastic surgeon was the perfectionist that she needed. Finally, the ordeal is over, and although the experience still haunts her, Sara no longer feels like a victim.

How did you react to your diagnosis of breast cancer?

This came out of the blue. No lumps, no fibrocystic disease. No nothing. It was a whirlwind, a nightmare. I felt like a victim; I mean I was only 36 years old. It just didn't make any sense. I had a 1½-year-old child and my life went topsy-turvy.

Why did you choose a mastectomy over a lumpectomy with irradiation?

My surgeon gave me a choice between a mastectomy and lumpectomy with irradiation and I didn't even hesitate. I just said mastectomy. I didn't want the uncertainty. I wanted it over. I felt a mastectomy was the safest approach. I was not worried about preserving my breast. I was just worried about getting rid of the cancer. Now that I know more, I still would do the same thing. I know of too many women who have had recurrences after lumpectomy, and it's horrid to face cancer a second time. I don't care what they say; if cancer recurs, it's probably tougher to deal with than the first time. So a week after I found the lump I had my mastectomy.

Did your surgeon tell you about the option of breast reconstruction before you had your mastectomy?

My surgeon didn't offer me reconstruction; he didn't work with a plastic surgeon. Later, when I read about reconstruction, I thought a lot about that. How would I have felt about that experience if I had a choice. God forbid it should happen to me again, but I would definitely have some kind of immediate reconstruction. The first time, however, I might have needed to adjust to what I was going through. I have such high expectations that I might have been easily disappointed with a less than perfect result.

How long did it take you to recuperate from your mastectomy? What was your emotional reaction to the surgery? Did you experience much pain?

I stayed in the hospital for 5 days; it was longer than I needed. Finally, my surgeon kicked me out. I was going home to three children and I had a lot to deal with. I was comfortable in the hospital. I pampered myself. I had private nurses. That was good for me. When I woke up in the middle of the night, there was somebody there. My night nurse was wonderful, very supportive; she helped me through it. I came home to a roomful of people staring at me: my parents, my sisters, my brothers-in-law, and my husband and children. They were all there and it was overwhelming.

I hung around the house for several weeks. I still had the drains in. Because I came home with my drains and those bags hanging from them, I did not look at myself. I hated those drains. The surgeon wanted me to look at myself before I left the hospital, but I couldn't. I also didn't deal with the bandages. I let my husband, who is a doctor, change the bandages. When I went back to the surgeon and he took the drains out, I almost fainted. I'm a very squeamish person. It wasn't that it hurt so much. It was just a horrible feeling, having these things snake through your body. I must have turned a strange shade of green. I went through the same thing with the stitches. I'm just not good with the medical part; I can't handle the scars, the stitches, the blood. When my surgeon took out the final stitches, I still had not looked at myself. My husband had; we were down to a very small bandage and he was still changing it for me. When I left the surgeon's office that day, he said, "You are going to have to deal with this. You are going to have to face it."

What was your reaction when you finally looked at your mastectomy?

The first time I looked at myself I went as far away from the mirror as I could and I kind of peered at myself through another mirror. It was terrible. It wasn't gory. It wasn't the scab or the scar or even the missing breast. I had pictured it flat, but fleshy. And instead it was bony and hard. That hard, flat surface was difficult to take. I went straight to the phone and called a plastic surgeon.

Did your mastectomy appearance prompt you to have breast reconstruction? Was it difficult to have another surgery, breast reconstruction, after your mastectomy?

Given my squeamishness about medical procedures, breast reconstruction was a big step for me. I decided to have breast reconstruction for my daughter and for me.

I was concerned about my daughter growing up seeing me like this. My little girl was 1½ and I didn't want to scare her. She's 5½ now and she looks at me and says, "Why are your nipples a little different? Why do you have that scar?" And I can just imagine how I would feel if she asked me "Why do you only have one?" I didn't want to scare her.

I also wanted normalcy in my life. I knew it was risky to have breast reconstruction; I might not like the results. I knew I didn't want more surgery. I wasn't sure that I was going to be happy. I talked to a friend of mine who had an implant reconstruction, and I realized that I needed to go for it. I needed to try to have a more normal appearance so that I could stop thinking cancer all of the time. I wasn't sure reconstruction would do it for me, but everything I had read and the few people I had talked to made me think that if I had this surgery I could put the trauma and the horror behind me. I wouldn't be confronted by it every day in the mirror. Everybody said I would feel more whole and back to normal.

The final reason was the prosthesis. It just wasn't comfortable. Every time I bent over this thing pulled my bathing suit away from my body, and you could see right down to my belly button. It was nerve racking. I actually had my prosthesis fall out once when I was out in public. It was hot and heavy, and even though I was grateful to have *something* to make me feel better about myself, I wasn't happy with the prosthesis.

How did you hear about reconstruction? How did you decide which technique of reconstruction was right for you?

My neighbor had breast reconstruction. I remember when I first heard about her reconstruction, I couldn't believe that she wanted to go through all of that surgery again. This was years before this ever happened to me. So I knew it was possible. I didn't know how they did it. A friend of mine had a mastectomy a year before I did and she had a TRAM flap reconstruction. I knew what that was about, and I knew I didn't want it. When she came to see me right before I went to surgery and then right after, she still couldn't stand up straight, and she was one of these tough cookies. She still is. She swears she never worried about cancer after her surgery, not for a day. She is just a very strong, determined person. Two days after her first mastectomy they told her that they needed to remove her other breast, and she said, "I have to go to a bar mitzvah. I'll come back." And she did. She was just tough. It seemed like nothing could phase her. When she had the TRAM flap, however, she had trouble with it. She was in a lot of pain. It was more than she had bargained for. So her experience biased me right away.

Probably the best thing I did to help me decide for sure which technique I wanted was to attend a breast reconstruction conference for nurses and patients that was sponsored by the American Cancer Society. They had an implant surgeon, a TRAM surgeon, and a free flap surgeon. I listened to those doctors and to the testimonial of their patients. I looked at slides all day, and I was in shell shock when I came out. But I knew what I wanted.

How did you select the plastic surgeon to perform your breast reconstruction? Did you consult more than one?

I went to see three doctors, The first plastic surgeon only did TRAM flaps, but I didn't know it at the time; he took my case knowing that I didn't want a TRAM flap. I told him I wanted an implant. I really felt that there was no special art to putting an implant in, but I went to him because he had a good reputation and would be up to date on nipple grafting. He accepted me as a patient for an implant reconstruction, and I had a surgery date set for January. Then in December he called me in. I went without my husband because I didn't know why he wanted to see me. He called me in and he made me undress. He took another set of humiliating pictures of me and then walked in while I was sitting there vulnerable, by myself, and told me I could not have an implant because it would fail. I did not have enough skin and my skin would not expand. The only choice I had was a TRAM flap reconstruction.

Had this first plastic surgeon already agreed to perform an implant reconstruction? Were you surprised when he changed his mind and recommended a TRAM flap?

I was totally shocked. I had gone in with lots of trepidation to begin with because I knew I had tight skin. He had led me on and I was very upset. I started crying. I was very mad at him. I said, "Well, then, I won't have anything at all if I can't have an implant. I won't have it. I don't want it. It's not for me. I have an 18-month-old daughter. I'm not going to walk around bent over, and I don't want all this major surgery right now." I was very angry. I said, "You've wasted 3 months of my time and I wanted to have this surgery at this time of year." I was very upset. When I left, he asked if there was anything he could do. I said, "I'll see." I went home and called two other plastic surgeons and made appointments.

How did you hear about these other plastic surgeons? Who suggested them?

I knew about the first one because my friend had been operated on by him for her TRAM and I had heard that he was a great name. And I knew about the other plastic surgeon, the one I finally went to, because my neighbor had implant surgery by him years ago. I called for an appointment and he was booked for a month. So I called the other plastic surgeon back, and I said, "Yes, you can do something for me. Get me an appointment with this plastic surgeon." And he did; I got an appointment the next week. I also made an appointment with another plastic surgeon at a small local hospital where I had my mastectomy. Both of these plastic surgeons said that tissue expansion with implant placement would work for me. One plastic surgeon compared the expansion process to what happens when you get pregnant and your skin stretches. They both assured me that nobody can tell you that your skin won't stretch as long as it hasn't been irradiated. That made me glad that I didn't have lumpectomy and irradiation.

How did you decide between these two plastic surgeons?

I finally decided between the last two plastic surgeons based on the hospitals where they practiced and their approaches to my opposite breast. One plastic surgeon wanted to operate on my normal breast because he needed to lift my nipple and put in a small implant so that I would get a good match. This plastic surgeon practiced at the university hospital, and he wanted to do my normal breast first and match the expander side to it. The other plastic surgeon wanted to do the expansion first and then operate on my other breast. This plastic surgeon was at the hospital where I had my mastectomy, and I didn't particularly want to go back there because I didn't want to relive that experience. When I thought about it and weighed the two approaches, I decided that the first plastic surgeon had the better approach.

Are you pleased with the plastic surgeon that you selected? Was he responsive to your needs?

I feel so fortunate that I found my way to my plastic surgeon. He is a perfectionist. I felt comfortable with that from the start. From a woman's standpoint, I was worried that this male plastic surgeon would be arrogant; he would give me this breast that wouldn't look anything like my other breast and would say I should be grateful for what I got. "Just what are you complaining about? It's better than what you had before." But he wasn't like that at all. He was so sensitive to my needs about my appearance and my desire for my breast to be perfect. He really listened to what I had to say. I always felt like I could walk in with a whole shopping list of questions and he would find the answers to solve my problems. He made me feel that he wouldn't be happy unless I was happy. That was such a relief to me. I brought a tremendous amount of tension into the plastic surgery experience. I had a lot of concerns; one woman I knew had problems with encapsulation. She had to go back and they had to break up the capsule; it was very painful. I kept hearing the TRAM plastic surgeon's voice in my head telling me, "It can't be done. It's going to fail. It's not going to look good; it's going to be a lump on your chest." So I went into my reconstructive surgery with more psychological baggage than most people do. I was terrified that I wouldn't be satisfied and that he would brush me off. He did what I needed done to make me feel good about myself with as few procedures as possible.

What was done during the first operation? Did you have any surgery on the remaining breast?

The hardest thing about the first surgery was that when my plastic surgeon came in to see me before the operation, he drew all over me with a pen and he had a resident with him. I guess he needed the markings to help guide him, but it was very humiliating. During this operation he raised the nipple and placed a small implant in my opposite (left) breast; then he placed an expander in my right side. When the plastic surgeon was finished, my gynecologist came in and I had my tubes tied. It seemed a good idea to get it all done at the same time since I was going under anesthesia.

How long were you in the hospital? Did you experience much pain?

I don't come out of anesthesia that well. I was very nauseous and uncomfortable after the operation. I ended up spending 2 days in the hospital instead of the usual one because I was vomiting and very weak. I was in pain, but it wasn't that bad. I don't remember feeling that it was more than I bargained for.

How did your breasts look and feel during the first few weeks after surgery? Did you have any surprises?

I had expected some pain, but I wasn't really prepared for the bruising after surgery. When I signed the informed consent, they had mentioned that I would probably be bruised from my chest to my waist, but I really hadn't pictured it. After the operation my reconstructed breast was slightly swollen and bruised. But it wasn't a problem. What was surprising to me, however, was the way my left side looked after he operated on it. It was my normal side and it was swollen and purple. It was alarming. It was distended, and I was more uncomfortable there than on the side where he put the expander in.

After the first stage of your breast reconstruction was your breast what you expected?

When they first put the expander in everybody said, "Oh, you are going in for a happy, positive thing. When you look down, you will have something on your chest and it will be wonderful." But when I looked down, all I saw was this shapeless lump, and I said, "This is not wonderful." I can only imagine what I would have thought if it had been done immediately. I would have said, "This is all I get?" I would have been in a total panic. When the surgeon checked me the next day, he looked under the bandages and said, "Oh, good, it's healing fine." He had been concerned because he barely had enough skin to close me. He took every bit of tissue I had. I was glad that I didn't need a skin graft like some women do when there isn't enough skin. I also had a terrible scar because the lesion was very high on my breast, so the scar forked up. Some women have these cute little slashes in an inconspicuous area, but I had a semicircular scar. It was so high that it would always show even when I had reconstruction.

How long did it take you to get your breasts expanded after the tissue expander was placed? Was expansion painful? Did you experience any problems?

It was just a little uncomfortable. The part when the needle was put into the port was uncomfortable. I felt a bit of tightness, but I don't remember it being unpleasant. I'm not a good one to ask, however, because I only went two or three times before I had a problem. After the first two times there wasn't much expansion. They couldn't seem to get my skin to stretch; it was so tight. It just looked bad. The third time I went they couldn't get any saline solution to go in through the expander. My plastic surgeon said, "It's one of two things—either the expander has failed because it has some defect in it or you've already formed some scar tissue, which would be unusual but is a possible complication." He made an appointment for me to go back into surgery the next week.

I had lots of fears that time because I didn't know what was wrong. I was shaking like a leaf; I kept telling them you need to give me something to calm me down. My plastic surgeon said that if he could get an implant in there, he would just go ahead and put it in and would not put in another expander. He was able to do that. That was great because it saved me an extra surgery. The expander had failed because the valve was clogged. So I walked out of there in much better shape than when I came in.

After your implant had been placed, were any adjustments needed?

I wasn't finished at that stage. Even though he had put the implant in, my breasts didn't match well enough. My breast wasn't large enough, so the implant served as it's own expander. He told me to wait at least 6 months before he adjusted my breasts to make them symmetric and to add the nipple. If necessary for symmetry he would exchange my implant for a larger one at that time. I also complained that there was no crease under my breast. My breast just sloped straight into my chest; there was no rounding.

He made all three adjustments in one outpatient surgery. He created a very nice crease. He was able to lift my breast up and build a nipple. I don't know how he did it—it is really a miracle.

The only negative aspect was that there was not enough skin there to use for the nipple. He had to extend my scar under my arm to get the tissue he needed to make the nipple. I still think maybe there was another way. That was uncomfortable for me. It was painful, a sticking pain. But it didn't last long. I worried about the scar showing in sleeveless clothes, but it turns out that it's not a problem. My bra covers it; bathing suits cover it. I can't wear a bathing suit that's cut out under the arm, but I wear one that comes right under my arm and then dips back. That was my only regret. I feel like we might have been able to solve that without going under my arm for the tissue. And the scar was kind of raggedy for a while because it's under your arm, which is not a good place for healing. It didn't hurt because I had no feeling under there. But I'm a little self-conscious about the scar, and I have to be careful when I buy certain kinds of clothes.

Now that the adjustments have been made, are you satisfied with the appearance of your reconstructed breast and nipple? Is your breast soft? Is it warm? Does it have sensation?

My reconstructed breast is not as soft as the other side, but it's soft enough. I've seen breasts that are hard, but some of those women had radiation therapy. For me, my reconstructed breast is soft enough and it's natural enough. I don't like its coldness and lack of sensation, but I realize that is the best I can do. And, from talking to other women, you realize that you don't have those sensations with a TRAM flap either.

I am pleased with my breast form and shape; it looks good. If I go too close to the mirror, I notice that one breast is a little fuller on top, the nipples don't exactly match, and the tattooing isn't perfect because the color isn't an exact match; my reconstructed one is lighter than my normal one. I could go back and have it retattooed and darkened, but I don't want the tape, I don't want the Polysporin, I don't want the blood. Even when I went back for the tattoo 5 months or more after the last phase of surgery, I was tired of being a patient and having a wound. Something major would have to happen to drag me back because I'm not a surgery person.

The nipple is great. It's not exactly the same shape as the other one, but that is okay. My only disappointment about the nipple is not the areola part, but the actual projection. When they first reconstruct your nipple, it projects out, then it collapses a little bit. I guess it's the nature of it. So it does protrude slightly, but my other nipple protrudes more. When I'm wearing a T-shirt, one nipple will be more noticeable than the other. I think that's something that nobody would ever notice. I'm not that concerned or self-conscious about it anymore. In the beginning, however, I would not wear a T-shirt or I would wear one with a pocket so that you couldn't actually compare the two nipples. The breast symmetry is now good.

Are you restricted now in any activity?

No. I play tennis, and I'm not at all uncomfortable. Every now and then I get a little muscle cramp, but that's no big deal.

What were your goals for breast reconstruction? Did you reach them?

I had higher goals than most. I had read somewhere that the goal of plastic surgery was to make you look good in a bra. I didn't think that was a high enough goal. I wanted to feel comfortable being naked. I knew I couldn't get an exact match. I didn't have unrealistic expectations, but I wanted to feel comfortable looking in a mirror. I definitely reached that goal. I got a very good result, especially considering what I started with. For implant surgery, I'm probably at the high end of good results.

Have you had second thoughts about the method of reconstruction that you selected?

I'm really glad I chose implant surgery. My doctor fully informed me before the operation about the implants. Currently I have no reason to doubt my decision despite all the negative publicity surrounding implants. I have called my plastic surgeon with my concerns and with any questions that I have, and he has been good about answering them. I like the technical information. Sometimes I'll even read the cancer journals that my husband subscribes to. Some people like a little pat on the hand. They want someone to say, "Honey, it's going to be okay; just trust us." I can't deal with that. I need to know. Any remaining questions should be answered by the ongoing clinical studies. I think I still will always worry about implants. I never felt 100% comfortable putting something foreign in my body, but I also didn't want the TRAM flap or something like it. I didn't want to carve my body up in the name of a breast. To me that was more barbaric and something I couldn't live with. But I had to weigh the two things because there is no miracle technique right now. We are not in "Star Trek" where they can just zap you and make you whole again. So I felt like I took the least invasive option, knowing that down the road they are going to be constantly revising and improving methods and I haven't closed my doors. Once you have had a TRAM flap you've closed the door. Now they are doing free flaps, which are better than TRAM flaps. I feel like I've left my options open and I'm not sorry. I'm happy with myself and I'm happy with the surgery. I know that I'm in good hands and my plastic surgeon will continue to follow me. If something needs to be done, I feel like he's the right person to do it.

Did your successful experience with breast reconstruction help you deal with your anger from your first encounter with the other plastic surgeon?

Yes, but I still needed closure, so I did something about it. I asked my plastic surgeon if he minded if I sent a picture of my reconstruction to the first plastic surgeon, the one who said I needed a TRAM. He said he wouldn't do it, but I did it anyway. I wrote him a long letter and enclosed my picture. I went through the whole story because I'm sure he didn't have it recorded in his chart about what he put me through that day. He wrote back to me and he said that he thought it was one of the finest examples of implant surgery that he had ever seen and asked if he could use my picture when he counseled patients. So it came full circle for me.

Was reconstruction worth the time, the pain, and the trouble?

Yes, yes. It was well worth it. It's not perfect. I never expected it to be perfect. But the ultimate result is that I look better in my clothes than

I did before. Now I even look great in bathing suits. The high point for me came one day when I was in this dress shop where the salesladies hover, which I hate. This saleswoman brought some clothes in for me. She was watching me try them on; she is a very high-pressure person. She was telling me how nice I looked in the dresses. She said, "You know, you're so thin, but you have such a nice bust." I just laughed and laughed the whole way home. I thought that's great. She said it totally out of the blue. If I had told her right then and there that I had had a mastectomy and breast reconstruction, I think she would have passed out.

Was your husband supportive during this experience?

My husband was great. He was very patient and he let me talk whenever and wherever. Normally he is not very patient; he is not one of these feeling, giving kinds of people. And he was really shaken up because he has had a lot of people die of cancer in his family. Cancer is not an easy thing for my husband. He was very scared and it brought us close together. He said something very sweet to me that showed me how he felt about it. He said, "If you can't sleep, just wake me up anytime and we'll talk." And sleeping was hard. After the mastectomy I couldn't roll on that side, and after the reconstruction I was uncomfortable again.

Were other people supportive of you through this experience?

The thing that helped me from the surgery through the prosthetic stage, through the plastic surgery stage, was the people—the doctors and the nurses. I was so blessed with supportive people all the way through. They were very personal with me. They treated me as an individual, not just as another patient. They knew my fears, my personality, and they made me feel like they really cared.

What questions do you think a woman should ask when she is considering breast reconstruction?

The most important thing a woman should do is talk to other women and see pictures. My plastic surgeon showed me pictures in a book. Another doctor showed me pictures of other patients. The before's and after's are very hard to look at, but they give you a better idea of what you are getting yourself into. You need to know all of the downsides. You need to ask about the pain, the scars, all the problems, so you know what to expect, both positive and negative.

What advice would you like to share with other women about your experiences with breast cancer and breast reconstruction?

Breast reconstruction made a difference in my life. I don't know if I could have gotten to the place I am now emotionally without the surgery. What happened to me can happen to any woman; it's one in nine right now. I see people with other kinds of disabilities and I feel grateful because I can hide my disability and I could reconstruct it. The reconstruction gave me a feeling of normalcy in my life. I'm not angry anymore. I don't feel like a victim.

INGRID: WE NEED TO TALK ABOUT IT

As I looked at Ingrid, I couldn't believe that this petite blond with her wide smile and ready laugh had undergone a mastectomy and immediate breast reconstruction with a TRAM flap only 8 short weeks before our interview. She was not bent over as I would have expected; and in fact, she was particularly bouncy and energetic. Her enthusiasm propelled our conversation.

Ingrid, a native of Sweden, has the blond good looks one associates with that part of the world. She is expressive and animated, and her speech is punctuated with short, clipped phrases, a type of verbal shorthand that lends emphasis to her words. A flight attendant working for one of the major airlines, she is 43 years old, married, and has a young daughter and son.

When her cancer was discovered, she and her family had recently relocated, and she knew few people to ask for advice. But for Ingrid, with her outgoing personality, being a stranger in a strange city was not an obstacle. Ingrid, as I was to learn, does not let things get in her way. Accustomed to responding quickly to difficult situations in her job, Ingrid approached her breast cancer and reconstruction with the same no-nonsense attitude. She investigated her options, interviewed everyone she could talk to, and then took the course of action that she felt was best for her and her family.

Because she didn't want anything unnatural in her body, TRAM flap breast reconstruction seemed the best long-term solution. She dealt with each problem as it arose, discussed it, and then solved it. As she explained, "My attitude is to bare it all as soon as possible and see the worst because then it will never be as bad again." That included telling her young children about her cancer and talking to her husband about the impact this surgery would have on their sex life. Her warmth was contagious. Her story is a heartwarming one.

How did you discover your breast cancer?

I went for a routine mammogram. I had no lump, no indication that anything was wrong. Two days later the doctor called and suggested that I have a biopsy. Right away I thought the worst. "Biopsy equals cancer. Be prepared . . . possible mastectomy." He made an appointment for me to see a general surgeon. I went to see him just to talk and get a general idea of what was going on. He looked at my mammograms and said this doesn't look like cancer, but we need a biopsy. I was not too happy with that particular surgeon. He was brand new. I didn't feel that he had enough experience. I didn't know if I had cancer or if I needed a mastectomy, but I wanted to be prepared—that meant seeing the best doctor possible. I felt that I wanted to get more opinions than just one. I saw another doctor a few days later. That weekend I called some neighbors and told them that I needed a breast biopsy. I was afraid I might have cancer and need a mastectomy. I asked if they knew of anybody in the area who had had a mastectomy. I wanted to find names of surgeons and hospitals. If in fact I had cancer, I had to act on it quickly. I couldn't sit around for months finding out. By Sunday afternoon people started returning my calls: strangers, friends, friends of friends. I got names of several general surgeons in the area at major hospitals; finally, I selected a woman surgeon.

When I went to the surgeon, she read my previous mammograms and took new ones to verify what she saw. Then she did a fine-needle biopsy. I was at the hospital all day. By the time I left they had diagnosed breast cancer. I was lucky. It was not invasive.

Did your surgeon offer you a choice between lumpectomy and modified radical mastectomy?

Because a large area of my breast was involved, my surgeon felt a modified radical mastectomy was a better choice for me. I have very small breasts and there wasn't much to work with; I would have very little breast remaining after lumpectomy and irradiation.

Why did you decide to have immediate breast reconstruction?

When I was diagnosed with cancer, I could only think mastectomy. I did not think immediate reconstructive surgery. That was secondary—for the future. Number one, get rid of the cancer. But when my surgeon said I was an excellent candidate for immediate reconstructive surgery, that was fantastic. I could get rid of my cancer and also walk out of the hospital with something that resembled a breast.

What were your goals for breast reconstruction? Why did you select a TRAM flap reconstruction?

My cancer surgeon gave me a copy of your book, and I read as much as I could about the different reconstructive options before I met with the plastic surgeon. I learned about implants and possible problems with scar tissue and maintenance and decided that I didn't want an implant if I could avoid it. Also, I didn't want my other breast touched. I wanted to have one that was still intact. I had never wanted to change my breast; I was happy with what I had. My goal was to have my reconstructed breast look and feel as similar as possible to what I had before. Considering my goals, my plastic surgeon suggested a TRAM flap. He saw I had a lot of extra tissue in my abdomen and felt that might be the best method for me. I was delighted when he told me that I wouldn't need an implant; my reconstructed breast could be all my own tissue. That was wonderful.

Why did you decide on that particular plastic surgeon?

When I discovered I needed a biopsy, I wanted the best, even if I had to go to another state or another country. From the women that kept calling me back that Sunday, I knew that the hospital had a good reputation. I was also confident with the expertise of my cancer surgeon, who has an excellent reputation as a breast surgeon. She referred me, and I trusted that she would only associate herself with the best plastic surgeon.

When I met with the plastic surgeon, I knew he was right for me. He's very human. As a man, he is surprisingly sensitive to a woman's feelings. He wants to make you feel like a woman. It's important to him to keep you as beautiful as possible and help you stay beautiful. He has a special quality that is hard to put into words. It's not given to everybody; you are born with it. He's a creator, an artist and that came across in our conversation.

Did he explain to you what he was going to do? Did he give you enough information?

He explained that he was going to use the tissue and muscle from my abdomen and move it up through my body cavity to build a breast. I asked how he would know how much tissue to put in there? He said that when the general surgeon takes out the breast tissue, they weigh and measure it. He would try to put the same amount back in and trim down any excess. He also explained that with the TRAM I could lose a lot of blood; he wanted me to donate 2 units of blood. That took 2 weeks.

Did you have any reservations about reconstruction?

I was afraid that it would cover up a possible cancer underneath; I also didn't know if it would be more difficult to detect a cancer recurrence after immediate reconstruction. I asked both my surgeons more than once if this was safe. I kept asking. That was my big worry. To me it was more important to live and not worry about the cancer than to look good; that was secondary. My general surgeon and plastic surgeon answered my questions. My surgeon said there was no need to wait because my cancer was caught so early. At a later stage reconstruction would have to be delayed until after chemotherapy and radiation.

How long were you in the hospital? Did you experience much pain?

The first 2 to 3 days in the hospital were painful and uncomfortable, even though I had the pain pump for the first 2 days. I had oral medication after that. The pain was mostly in the abdomen, not much in the breast at all. I was surprised that I could move my arm on the side of the mastectomy. I was happy with that. I was out of bed on the third day.

Can you describe the pain that you had in your abdomen?

The first couple of days I ached badly. After that my abdomen felt very, very tight. It is still tight, and it has been 8 weeks since I had my breast reconstruction. It is not uncomfortable; it just feels strange. It's like wearing a belt that is a little too tight. That's how I feel in an area 4 to 5 inches wide from between my breasts down to the pubic area. I can pinch myself and even stick a needle there, but I don't feel anything.

How long did it take you to recuperate before you could return to work and resume your normal activities?

I'm a flight attendant, and my plastic surgeon didn't want me to go back to work for 3 months. If I had an office job, I probably could have been back at work after 4 weeks. The first day home from the hospital I started doing laundry, dishes, cooking…just everything. In the beginning there was a restriction on lifting my arm. The first 2 weeks I could lift it only at the shoulder. Now I have no restrictions; even so, I don't try to lift more than 20 pounds. Otherwise I do everything. I exercise. I take brisk walks. Considering how tight my abdomen is, I am surprised that I still have the control to inhale and exhale.

Are you satisfied with the appearance of your reconstructed breast? Is it soft? Does it have sensation? Is it warm?

My breast is becoming much softer; I can see it change every week. It still is not quite as soft as the other breast. My breast feels warm to the touch, but it has no sensation; it is numb when you pinch it. Originally my underarm was numb also, but the feeling is coming back. That's probably because they only removed nine lymph nodes; I think if they take more you don't feel as much. It still feels strange when I shave under the arm.

The new breast is a little big right now; I don't know exactly how the finished product with the nipple is going to look. My plastic surgeon is going to make an adjustment when he reconstructs my nipple so my breasts match more closely. But I am happy with what I have right now because I can wear regular clothes. I can wear open sundresses, I can wear bathing suits, I look nice in a bra and underwear.

What are the scars like?

I have a big scar across my abdomen and a circular scar on my breast where the stomach tissue was inset. I read somewhere that vitamin E oil helps the scars, so I've been putting it on. It softens them. I think that makes them look nicer. I also use it in both areas to alleviate the dryness. I don't think my scars are bad at all; they are pretty good. After 8 weeks I look fine. With this particular incision, my scars don't show in a bathing suit.

Did you have any problems or complications from your breast reconstruction?

No. Everything has gone very smoothly.

Are you happy that you had your reconstruction immediately or would you have preferred to have some time to recover between the mastectomy and the breast reconstruction?

After I absorbed the shock of cancer, it was nice knowing that I would come home with something that looked like a breast. It was summertime and I always like to wear little sundresses and bathing suits; without a breast I couldn't wear those clothes. So it was great to be able to go home right out of the hospital and put on an open sundress and nobody could tell that there wasn't a regular breast there. That was fantastic. I am very happy I did it immediately. Maybe some women would not be as appreciative of a reconstructed breast that isn't quite like the other breast—unless they are without a breast for a time. I felt that whatever I ended up with would be better than nothing. This is much better than nothing; this is almost like the other one. So I am very, very pleased. But I was prepared for the difference. That is important. You are not going to come out with a breast that is identical to what you lost. That will never be. But it will be very good and very acceptable.

If you had it to do over, would you have a TRAM flap again or would you select another technique?

I know the TRAM is major surgery with more potential for problems, but I would still choose it without hesitation. It takes more hours in the operating room, longer to recuperate, and of course my stomach is still stiff. But there is nothing artificial; it's all me. I don't have this maintenance business with an implant to worry about. I am planning to live for many years. In the long run I'm better off with this approach. That's why there was no other choice for me.

Was your plastic surgeon responsive to your needs?

I don't think that he could have done anything better than he has done for me. I am very satisfied. I chose him because of the way I felt about him. I felt confident that he would do the best possible for me, and he did.

How did your children react to this experience?

I wanted to tell them what was going on, but I didn't know how. My children are so young. Before I had a chance to talk to them about it, somebody that my husband works with told the mother of a child in my son's class that I had breast cancer. The next day at school the little boy goes to my son and says, "Your mother has breast cancer and she is going to die." That night at the dinner table, my son says, "Mommy, Johnny says that you have breast cancer and you are going to die." I said "Yes, I have breast cancer. That's why I'm going to have surgery. I'm going to have my breast taken off and the cancer removed and I am not going to die." I told them straight out, just like that, and that was fine. The next day I explained further. I said, "One doctor is going to take the old breast off with the cancer in it so that the cancer will be gone; then another doctor is going to make a new breast. And you know Mommy has a little tummy and that is what the doctor is going to use. When I come home from the hospital, I will not have a nipple, but I'm going to get one later. I am going to have a scar on my stomach and a scar on the new breast." I told them this because sometimes when I'm in the shower they come in with "Mommy this, and Mommy that." This way they will not be shocked because they already know about my scars and stomach and that my breast is without a nipple. As soon as I came home from the hospital, my kids asked to see the new breast and the scar on my tummy. So I showed them, and it was fine, because they knew what to expect.

Was your husband supportive? How did he feel about your having reconstructive surgery?

My husband Eric and I looked at a book of pictures of women who had breast reconstruction. He wasn't so worried about the breast; he was more concerned about this big ugly scar on the abdomen. That to him was grotesque. Before the surgery Eric asked me if I was sure I wanted to do this. I wasn't going to worry about what he said. I was going to do what I felt was the right thing. The second day after the surgery when I was in the hospital one of the nurses came in to check on the flap. Eric was sitting right there. She asked if he had seen my surgery yet. She undressed me completely and showed him. I had planned to wait until the scars, especially the one on the stomach, looked a little nicer and not as red as they do the day after surgery. This early unveiling was actually a wonderful idea; he saw the scars at their worst. Now he thinks they looks nice. He says, "Hey, they're looking better."

Has reconstruction affected your sex life?

Many couples have concerns about their sex life after mastectomy, and they don't talk about it. It is important to talk. Eric and I talked through our worries. After the surgery he was concerned that I would feel rejected if he didn't always want to have sex when I was in the mood for lovemaking. He worried that if he were tired or not in the mood, I would interpret it as a negative and think he didn't find me attractive anymore because of my breast. He felt that he would always have to be on call, responsive to any indications I would give him that I wanted to make love. He didn't know if he could cope with having to make love all the time. Eric was also concerned that I would want to test him, and even when I didn't really want sex I would suggest it just to see what his response would be. So we talked about it, got our concerns out in the open, and now everything is okay. It is essential for couples to discuss these issues.

I think something else helped our initial adjustment. Since I knew that my husband was not too excited about the big scar on my abdomen, I figured that I could still be sexy without being stark naked, at least until the scars looked a little better. I bought some pretty sexy nighties that were revealing but still covered up the scars.

What advice would you care to share with other women about breast cancer or breast reconstruction?

People came out of the woodwork to provide support to me. Women would come up to me on the street and say, "I know what you're going through. I had breast cancer too, but nobody knows." One woman had a lumpectomy and never even told her husband. Two women on my street told me that they also had mastectomies. There are many women around us who have had breast cancer. I think it is important to talk about it. I share it with everybody because I was very fortunate. I found my cancer because of a mammogram. Many women believe that a mammogram hurts so much that they don't dare go for one.

More information and openness is needed. For a while it was hush-hush to have a hysterectomy. All of a sudden that's the thing to talk about. Everybody is talking about hysterectomies. You find out every other women has had a hysterectomy and that it's acceptable. Now I think it is time to talk about breast cancer because there are so many of us out there; we are everywhere. So it is important to talk about it and I do. I tell people, "Yes, I had breast cancer. I had a mastectomy, and I was fortunate enough to have had reconstructive surgery." And they want to know more, and then I find out that they haven't had a mammogram for 5 years. They keep running away from it. I must have sent at least 100 women for mammograms because they discovered that's how I found my cancer. I didn't even have a lump. Because the mammogram detected my cancer early, it did not have time to become invasive. My surgeon said if I had come 6 months later my prognosis would have been different. And now it's life after cancer; it's life after a mastectomy, it's life after reconstructive surgery. Life goes on.

APPENDICES

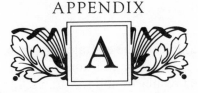

BREAST CANCER
AND RECONSTRUCTION
SUPPORT SERVICES

One of the major advances in the care of cancer patients in recent years has been the development of effective and widely available cancer information and support services. The American Cancer Society and the National Cancer Institute have both been instrumental in improving the quality of communication and overall care for patients with breast cancer.

Today a woman who seeks information on breast care, breast cancer, or breast reconstruction has a variety of sources to investigate. Updated literature written for patients can be obtained from physicians' offices, hospitals, cancer information services, and local American Cancer Society offices or by telephone from the National Cancer Institute. The popular literature has also grown to meet information needs, and a plethora of books and articles are now available in bookstores and libraries.

Many hospitals or communities have established cancer information centers that provide a variety of publications, audiocassettes, and videotapes for easy patient access. These centers are usually staffed by nurses, social workers, or volunteers who are knowledgeable about breast cancer and the many emotional and physical effects of this illness and its treatment. Support services are often coordinated with or through these cancer information (or support) centers.

Computer networks are another source of information. One of the best of these is the Physician Data Query (PDQ), an international computer network supported by the National Cancer Institute and its International Cancer Information Service, that helps to coordinate and update the information provided to patients and health care professionals. The computer system contains material written for patients and their families, physicians, and nurses. The content of the computer files is updated regularly, and research studies are also listed by disease, stage, and even geographic area. PDQ may be reached by online computer, telefax (CancerFax No. 301-402-5874), or telephone (800-422-6237 or 800-4-CANCER).

While factual information is critical to a woman confronting breast cancer and its treatment, she needs more than facts to cope with the trauma that accompanies this disease. Support groups of women who have experienced similar problems provide an enormous service and their value has become increasingly evident with time. Several years ago David Spiegel, a psychiatrist at Stanford University, published the results of a study that examined the value of support groups on the survival of women with metastatic breast cancer. His study confirmed what many have long suspected. He found that the value of these groups extended beyond ministering to a woman's emotional needs—women who participated in the support groups survived almost twice as long as those who had not participated.

Support groups are now available to address a variety of needs of women and their loved ones. Although not all women avail themselves of these groups, those who do praise these groups for their educational value and the opportunity they provide to learn from others who have had similar experiences and from the experts that they recruit to educate them about the latest developments in research and treatment. As one woman explained during an interview, "When I am with my group, I can express my fears openly because these women know what I am talking about. They have walked in my shoes. We can discuss sex, children, anything. It is a wonderfully liberating and empowering experience."

Some groups such as the I Can Cope program, developed by the American Cancer Society, emphasize cancer information and introduce the range of support services. Reach to Recovery, one of the original and most successful efforts, has emphasized the practical and emotional aspects of supporting women who have had mastectomies. CanSurMount is another patient support mechanism from the American Cancer Society.

Organized breast cancer support groups have developed across this country and internationally and are often coordinated by hospitals, treatment centers, the American Cancer Society, or even freestanding community-based centers. Support groups are usually led by a health care professional such as a nurse or social worker but are dependent on those women who attend for the daily activities. There is a trend toward the development of groups that are targeted to women or family members with specific needs. Mastectomy and lumpectomy patients, individuals interested in reconstructive surgery, women with young children, patients with metastatic disease, or even spouses may each have their own support groups.

Some women require emotional support and counseling that cannot be provided by a support group, gynecologist, oncologist, or oncology nurse. Those individuals may be best served by referral to psychologists, social workers, and counselors who have developed expertise with cancer patients. Patients with specific emotional or psychiatric problems might be helped by referral to psychiatrists as well.

As physicians study and refine the scientific aspects of treating cancer with drug therapy, surgery, and radiation, there is an increasing amount of research being done on the supportive care needs of the cancer patient. Recent work has emphasized the emotional aspects of cancer treatment and even evaluated improvements in the quality of life possible with treatment. New drugs have been introduced that help to control anxiety, pain, and nausea. All of these efforts have improved the ability to comfortably treat cancer and best support the patient through a difficult illness.

The following appendices incorporate a range of supportive services and facts and suggestions that may be helpful to a woman and her loved ones as they seek to cope with this disease.

800 NUMBERS/HOTLINES

American Cancer Society
800-ACS-2345
800-227-2345

Appearance Concepts Foundation
800-227-7730

Cancer Care Line
800-622-8922

Cancer HelpLink
800-999-LINK
800-999-5465

Cancer Information & Counseling
Line
800-525-3777

Cancer Information Service
800-422-6237
800-4-CANCER

Hospice Association of America
800-232-3442

Hospice Link
800-331-1620

The Komen Alliance
800-IM-AWARE

Look Good, Feel Better
800-558-5005

National Cancer Institute
800-638-6694

National Health Information
  Clearinghouse
800-336-4797

National Hospice Organization
800-658-8898

National Insurance Consumer Help
  Line
800-942-4242

National Rehabilitation Information
  Center
800-346-2742

Y-Me Breast Cancer Support Program
800-221-2141

NATIONAL CANCER SUPPORT SERVICES

American Cancer Society
National Office
1599 Clifton Rd., NE
Atlanta, GA 30329
800-ACS-2345
404-320-3333

The American Cancer Society, Inc. (ACS), is a national organization fighting cancer through numerous research and educational programs. Fifty-eight chartered divisions and nearly 3000 local units offer patient service and rehabilitation programs for cancer patients and their families, including information and guidance, donated and loaned equipment, rehabilitation programs (Reach to Recovery), literature, films, and speakers.

The ACS has a variety of excellent programs for cancer patients and their families, such as I Can Cope, CanSurmount, Reach to Recovery, and Look Better, Feel Good. Patients can call the national office or their local ACS for further information on where to obtain low-cost mammograms and breast self-examination training.

Cancer Response System
The CRS, sponsored by the ACS, provides telephone information and publications on cancer and refers callers to local chapters of the society for support services. Call 800-ACS-2345.

CanSurmount
CanSurmount is a patient visitor program in which trained volunteers make home and hospital visits to patients with various types of cancer, including breast cancer, and provide counseling and practical advice. For information, contact your local ACS chapter.

I Can Cope
This information seminar is sponsored by the ACS through area hospitals and offers (free of charge) eight sessions for cancer patients and their families on living with various aspects of cancer. The local ACS can be contacted for times, dates, locations, and registration information.

Reach to Recovery

This ACS rehabilitation program for women who have had breast surgery is designed to help them meet their physical, psychological, and cosmetic needs. No meetings are held. On written referral from a physician, a trained volunteer who has had a mastectomy makes a hospital visit a few days after surgery, bringing a temporary breast form and providing information about rehabilitation. Information on breast reconstruction and breast-conserving treatments is usually available through this program. For more information, contact your local ACS chapter.

Reconstruction Education for National Understanding

RENU is a breast reconstruction support group sponsored by the ACS that provides volunteers who will discuss reconstruction options and related issues. Call 216-356-2683.

Road to Recovery

This group enlists volunteers to drive cancer patients to and from medical facilities for treatment and rehabilitation. For information, contact your local ACS chapter.

Cancer Research Council

4853 Cordell Ave., Ste. 11
Bethesda, MD 20814
301-654-7933
This organization will send information regarding new medical treatments currently in the experimental stage.

Cancer Research Institute

133 East 58th St.
New York, NY 10022
800-223-7874
This independent organization directs its efforts to selecting and supporting the most significant advances in cancer immunology research. It is a good resource for medical and research questions.

Corporate Angel Network

10604 Westchester County Airport
Bldg. #1
White Plains, NY 10604
914-328-1313
This nationwide volunteer program provides free long-distance air transportation by using available space on corporate and private jets for cancer patients (and one accompanying family member) who need to travel for their treatment. To inquire about the availability of flights, a patient should call at least 5 days before she needs to travel.

Encore (YWCA)
National Headquarters
610 Lexington Ave.
New York, NY 10022
212-735-9755
This group provides supportive discussion and rehabilitative exercise for women who have been treated for breast cancer. To find the location of the nearest program, a woman can contact the national office.

The Hereditary Cancer Institute
PO Box 3266
Omaha, NE 68103-9990
800-648-8133
The Hereditary Cancer Institute at Creighton University is a nonprofit institution dedicated to research about hereditary cancers. It also disseminates information on cancer genetics and research and evaluates families to identify hereditary cancer and to predict cancer risk to family members and their offspring. This group maintains a registry of families with a pattern of familial cancer.

The Komen Alliance
3500 Gaston Ave.
Baylor University Medical Center
Dallas, TX 75246
The Komen Alliance offers a comprehensive program for the research and treatment of breast disease. Information on screening, BSE, treatment, and support is available by calling 1-800-IMA-WARE or The Susan G. Komen Foundation, 6820 LBJ Freeway, Ste. 130, Dallas TX 75240, at 214-980-8841.

National Alliance of Breast Cancer Organizations
NABCO is a central information network for breast cancer interest groups, organizations, and individuals; it is also involved with research and legislative issues. This not-for-profit central resource provides individuals and health organizations with accurate, up-to-date information on all aspects of breast cancer and promotes affordable detection and treatment. This association is also active in efforts to influence public and private health policy on issues that pertain directly to breast cancer, such as insurance reimbursement, health care, and funding priorities. Individuals and organizations who join NABCO receive the quarterly *NABCO News*, resource lists, and other important information such as *Breast Cancer: Your Best Protection . . . Early Detection and Partner's Guide*, which is available free of charge on written request. NABCO is an excellent resource organization for any breast cancer patient. (Membership fee to join.)

National Cancer Institute
Publications Order—Office of Cancer Communications
National Cancer Institute
Bethesda, MD 20892
301-496-5583
800-422-6237 (cancer information specialist)
800-4-CANCER (pub order line)
The NCI is the federal government's principal agency for research on cancer prevention, diagnosis, treatment, and rehabilitation and for dissemination of information for the control of cancer. This organization offers free information to the general public and to professionals about cancer detection, diagnosis, and treatments, NCI-supported clinical trials, and research programs. NCI supports treatment centers around the country and conducts research on the causes, prevention, diagnosis, and treatment of breast cancer. In addition to its Cancer Information Service, NCI also conducts clinical studies. If a woman wishes to learn more about participating in these clinical studies, she can ask her physician, write NCI, or call the Cancer Information Service. Free literature is available on request.

Cancer Information Service

The NCI conducts its own breast cancer research. Especially useful and valuable to breast cancer patients and their families is NCI's information and referral service. This service is called the Cancer Information Service (CIS). The toll-free phone numbers are:
   800-4-CANCER (continental U.S., except Washington, DC)
   808-524-1234 (local in Oahu, Hawaii; call collect from neighboring islands)
   202-636-5700 (Washington, DC, and suburbs in Maryland and Virginia)
   800-638-6070 (Alaska)
   When you call the CIS number, you are connected with the regional office serving your area. They can give you accurate, personalized answers to your breast cancer questions and can tell you about various community agencies and services available. In many places the CIS offices are affiliated with Comprehensive Cancer Centers (specialized research and treatment centers designated by the NCI) and with the American Cancer Society.

Physician Data Query

The CIS's PDQ system is a computer system that gives up-to-date information on treatment for over 80 types of cancer. This NCI service is for doctors and for people with cancer and their families. PDQ tells about the current treatments for most cancers. The information in PDQ is reviewed each month by cancer experts and is updated when there is new information.

PDQ also tells about clinical trials (research on treatments) and lists doctors who treat cancer and hospitals with cancer programs. For the latest information, call:

800-4-CANCER

808-524-1234 (local in Oahu, Hawaii; call collect from neighboring islands)

800-638-6070 (Alaska)*

National Coalition for Cancer Survivorship
323 Eight St., SW
Albuquerque, NM 87102
505-764-9956

The National Coalition for Cancer Survivorship is a network of independent groups and individuals offering support to cancer survivors and their loved ones. It provides information and resources on support for those persons diagnosed as having cancer. This organization publishes a quarterly newsletter, *The Networker*, for its members.

National Consortium of Breast Centers
c/o Robert Wood Johnson Medical School
Comprehensive Breast Center
1 Robert Wood Johnson Place CN-19
New Brunswick, NJ 08903-0019

NCBC is a professional membership organization of comprehensive breast centers throughout the nation. To locate a comprehensive breast center near you, write for further information or check local phone listings. Comprehensive breast centers are full-service facilities that offer detection, diagnosis, and treatment services.

The National Health Information Center
PO Box 1133
Washington, DC 20013-1133
800-336-4797
301-565-4167 (Maryland)

This center is a health information referral organization that puts people with health questions in touch with those organizations best able to answer them. The center's main objectives are to identify health information resources, channel requests for information to these resources, and develop publications on health-related topics of interest to health professionals, the health media, and the general public.

---

*Spanish-speaking staff are available to callers from California, Florida, Georgia, Illinois, New Jersey (area code 201), New York, and Texas.

The National Women's Health Network
1325 G St., NW
Washington, DC 20005
202-347-1140
This organization is a national consumer group devoted to women and their health needs and concerned with protecting the rights of women in areas of health care. This group acts as a strong advocate for legislative and medical issues, including breast cancer. They have produced pamphlets on breast cancer and diet-related issues. They also produce newsletters (*Network News*) providing current information on a variety of women's health issues. Anyone may join this group, but there is a membership fee to join. Staff personnel will answer questions on the phone or send out an information package on breast cancer for $5.

Y-ME National Organization for Breast Cancer Information and Support, Inc.
National Headquarters
18220 Harwood Ave.
Homewood, IL 60430
708-799-8338 (office No.)
708-799-5937 (fax)
800-221-2141 (weekday hotline, 9 to 5 CST)
708-799-8228 (24-hr hotline)
Y-ME is a nonprofit consumer-oriented organization that provides information, referral, and emotional support to individuals concerned about breast cancer and reconstruction. Its national toll-free hotline is staffed by trained counselors and volunteers who have experienced breast cancer.

Y-ME national and its chapters conduct support meetings in many states. The organization promotes breast cancer awareness through educational workshops and its bimonthly award-winning newsletter. A wig and prosthesis bank is available for those in need. The medical information provided by Y-ME is monitored by a prestigious medical advisory board for accuracy.

REGIONAL CANCER SUPPORT GROUPS

Alaska
Anchorage Women's Breast Cancer
   Support Group
Anchorage, AK
907-261-3151

Arizona
Bosom Buddies
Phoenix, AZ
602-231-6648

Y-ME Breast Cancer Network of
   Arizona
Scottsdale, AZ
602-867-4760

Arizona Cancer Center
Tucson, AZ
602-626-6372

Arkansas
Breast Cancer Support Group
Ft. Smith, AR
501-782-9929

CARTI CancerAnswers
Little Rock, AR
501-664-8573

California
Breast Care for Life Program
   Anaheim Memorial Hospital
Anaheim, CA
714-999-6035

Woman's Cancer Resource Center
Berkeley, CA
510-548-9272

Beyond Breast Cancer Support Group
Chico, CA
916-891-7445

Enloe Hospital Beyond Breast Cancer
Chico, CA
916-893-1152

Scripps Breast Cancer Support Group
Encinitas, CA
619-942-7768

The Health Concern
Escondito, CA
619-746-0700

Breast Cancer Support Group
Freemont, CA
415-357-1961

Breast Surgeries Support Group
Fresno, CA
209-449-5222

Family Service Center
Fresno, CA
209-227-3576

Uniquely You
Fresno, CA
209-442-6520

Uniquely You—Breast Evaluation
   Center
Fresno, CA
209-221-5766

Y-ME of Orange County
B.L.O.O.M.E.R.S.
La Habra, CA
714-447-6975
   (after 5:00 P.M.)

After Breast Cancer
Lancaster, CA
805-945-7585

Y-ME/Ladies of Courage
Lancaster, CA
805-943-1054 or 805-948-5895

Long Beach Memorial Breast Center
Long Beach, CA
213-595-3838

Y-ME South Bay/Long Beach,
   California
Long Beach, CA
310-984-8456

Breast Cancer Recovery Plus
Los Angeles, CA
213-478-9463 or 213-452-0200

Bosom Buddies
Napa, CA
707-257-4047

Desert Hospital Breast Cancer
   Support
Palm Springs, CA
619-323-6831

Y-ME Save Our Selves, Sacramento
Sacramento, CA
916-334-2273

Women's Cancer Task Force
San Diego, CA
619-586-7858

Y-ME San Diego Chapter
Women's Cancer Task Force
San Diego, CA
619-586-7858 or 619-578-6282

Breast Cancer Action
San Francisco, CA
415-922-8279

The Cancer Support Community
San Francisco, CA
415-929-7400

Y-ME Bay Area Breast Cancer
   Network
San Jose, CA
408-261-1425

Woman's Breast Center
Santa Monica, CA
310-829-2931

Vital Options (young adults)
Studio City, CA
818-508-5657

The Breast Center Support Group
Van Nuys, CA
818-787-9911

Connecticut *(CT, RI, Lower NY)*
Y-ME of New England
Branford, CT 06405-3770
203-483-8202 (business)
203-483-8200 (hotline)
800-933-4963 (state [CT] hotline)

I Can
Danbury, CT
203-790-9151

St. Francis Hospital and Medical
   Center
Hartford, CT
203-548-4929

District of Columbia
Betty Ford Comprehensive Breast
   Center
Washington, DC
202-293-6654

Lombardi Breast Cancer Support
   Group
Washington, DC
02-784-3750

The Mary-Helen Mautner Project
   for Lesbians With Cancer
Washington, DC
202-332-5536

Florida
Y-ME of Florida
Coral Springs, FL
305-752-2101

Halifax Medical Center Women's
   Services
Daytona Beach, FL
904-254-4211

Bosom Buddies
Jacksonville, FL
904-396-5973

South Florida Comprehensive
   Cancer Center
Miami, FL
305-227-5582

Center for Women's Medicine at
   Florida Hospital
Orlando, FL
407-897-1617

Ann L. Baroco Center for Women's
   Health
Pensacola, FL
904-474-7878

Vital Alternatives
Sunrise, FL
305-424-6412

FACTORS/H. Lee Moffit Cancer
   Center
Tampa, FL
813-972-8407

Georgia
Bosom Buddies
Decatur Hospital
Atlanta, GA
404-978-0543 or 404-377-4851

Bosom Buddies
Douglas General Hospital
Atlanta, GA
404-920-6337

Bosom Buddies
Emory Clinic
Atlanta, GA
404-634-3416

Image Reborn
Breast Reconstruction Support Group
Atlanta, GA
Crawford Long Hospital
404-686-8143

Bosom Buddies
Northside Hospital
Atlanta, GA
404-851-1894 or 404-851-6100

Bosom Buddies
Peachtree Corners Planning Stage
Atlanta, GA
404-448-5844

Bosom Buddies
St. Joseph's Hospital
Atlanta, GA
404-934-2308, 404-451-4115,
   or 404-394-4276

Bosom Buddies
Atlanta, GA
Spanish Self-Help Group
404-239-0287

Bosom Buddies
Stone Mountain/DeKalb
Atlanta, GA
404-469-0272, 404-469-2409,
   or 404-294-7983

Bosom Buddies
Duluth Planning Stage
Duluth, GA
404-623-0913

Bosom Buddies
Fayetteville, GA
404-461-7988

Bosom Buddies
North Fulton Hospital
Roswell, GA
404-998-3552

St. Thomas General Cancer Support
   Group
Smyrna, GA
404-973-3468

Bosom Buddies
Humana Hospital
Snellville, GA
404-979-1921

Bosom Buddies
Tucker/DeKalb, GA
404-493-7517 or 404-633-5256

Idaho
Mountain States Tumor Institute
Boise, ID
208-386-2760

Women's Life
Boise, ID
208-386-3033

North Idaho Cancer Care
Coeur d'Aline, ID
208-667-8818

Illinois
A Time for Healing
Wellspring Women's Health Center
Barrington, IL
708-705-6700

Cancer Support Network
Bloomington, IL
309-829-2273

After Breast Cancer Elmhurst
  Memorial Hospital
Elmhurst, IL
708-833-1400, ext 4445

McDonough District Hospital
  Women's Health Resource Center
Macomb, IL
309-833-4101, ext 3198

Lisa Madonia Memorial Fund (young
  adults)
Oak Park, IL
708-524-4879

Susan G. Komen Breast Center
Peoria, IL
309-693-6800

Indiana
Caylor-Nickel Medical Center
Bluffton, IN
800-552-2923, ext 6181

Y-ME of Central Indiana
Indianapolis, IN
317-887-7740

The Center for Women's Health
Indianapolis, IN
317-887-7740

Y-ME of the Wabash Valley YWCA
Terre Haute, IN
812-877-3025 or 812-877-3266

Women Winning Against Cancer
Warsaw, IN
219-269-9911

Iowa
"ESPECIALLY FOR YOU" After
  Breast Cancer
Cedar Rapids, IA
800-642-6329 or 319-398-6452

Marshalltown Cancer Support Group
Marshalltown, IA
515-752-8775

Louisiana
Bosom Buddies
West Jefferson Medical Center
Marrero, LA
504-349-1640

Center for Living With Cancer
Metairie, LA
504-454-5500

Humana Hospital
New Orleans, LA
504-245-4855

Patricia Trost Friedler Cancer
  Counseling Center
New Orleans, LA
504-588-2317

Tulane/Friedler Cancer Counseling
New Orleans, LA
504-587-2120

Understanding Life With Cancer,
  Touro Infirmary
New Orleans, LA
504-897-8263

Northshore Regional Medical Center
Slidell, LA
504-646-5127

Maryland *(Western MD, Eastern WV, Southern PA)*
Y-ME of the Cumberland Valley
Hagerstown, MD
301-791-5843

Arm-in-Arm
Baltimore, MD
301-828-3301

Arm-in-Arm
Timonium, MD
301-561-1650

Massachusetts *(Western MA, Eastern NY)*
New England Medical Center Breast
    Health Center
Boston, MA
617-956-5757

Lahey Clinic
Burlington, MA
617-273-8989

Framingham Union Hospital
Framingham, MA
508-626-3543

Faulkner Breast Centre Support
    Group
Jamaica Plain, MA
617-983-7777

Y-ME of the Berkshires
Lee, MA
413-243-4822 (business)
800-439-4821 (hotline, area code
    413 only)

Michigan
Comprehensive Breast Center
Detroit, MI
313-745-2754

Michigan Cancer Foundation
Meyer L. Prentis Cancer Center
Detroit, MI
313-541-8162

"EXPRESSIONS" for Women
E. Grand Rapids, MI
616-957-3223

McLaren Mastectomy Support Group
Flint, MI
313-762-2375

Woman to Woman
St. Mary's Breast Center
Grand Rapids, MI
616-774-6756

Sparrow Hospital
WINS Support Group
Lansing, MI
517-483-2135

Midland Community Cancer Services
Midland, MI
517-835-4841

Minnesota
Duluth Clinic
Duluth, MN
218-725-3195

Missouri
Cancer Hotline
Kansas City, MO
816-932-8453

Mid-America Cancer Center
Springfield, MO
800-432-CARE or 417-885-CARE

St. Joseph Health Center—Hospital
    West
St. Charles, MO
800-835-1212 or 314-947-5000

SHARE Breast Cancer Support
    Program
St. Louis, MO
314-991-4424

St. John's Mercy Cancer Center
St. Louis, MO
314-569-6400

St. Luke's Hospital
FOCUS Breast Cancer Support
   Group
St. Louis, MO
314-851-6090

"We Can" Missouri Baptist Medical
   Center
St. Louis, MO
314-569-5266

North Carolina
CANCARE
Charlotte, NC
704-372-1232

Duke University Comprehensive
   Cancer Center
Durham, NC
919-684-4497

Triangle Breast Cancer Support
   Group
Raleigh, NC
919-881-9754

Tri-County Breast Cancer Support
Rocky Mount, NC
919-443-1018

Pink Broomstick Cancer Services Inc.
Winston-Salem, NC
800-228-7421 or 919-725-7421

New Jersey
B.E.S.T. CARE
Ruth Newman Shapiro Regional
   Center
Atlantic City, NJ
609-652-3500

Comprehensive Breast Care Center
Cooper Hospital University Medical
   Center
Camden, NJ
609-342-2474

Dover General Hospital and Medical
   Center
Dover, NJ
201-989-3643

YWCA Post-Mastectomy Program
Hackensack, NJ
201-487-2224

Concern—St. Barnabas Medical
   Center
Livinston, NJ
201-533-5633

Monmouth Medical Center
Long Branch, NJ
908-890-5429

Beyond Cancer
Princeton, NJ
609-497-4191

Breast Cancer Resource Center (for
   men and women)
Princeton, NJ
609-497-2126

Post Breast Surgery Support Group
Somerville, NJ
201-725-4664

CHEMOcare
Westfield, NJ
908-233-1103
800-55-CHEMO (outside of New
   Jersey)
908-233-7510 (hearing impaired
   TDD)

New Mexico
Living Through Cancer
Albuquerque, NM
505-242-3263

New York
The Brass Ears
Binghamton, NY
607-797-4222

Support for Women With Breast
  Cancer
Buffalo, NY
716-836-6460

Adelphi Breast Center Information
  HOTLINE
Garden City, NY
516-877-4444

After Breast Cancer
Glen Falls, NY
518-251-3126

Women's Health Connection
Wilson Hospital
Johnson City, NY
607-763-6546

Long Island Jewish Medical Center
Post Lumpectomy Support Group
New Hyde Park, NY
718-470-7188

Cancer Care Inc.
New York, NY
212-302-2400

New York Hospital Hematology-
  Oncology Clinic
New York, NY
212-746-3114

NYU/Rusk Institute CRS
New York, NY
212-263-6847

Post-Treatment Resource Program
Memorial Sloan-Kettering Cancer
  Center
New York, NY
212-639-3292

SHARE: Self-Help for Women With
  Breast Cancer
New York, NY
212-719-0364

Cancer Action Inc. Breast Cancer
  Support
Rochester, NY
716-423-9700

Cancer Support Team
Rye Brook, NY
914-253-5334

Ohio
Bethesda Oak Hospital Cancer
  Center
Cincinnati, OH
513-569-6111

Cancer Family Care
Cincinnati, OH
513-731-3346

Y-ME of the Greater Dayton Area
Dayton, OH
513-274-9151 (evenings)

Breast Cancer Support Group
St. Elizabeth Regional Cancer
  Center
Dayton, OH
513-229-7474

Lima Memorial Hospital
Lima, OH
800-227-3564

HERS—Breast Cancer Support
  Network
Mercy Medical Center
Springfield, OH
513-390-5030

Young Women's Breast Cancer
  Support Group
Westerville, OH
614-475-7202 or 614-846-2052

Southside Medical Center
Youngstown, OH
216-740-4176 or 216-788-5048

Oklahoma
Central Oklahoma Cancer Center
Oklahoma City, OK
405-636-7104

Oklahoma Breast Care Center
Oklahoma City, OK
405-755-2273

Oregon
Breast Cancer Outreach
Portland, OR
503-291-4671

St. Vincent Hospital and Medical
   Center
Portland, OR
503-291-4673

Meridian Park Hospital
Tualatin, OR
503-778-7631

Pennsylvania
"A New Beginning" Self Help Group
Abington Memorial Hospital
Abington, PA
215-646-4954

Woman Care Resource Center—
   Harrisburg Hospital
Camp Hill, PA
717-731-4035

Nesbitt Memorial Hospital
Breast Cancer Support Group
Kingston, PA
717-288-1411, ext 4300

Montgomery Breast Cancer Support
   Program
Norristown, PA
215-270-2700

Fox Chase Cancer Center
Philadelphia, PA
215-728-2668

Linda Creed Foundation
Philadelphia, PA
215-955-4354

The Lesbian Cancer Network
Philadelphia, PA
215-242-3323

Thomas Jefferson University
   Hospital
Philadelphia, PA
800-Jeff Now

Cancer Guidance Institute
Pittsburgh, PA
412-261-2211

Cancer Support Network
Pittsburgh, PA
412-361-8600

Magee-Women's Hospital
Breast Cancer Support Group
Pittsburgh, PA
412-647-4255

Rhode Island
Breast Health
Providence, RI
401-751-6890

Hope Center for Life Enhancement
Providence, RI
401-454-0404

Roger Williams Psychosocial
   Oncology
Providence, RI
401-456-2000

South Dakota
St. Luke's Midland Regional Medical
   Center
Aberdeen, SD
605-622-5588

Y-ME of South Dakota
Friends Against Breast Cancer
Sioux Falls, SD
605-331-1111

Tennessee
Y-ME of Chattanooga
Chattanooga, TN
615-886-4171

Knoxville Breast Center
Knoxville, TN
615-546-4661 or 800-456-8169

The Breast Concerns Mastectomy
   Support Group
Nashville, TN
615-665-0628

Texas
Women Helping Women
Don & Sybil Harrington Cancer
   Center
Amarillo, TX
806-359-4673

Between Us
Dallas, TX
214-521-5225

Komen Kares Support System
Dallas, TX
214-692-8893

Woman to Woman
Presbyterian Hospital of Dallas
Dallas, TX
214-345-2600

Women's Information Network
Medical City Dallas Hospital
Dallas, TX
214-387-2504

Not Alone
Y-ME of El Paso
El Paso, TX
915-584-6063

Doris Kupferle Breast Center
Fort Worth, TX
817-882-3650

Spring Shadows/ACS
Houston, TX
713-895-7722

The Joan Gordon Center Support
   Group
Houston, TX
713-668-2996

The Rose Garden
Houston, TX
713-484-4708

Utah
Holy Cross Hospital Breast Care
   Services
Salt Lake City, UT
801-350-4012

Ashley Valley Breast Care Center
Vernal, UT
801-789-3342

Virginia
My Image After Breast Cancer
Alexandria, VA
703-461-9616 (hotline)
703-461-9595, 703-461-9596 (office)

Fairfax Hospital
Annandale, VA
703-698-3201

Sentara Leigh Hospital
Norfolk, VA
804-466-6837

Bone Marrow Transplant/Breast
   Cancer Support Group
Richmond, VA
804-530-2817

Breast Cancer Support Group
Richmond, VA
804-225-4164

Massey Cancer Center
Richmond, VA
804-786-9901

Lewis-Gale Regional Cancer Center
Salem, VA
800-543-5660

Washington
A Touch of Strength
St. Peter Hospital Regional Cancer
   Center
Olympia, WA
206-493-7510

Operation Uplift
Port Angeles, WA
206-457-5141

CANHELP, Inc. (treatment
   decisions—fee)
Port Ludlow, WA
206-437-2291

Cancer Lifeline
Seattle, WA
206-461-3866

West Virginia
CAMC Family Resource Center
Women & Children's Hospital
Charleston, WV
304-347-9229

CAMC Family Resource Center
Scott Depot, WV
304-757-3095

• • •

Canada
Burlington Breast Cancer Support
   Services
Burlington, Canada
416-637-7738

England
Breast Care and Mastectomy
   Association
London, England
071-867-1103

Scotland
Breast Care and Mastectomy
   Association
Glasgow, Scotland
041-353-1050
Edinburgh, Scotland
031-458-5598

National Self-Help Clearinghouse
Any individual who is looking for a self-help group in their region can find it by calling this organization at 212-642-2944. Also check for listings of statewide self-help clearinghouses. Call 800-555-1212 for information. If you cannot locate a convenient support group from this listing or from the National Self-Help Clearinghouse:
   • Inquire at a local major hospital's Breast Center or Departments of Social Work or Psychiatry.
   • Call the National Cancer Institute's Cancer Information Service at 800-4-CANCER for names of American College of Radiology (ACR)–accredited mammography providers in your area and ask these providers for support group suggestions.

- Contact your local American Cancer Society office for local groups that they or others sponsor.
- Call a group on the list in your state and ask if they know of any groups located nearer to you.

For information on starting your own support group, contact your local American Cancer Society office or call Y-ME (see p. 483).

SOURCES FOR CERTIFIED SPECIALISTS AND CANCER FACILITIES

American Cancer Society
800-ACS-2345
Will provide the names of breast and cancer specialists and approved hospital programs.

American College of Radiology
1891 Preston White Dr.
Reston, VA 22091
703-648-8900
Will provide names of certified radiologists for mammography and a list of accredited mammography facilities by geographic area as well as the ACR resource materials listed previously. A fee is charged for bulk orders. 800-ACR-LINE (8:30 A.M. to 5 P.M., EST, Monday-Friday)

American College of Surgeons
55 East Erie St.
Chicago, IL 60611
312-664-4050
Will provide names of certified surgeons specializing in breast surgery by geographic area.

American Medical Association
535 N. Dearborn
Chicago, IL 60610
312-645-5000
Will provide a list of member doctors in your area or refer you to a local service that can do the same. Can also give you information on the educational background and credential of any doctor who is a member.

American Psychiatric Association
1700 18th St., NW
Washington, DC 20009
202-232-7878
This national organization of psychiatric specialists will be able to put you in touch with a local group.

American Psychological Association
1200 17th St., NW
Washington, DC 20036
202-833-7600
This national organization of psychologists will be able to put you in touch with a local group.

American Society of Plastic and Reconstructive Surgeons
444 East Algonquin Rd.
Arlington Heights, IL 60005
312-228-9900
800-635-0635 (referral message tape only)
This association's referral operators provide listings of up to 10 certified plastic surgeons within the caller's geographic area; also provides written materials.

Cancer Research Council
4853 Cordell Ave.
Ste. 11
Bethesda, MD 20814
301-654-7933
Will send information regarding new medical treatment concepts currently in the experimental stage.

Clinical Cancer Centers

Clinical Cancer Centers are medical centers that have support from the National Cancer Institute for programs to investigate promising new methods of cancer diagnosis and treatment.

Arizona
University of Arizona Cancer Center
1501 North Campbell Ave.
Tucson, AZ 85724
602-626-6372

California
Northern California Cancer Center
(consortium)
1301 Shoreway Rd.
Belmont, CA 94002
415-591-4484

City of Hope National Medical
    Center
Beckman Research Institute
1500 East Duarte Rd.
Duarte, CA 91010
818-359-8111, ext 2292

Charles R. Drew University of
    Medicine and Science
    (consortium)
12714 South Avalon Blvd., Ste. 301
Los Angeles, CA 90061
213-603-3120

University of California at San Diego
   Cancer Center
225 Dickinson St.
San Diego, CA 92103
619-543-6178

Colorado
University of Colorado Cancer
   Center
4200 East 9th Ave., Box B190
Denver, CO 80262
303-270-3019

Kentucky
Lucille Parker Markey Cancer
   Center
University of Kentucky Medical
   Center
800 Rose St.
Lexington, KY 40536
606-257-4447

Michigan
University of Michigan Cancer
   Center
101 Simpson Dr.
Ann Arbor, MI 48109-0752
313-936-2516

New Hampshire
Norris Cotton Cancer Center
Dartmouth-Hitchcock Medical
   Center
2 Maynard St.
Hanover, NH 03756
603-646-5505

New York
Albert Einstein College of Medicine
1300 Morris Park Ave.
Bronx, NY 10461
212-920-4826

Mt. Sinai School of Medicine
1 Gustave L. Levy Place
New York, NY 10029
212-241-8617

New York University Cancer Center
462 First Ave.
New York, NY 10016
212-340-6485

University of Rochester Cancer
   Center
601 Elmwood Ave., Box 704
Rochester, NY 14642
716-275-4911

North Carolina
Lineberger Cancer Research Center
University of North Carolina School
   of Medicine
Chapel Hill, NC 27599
919-966-4431

Bowman Gray School of Medicine
Wake Forest University
300 South Hawthorne Rd.
Winston-Salem, NC 27103
919-748-4354

Ohio
Case Western Reserve University
University Hospitals of Cleveland
Ireland Cancer Center
2074 Abington Rd.
Cleveland, OH 44106
216-844-8453

Pennsylvania
Pittsburgh Cancer Institute
230 Lothrop St.
Pittsburgh, PA 15213-2592
800-537-4063

Rhode Island
Roger Williams General Hospital
825 Chalkstone Ave.
Providence, RI 02908
401-456-2070

Tennessee
St. Jude Children's Research Hospital
332 North Lauderdale St.
Memphis, TN 38101
901-522-0694

Utah
Utah Regional Cancer Center
University of Utah Medical Center
50 North Medical Dr.
Room 2C10
Salt Lake City, UT 84132
801-581-4048

Vermont
Vermont Regional Cancer Center
University of Vermont
1 South Prospect St.
Burlington, VT 05401
802-656-4580

Virginia
Massey Cancer Center
Medical College of Virginia
Virginia Commonwealth University
1200 East Broad St.
Richmond, VA 23298
804-786-9641

Comprehensive Cancer Centers

The National Cancer Institute has designated 27 comprehensive cancer centers that are devoted to investigating new methods for cancer diagnosis and treatment. These medical research centers generate scientific information that can then be used by doctors treating cancer patients. Comprehensive Cancer Centers have teams of experts combining their expertise in cancer research, patient care, and education. They treat cancer patients and provide second opinions. They also participate in clinical trials to test new treatments to determine if they are more effective than the standard ones. They are knowledgeable about the latest developments in cancer treatment.

Alabama
University of Alabama
    Comprehensive Cancer Center
1918 University Blvd.
Room 108
Birmingham, AL 35294
205-934-6612

Arizona
Arizona Cancer Center
University of Arizona
1515 N. Campbell Ave.
Tucson, AZ 85724
602-626-7935
1-800-622-COPE (Arizona residents
    only)

California
Kenneth T. Norris, Jr., Comprehensive
    Cancer Center
Kenneth T. Norris, Jr., Cancer Hospital
    and Research Institute
University of Southern California
1441 Eastlake Ave.
Los Angeles, CA 90033-0804
213-226-2370

Jonsson Comprehensive Cancer
    Center
UCLA Medical Center
10-247 Factor Bldg.
10833 Le Conte Ave.
Los Angeles, CA 90024-1781
213-825-8727

Connecticut
Yale University Comprehensive
    Cancer Center
333 Cedar St.
New Haven, CT 06510
203-785-6338

District of Columbia
Vincent T. Lombardi Cancer
    Research Center
Georgetown University Medical
    Center
3800 Reservoir Rd., NW
Washington, DC 20007
202-687-2110

Florida
Sylvester Comprehensive Cancer
    Center
University of Miami Medical School
1475 Northwest 12th Ave.
Miami, FL 33136
305-548-4850

Maryland
The Johns Hopkins Oncology
    Center
600 North Wolfe St.
Baltimore, MD 21205
301-955-8638

Massachusetts
Dana-Farber Cancer Institute
44 Binney St.
Boston, MA 02115
617-732-3214

Michigan
University of Michigan Cancer Center
101 Simpson Dr.
Ann Arbor, MI 48109-0752
313-936-9583

Meyer L. Prentis Comprehensive
    Cancer Center of Metropolitan
    Detroit
110 East Warren St.
Detroit, MI 48201
313-745-4329

Minnesota
Mayo Comprehensive Cancer Center
Mayo Clinic
200 First St., SW
Rochester, MN 55905
507-284-3413

New Hampshire
Norris Cotton Cancer Center
Dartmouth-Hitchcock Medical
    Center
1 Medical Center Dr.
Lebanon, NH 03756
603-650-4141

New York
Roswell Park Cancer Institute
666 Elm St.
Buffalo, NY 14263
716-845-4400

Memorial Sloan-Kettering Cancer
  Center
1275 York Ave.
New York, NY 10021
800-525-2225

Kaplan Cancer Center
New York University Medical Center
550 1st Ave.
New York, NY 10016
212-263-5349

North Carolina
UNC Lineberger Comprehensive
  Cancer Center
University of North Carolina at
  Chapel Hill
Campus Box No. 7295
Chapel Hill, NC 27599
919-966-1101

Duke University Comprehensive
  Cancer Center
PO Box 3843
Durham, NC 27710
919-286-5515

The Comprehensive Cancer Center
  of Wake Forest University
Medical Center Blvd.
Winston-Salem, NC 27157-1082
919-716-7972

Ohio
Ohio State University
  Comprehensive Cancer Center
410 West 12th Ave.
Columbus, OH 43210
614-293-08619

Pennsylvania
Fox Chase Cancer Center
7701 Burholme Ave.
Philadelphia, PA 19111
215-728-2570

University of Pennsylvania Cancer
  Center
3400 Spruce St.
Philadelphia, PA 19104
215-662-6364

University of Pittsburgh Medical
  Center
369 Victoria Bldg.
Philadelphia, PA 15261
800-537-4063

Texas
The University of Texas
  M.D. Anderson Cancer Center
1515 Holcombe Blvd.
Houston, TX 77030
713-792-3245

Vermont
Vermont Cancer Center
1 South Prospect St.
University of Vermont
Burlington, VT 05401
802-656-4414

Washington
Fred Hutchinson Cancer Research
  Center
1124 Columbia St.
Seattle, WA 98104
206-467-4675

Wisconsin
University of Wisconsin
Comprehensive Cancer Center
600 Highland Ave.
Madison, WI 53792
608-263-6872

Second Opinion Centers

A number of major hospitals throughout the country offer second-opinion consultation services at varying costs. A multidisciplinary team of specialists will meet with the patient and the family to review the diagnosis and other diagnostic tests in order to provide the patient with a recommended second opinion for the course of treatment. Call the Cancer Information Service at 800-4-CANCER to locate the center nearest you.

INFORMATION ON BREAST IMPLANTS

American Society of Plastic and Reconstructive Surgeons
444 East Algonquin Rd.
Arlington Heights, IL 60005
800-635-0635 or 312-228-9900

Breast Implant Manufacturers
Women can call these numbers to get information about specific types and models of breast implants.

Bioplasty*	800-328-9105
Bristol-Myers Squibb (Surgitek)*	800-634-4397
CBI Medical, Inc.*	800-527-1213
CUI Corporation*	800-872-4749
Dow Corning*	800-442-5442
Mentor Corporation	800-235-5731
McGhan Medical Corporation (Inamed Corporation)	800-624-4261

Food and Drug Administration
FDA/CDRH, HFZ-210
5600 Fishers Lane
Rockville, MD 20857
303-443-5006
800-532-4440
Provides over-the-phone and print information on current breast implant issues and findings; consumer information package also available by sending a postcard or letter.

*No longer manufactures silicone gel—filled implants.

International Breast Implant Registry
800-892-9211
An information database run by Medic Alert that keeps women and their physicians informed about health and safety issues concerning breast implants. If
you phone, they will send information and instructions on how a woman who
has had implant surgery can register her implant. The fee is $25 for the first year
and $15 every year thereafter.

U.S. Pharmacopeia
800-638-6725
301-881-0256 (Maryland)
FDA product problem reporting program. Patients can report implant problems
to this agency. When making a report, a woman needs to know specific information about her implant type, manufacturer, size and lot number, as well as the
name and address of her surgeon and the facility.

INFORMATION ON HEALTH INSURANCE

The Health Insurance Association of America
Fulfillment Department
PO Box 41455
Washington, DC 20018
202-866-6244
This association will answer questions concerning insurance coverage as it ap-
plies to breast cancer prevention and treatment.

Local Social Security Office
A patient's local social security office distributes single copies of a "Guide to
Health Insurance for People with Medicare," which explains what Medicare
does not pay for and what to look for in private health insurance.

Medicaid/Medicare
Health Financing Administration
Department of Health and Human Services
Washington, DC 20201
202-245-0312
The home office can provide women with the address and telephone number of
their regional office.

The National Insurance Consumer Organization
121 North Payne St.
Alexandria, VA 22314
703-549-8050
This nonprofit public interest advocacy and educational organization promotes the interests of insurance buyers and helps consumers buy insurance wisely.

The People's Medical Society
14 East Minor St.
Emmaus, PA 18049
This society acts as a consumer advocate in the health care field; it also helps consumers evaluate and select health insurance.

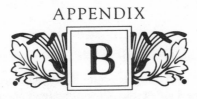

THE PATIENT'S RIGHTS

The three documents that follow confirm the rights and standard of care that women should expect from their doctors and from the medical personnel who treat them.

A BREAST CANCER PATIENT'S OPTIONS AND RIGHTS*

- To receive a simple and clear diagnosis of her condition.
- To receive all available diagnostic procedures and a complete workup prior to surgery.
- To have the consent form clearly explained to her before she signs it.
- To have the biopsy performed first (under local anesthesia), including the right to see the pathologist's report and have it explained to her. Surgery may be performed at a later date.
- To be aware that for certain patients the future option of reconstructive plastic surgery exists and to have the surgeon take that option into consideration.
- To receive consideration from the surgeon and other medical personnel for the physical and emotional trauma she is undergoing.
- To receive an explanation of any viable alternative treatments—including biopsy with radiation therapy as primary treatment, chemotherapy, mastectomy, etc.—risks, disadvantages, and advantages of each treatment.
- To receive a satisfying explanation as to why the surgeon has decided on a particular surgical procedure rather than a less mutilating one.
- To be referred to a therapist for physical or psychiatric therapy following surgery.
- To receive competent follow-up care after surgery and to know who is going to be responsible for that care.
- To be referred to a support group for information and assistance with her personal concerns.
- To be always treated as an adult.

*Prepared by Women for Women, a nonprofit West Coast organization.

A PATIENT'S BILL OF RIGHTS*

During the 1970s the board of trustees and house of delegates of the American Hospital Association developed the following statement on patients' rights with the expectation that observation of these rights would contribute to more effective patient care and greater satisfaction for the patient, her physician, and the hospital organization. It defines the responsibilities of the physicians and medical staff. Implicitly, it expects the patient to share in her own health care by first knowing her rights, then exercising them.

1. The patient has the right to considerate and respectful care.
2. The patient has the right to obtain from her physician complete current information concerning her diagnosis, treatment, and prognosis in terms the patient can be reasonably expected to understand. When it is not medically advisable to give such information to the patient, the information should be made available to an appropriate person on her behalf. She has the right to know, by name, the physician responsible for coordinating her care.
3. The patient has the right to receive from her physician information necessary to give informed consent prior to the start of any procedure and/or treatment. Except in emergencies, such information for informed consent should include, but not necessarily be limited to, the specific procedure and treatment, the medically significant risks involved, and the probable duration of incapacitation. Where medically significant alternatives for care or treatment exist, or when the patient requests information concerning medical alternatives, the patient has the right to such information. The patient also has the right to know the name of the person responsible for the procedures and/or treatment.
4. The patient has the right to refuse treatment to the extent permitted by law and to be informed of the medical consequences of her action.
5. The patient has the right to every consideration of her privacy concerning her own medical care program. Case discussion, consultation, examination, and treatment are confidential and should be conducted discreetly. Those not directly involved in her care must have the permission of the patient to be present.
6. The patient has the right to expect that all communications and records pertaining to her care should be treated as confidential.
7. The patient has the right to expect that within its capacity a hospital must make reasonable response to the request of a patient for services. The hospital must provide evaluation, service, and/or referral as indicated by the urgency of the case. When medically permissible, a patient may be transferred to another facility only after she has received complete information and explanation concerning the need for and alternatives to such a transfer. The institution to which the patient is to be transferred must first have accepted the patient for transfer.

*Prepared by the American Hospital Association.

8. The patient has the right to obtain information as to any relationship of her hospital to other health care and educational institutions insofar as her care is concerned. The patient has the right to obtain information as to the existence of any professional relationships among individuals, by name, who are treating her.
9. The patient has the right to be advised if the hospital proposes to engage in or perform human experimentation affecting her care or treatment. The patient has the right to refuse to participate in such research projects.
10. The patient has the right to expect reasonable continuity of care. She has the right to know in advance what appointment times and physicians are available and where. The patient has the right to expect that the hospital will provide a mechanism whereby she is informed by her physician of the patient's continuing health care requirements following discharge.
11. The patient has the right to examine and receive an explanation of her bill, regardless of source of payment.
12. The patient has the right to know what hospital rules and regulations apply to her conduct as a patient.

CANCER SURVIVORS' BILL OF RIGHTS*

The American Cancer Society has presented "Cancer Survivors' Bill of Rights" to call attention to the needs of survivors and to enhance cancer care:

1. Survivors have the right to assurance of lifelong medical care, as needed. The physicians and other professionals involved in their care should continue their constant efforts to be:
   • sensitive to the cancer survivors' lifestyle choices and their need for self-esteem and dignity;
   • careful, no matter how long they have survived, to have symptoms taken seriously, and not have aches and pains dismissed, for fear of recurrence is a normal part of survivorship;
   • informative and open, providing survivors with as much or as little candid medical information as they wish, and encouraging their informed participation in their own care;
   • knowledgeable about counseling resources, and willing to refer survivors and their families as appropriate for emotional support and therapy which will improve the quality of individual lives.
2. In their personal lives, survivors, like other Americans, have the right to the pursuit of happiness. This means they have the right:
   • to talk with their families and friends about their cancer experience if they wish, but to refuse to discuss it if that is their choice and not to be expected to be more upbeat or less blue than anyone else;

*Prepared by the American Cancer Society.

- to be free of the stigma of cancer as a "dread disease" in all social relations;
- to be free of blame for having gotten the disease and of guilt for having survived it.

3. In the workplace, survivors have the right to equal job opportunities. This means they have the right:
   - to aspire to jobs worthy of their skills, and for which they are trained and experienced, and thus not to have to accept jobs they would not have considered before the cancer experience;
   - to be hired, promoted and accepted on return to work, according to their individual abilities and qualifications, and not according to "cancer" or "disability" stereotypes;
   - to privacy about their medical histories.

4. Since health insurance coverage is an overriding survivorship concern, every effort should be made to assure all survivors adequate health insurance, whether public or private. This means:
   - for employers, that survivors have the right to be included in group health coverage, which is usually less expensive, provides better benefits, and covers the employee regardless of health history;
   - for physicians, counselors, and other professionals concerned, that they keep themselves and their survivor clients informed and up-to-date on available group or individual health policy options, noting, for example, what major expenses like hospital costs and medical tests outside the hospital are covered and what amount must be paid before coverage (deductibles).

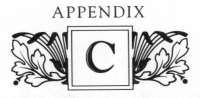

THE BREAST CANCER INFORMED CONSENT SUMMARY

Currently, several states require physicians to inform their patients of alternative treatments for breast cancer. In California physicians must provide that information in printed form: a seven-page pamphlet written in simple, nonmedical language, describing the various options (advantages and disadvantages) for breast cancer treatment with surgery, radiation, and chemotherapy.

The form is reprinted below.

BREAST CANCER TREATMENT: SUMMARY OF EFFECTIVE METHODS, RISKS, ADVANTAGES, DISADVANTAGES

Introduction

Breast cancer is a treatable disease, and you should know about the treatment options that are available, including surgical treatment, x-ray (radiation) therapy, and chemical and hormone treatment procedures. This brochure has been written to help you understand the various treatments with their advantages, disadvantages, and risks.

The treatment of breast cancer is complex and must be individualized. Choosing the best therapy for you may be difficult. It is important for you to have basic information about the methods of treatment so that you may discuss them with your physician. Using this information, you and your physician will be able to make the best choice for your stage or extent of the disease.

It may be appropriate for either you or your physician to seek additional opinions if either of you desire. Your consent is required before any treatment is carried out, and you have the right to make the final choice of the treatment procedure(s). Your physician has a corresponding right to withdraw from the case if the two of you cannot agree on a treatment plan.

Although a long delay may interfere with the ultimate success of your treatment, it is very important to take two to four weeks to obtain enough medical information and consultation to make a final and informed decision. Once that final and informed decision is made by you and your physician, you will be ready to begin treatment. A positive attitude will help you as you and your physician work together to carry out the treatment of your cancer. Because progress is being made in the management of breast cancer, your doctor may have new suggestions that have not been included in this brochure.

Plans and procedures to try out new methods of treatment are called protocols or clinical trials. Such trials often compare the current standard of care (the best treatment widely available) to a new treatment that is expected to increase the number of persons cured. The new treatment method is put into general use only after long-term evaluation by cancer experts shows that the new treatment is better than the current ones. The National Cancer Institute endorses the participation of patients and their physicians in clinical trials of new treatments.

Management of Breast Cancer

Management of breast cancer is achieved with the cooperation of appropriate specialists in the field which include:
• The primary (personal) physician for diagnosis, support, and coordination.
• The surgeon for diagnosis by biopsy and specific surgical procedures for removal of the breast tumor and/or axillary lymph nodes.
• The pathologist for examining the biopsy tissue under the microscope.
• The radiation oncologist for supervising and administering radiation treatment.
• The medical oncologist for administering and monitoring chemotherapy.
These health professionals proceed fairly independently once a treatment plan has been decided, but maintain communication with each other by telephone and written correspondence.

Diagnosis

While signs and symptoms of abnormal breast conditions such as presence of a lump, skin dimpling, red discoloration of the nipple, or thickening in the breast felt by self examination or seen in a mammogram all may be suggestive of cancer, the final diagnosis is the scientific determination made by the pathologist of the nature of the tumor. It is done by examining biopsied material from the breast lump under a microscope.

A breast biopsy is the procedure performed to find out (diagnose) if the abnormal breast tissue (lump or change on a mammogram) is cancer. Biopsies can be performed by inserting a needle into the lump, if it can be felt, and removing a small piece of tissue or opening the skin and removing all or part of the abnormal tissue. The pathologist then examines the biopsy material under a microscope. In addition to making a diagnosis of cancer, the pathologist may also prepare the tissue for analysis of other characteristics of the cancer such as hormone receptor concentration (proteins inside cancer cells that link up with the female hormones estrogen and progesterone), genetic studies, DNA analysis, epidermal growth factors, and others.

When the diagnosis of breast cancer can be made with a needle aspiration of the lump (through the skin), you and your doctor can discuss the various treatment options before any surgery is performed. If the biopsy requires surgery, the cancer operation may be done at the same time (one-step procedure) or at a later date (two-step procedure). The two-step procedure is considered preferable by many professionals in the field. Because your final choice for treatment may influence the biopsy technique to be used, you and your surgeon should discuss your decision for cancer treatment prior to the biopsy.

Prior to any surgical procedure, a general medical evaluation should be performed. It may include your medical history (including family history of cancer), physical examination, blood tests that evaluate the function of various systems (e.g., liver, kidney, etc.), chest x-ray and breast x-ray (mammography). Additional tests to assess the spread of the disease may be indicated, such as radioisotope scan (bones, liver, etc.), computerized tomographic (CT) or magnetic resonance (MRI) body scans (specialized views of internal organs and bones), or sonograms (pictures of internal organs made with ultrasound waves).

Surgery

Surgery for breast cancer can be divided into two parts: (1) operations to remove part or all of the diseased breast and (2) operations to remove the lymph nodes under the arm. The portion of the operation performed on the breast is designed to treat the cancer. The portion of the operation performed on the lymph glands in the armpit (axilla) is designed to evaluate whether or not the cancer has spread, as well as to remove the nodes into which the cancer has spread. This information is needed for further treatment decisions.

Segmental Mastectomy, Partial Mastectomy, Lumpectomy

These operations are designed to remove the breast cancer and preserve the breast shape. To be effective in controlling cancer in the breast, radiation therapy lasting five to six weeks is often given after any of these breast-preserving operations, but particularly after a lumpectomy, which is not adequate in most cases.

Advantages. There is only partial loss of breast tissue. No reconstruction is required. The chances of cure for certain types and stages of breast cancer, when combined with radiation therapy, are equal to having a total mastectomy.

Disadvantages. This method of treatment requires an operation and also five to six weeks of radiation therapy. Partial surgery may not be an option for all women, depending on the type and size of the cancer, the location of the tumor in the breast, and the size of the breast. Sometimes the cancer is in a part of the breast that cannot be removed without significantly changing the shape and appearance of the breast (for example, right under the nipple). Radiation therapy does not eliminate the possibility of a new or recurrent cancer in the treated breast. In addition, sensations in the breast may change or be experienced differently than before treatment.

Modified Radical Mastectomy, Total Mastectomy

The term "mastectomy" includes many different types of operations. In general, all breast tissue and the skin over the breast including the nipple and lymph nodes from the armpit are removed. Sometimes the smaller muscle of the chest wall (pectoralis minor) is removed or cut, but the larger muscle (pectoralis major) is left in place.

Advantages. This operation provides treatment for the cancer in the breast and evaluates the armpit lymph nodes for removing additional tumor tissues if present. There is minimal loss of arm strength or mobility due to muscle weakness. No radiation exposure is required.

Disadvantages. Some women experience shoulder stiffness, numbness of the skin on the inner side of the upper arm, and arm swelling. The entire breast is removed, and reconstructive surgery or an external prosthesis is required for those who wish to rebuild the breast form.

Radical (Halsted) Mastectomy

This operation is reserved for patients with extensive cancers of the breast that invade the underlying large muscle of the chest (pectoralis major). In addition to the entire breast, the lymph nodes in the armpit, the muscle of the chest wall, and large amounts of skin are also removed.

Advantages. In selected cases, this operation may increase the chances of controlling the cancer on the chest wall.

Disadvantages. Compared to the other operations already described, the radical mastectomy does not increase cure rates for most stages of breast cancer. This operation removes the entire breast and underlying chest muscles. It leaves a long scar and a hollow area where the muscles were removed. The operation may result in arm swelling, some loss of muscle power in the arm, and restricted shoulder motion and numbness in some individuals. Reconstructive (plastic) surgery and fitting of breast prosthesis are more difficult.

Lymph Node Dissection

This procedure is the removal of some (lymph node sampling) or most (lymph node dissection) of the lymph nodes in the armpit and behind the large muscles of the chest. It is done to find out if the cancer has spread and for further treatment to prevent recurrence of the cancer in the axilla. When this operation is combined with a segmental mastectomy, a separate incision may be used.

Radiation (X-Ray) Therapy

Radiation treatment of local tissues of the body, known as radiotherapy, can destroy cancer cells while producing minimal injury to surrounding tissues. The radiation may come from a number of devices (e.g., linear accelerator, betatron, cobalt-60, and radioactive isotopes). The source and type of radiation are chosen to suit the requirements of the individual. Radiation to the breast does not cause loss of hair from the head.

Breast-Preserving Treatment of Early Breast Cancer

This approach has been used for about 20 years in the United States and 30 years in Europe for the treatment of early breast cancer. Recent scientific studies involving thousands of breast cancer patients in the United States and in Europe demonstrate that the breast-preserving treatment is as effective as either modified radical mastectomy or radical mastectomy for tumor control and survival. Breast-preserving treatment involves both surgery (segmental mastectomy, partial mastectomy, lumpectomy) and radiation therapy to achieve the best possible results. Initially, surgery is performed to remove the tumor in the breast (and usually the lymph nodes in the armpit). Following healing from surgery, external radiation therapy is used to treat the breast and the chest wall. In some patients, the lymph nodes behind the collar bone and the breast bone may need treatment. Treatment usually consists of a few minutes each day, four or five days a week, for approximately six to seven weeks. Following this, some patients will need a radiation "boost" to the biopsy site. This can be accomplished by continuing treatment for approximately one to two weeks with external radiation or a temporary placement of radioactive seeds (implants) in the breast at the biopsy site. The implant requires a minor procedure under general anesthesia in the operating room and a hospital stay of two to three days.

Advantages. The breast is preserved, though it may be mildly to moderately firmer. Usually, there is minimal or no visible deformity of surrounding tissues. After completion of the treatment, the skin usually regains a nearly normal appearance. In early breast cancer, lumpectomy or segmental resection, with radiation as the primary treatment, has demonstrated results that are equal to more extensive, long established surgical procedures.

Disadvantages. A full course of treatment requires daily outpatient visits for five to eight weeks. Treatment may produce mild tiredness and a skin reaction similar to a mild to severe sunburn. If the lymph nodes behind the breast bone are treated, there may be a temporarily mild swallowing discomfort. Radiation therapy may affect the bone marrow where blood cells are made. This usually occurs only to a mild degree and is temporary. If chemotherapy is given at the same time, a small area of the bone marrow may be affected to a greater degree and may, in some cases, limit the dosage of chemotherapy that can be given. This is rarely a significant problem. A small portion of the lung behind the breast and chest wall will develop scar tissue from radiation therapy. This may be visible on x-ray examination but usually causes no breathing difficulties or other problems.

Radiation Therapy as a Supplement (Adjuvant) to Surgery

Following modified radical mastectomy or radical (Halsted) mastectomy, examination of the surgical specimen by the pathologist may show that all of the cancer cells were not completely removed. Postoperative radiation therapy may be recommended in this instance, particularly if the cancer is large, or the cancer has spread beyond the tumor which was removed. Radiation therapy will usually control cancer cells remaining in these areas. The treatment of advanced cancer requires the consultation and coordination of efforts of the surgeon, radiation oncologist, and the medical oncologist.

Advantages. The goal of radiation therapy is to destroy cancer cells in the tissue of the irradiated area. Modern equipment gives precise control of the x-ray treatment. Radiation therapy may be used to treat the spread of cancer to a specific part of the body; for example, the bones.

Disadvantages. The major side effects are the same as those listed under radiation (x-ray) therapy. When cancer is treated by radiation therapy as a supplement to surgery, there may be wide variations in the extent of the treatments required, depending on the problem or site of the disease being treated.

Chemotherapy (Anti-Cancer Drug Therapy)

The medical oncologist is an internal medicine specialist who plans and administers the chemotherapy or hormone therapy and may coordinate the patient's management with other physicians. Anti-cancer drugs or hormone drugs are given orally or by injection into the vein (intravenous) to destroy cancer cells that cannot be removed by surgery, by radiation, or by their combination.

In recent years, important and effective advances in breast cancer treatment have been made in the area of medical oncology, especially in treatment of patients with advanced cancer. Each treatment, however, must be selected to the individual patient. The decision to treat a patient with either hormonal therapy, chemotherapy, or a combination is complex and can be made only after a thorough medical evaluation.

Adjuvant (Supplemental) Chemotherapy

In this type of treatment, chemotherapy and/or hormone drugs supplement the initial surgical or radiation treatment when it is likely or possible that the cancer will recur. Certain characteristics may predict a higher risk of spread: involvement of the axillary lymph nodes with cancer, the microscopic characteristics of the cancer cells, the patient's age, and the lack of sensitivity of the cancer to female hormones. In certain groups of women with breast cancer, supplemental therapy may reduce the likelihood or recurrence slightly. Adjuvant chemotherapy may continue for six months to two years or longer, depending on several factors, including the cancer being treated and the drug program being used. It is almost always given on an outpatient basis.

Advantages. Adjuvant treatment may increase the effectiveness of surgery or radiation therapy and reduce or delay the recurrence of breast cancer. Because the drugs are blood borne and have a systemic (total body) effect, they work to stop cancer growth at distant sites (bones, lungs, liver) in the body. Every drug has specific effects (benefits) that vary for each patient.

Disadvantages. Most chemotherapy drugs have temporary side effects. Some are minimal while others can cause discomfort, including nausea, temporary loss of hair, blood count suppression (resulting in temporary susceptibility to infection, bleeding tendency, and anemia), loss of appetite, fatigue, and rarely, damage to heart muscles. The medication may also depress reproductive function and cause change of life (menopause) symptoms. Newer techniques of administration and more precise dosage reduce the side effects of chemotherapy. Most side effects are tolerable and do not interfere greatly with daily activities.

Chemotherapy for Recurrent or Metastatic (Widespread) Breast Cancer

Anti-cancer drugs, taken alone or in combination with other treatment, can arrest cancer growth or shrink the tumors, thereby helping to relieve symptoms and prolonging the life of a patient who has recurrent or metastatic breast cancer.

Hormonal Therapy

Some breast cancers are sensitive to and can be affected by the female hormones estrogen and progesterone. A fresh piece of the tissue from the tumor biopsy can be tested to measure hormone sensitivity (estrogen or progesterone receptor assay). In some breast cancer patients, beneficial effects can be produced by hormonal therapy. Treatment may consist of oral administration of hormones or anti-hormone pills that counteract the effects of hormones produced by the body or by surgically removing female hormone-secreting glands (ovaries).

Hormonal therapy can be effective by itself in recurrent or metastatic disease or may be used following primary therapy as an adjuvant treatment to decrease the likelihood of cancer recurrence.

Unproven Treatments

Although the great majority of the therapies offered to patients with breast cancer have well-recognized benefits, some practitioners offer and promote unproven therapies which are ineffective and possibly dangerous.

If you are offered a treatment which you suspect is unproven, you may consult either the American Cancer Society at 1-800-227-2345, or the California Department of Health Services' Food and Drug Branch for information and assistance. The two national organizations available for guidance are the National Council Against Health Fraud and the U.S. Food and Drug Administration.

Restoration of the Breast Forms

External prostheses are worn beneath clothing to restore the bustline. They either fit in a brassiere or adhere to the skin. They are made of a variety of substances such as silicone, foam rubber, glycerin, or other viscous fluid.

Reconstructive Surgery

Reconstructive surgery is an option a patient may choose to assist in restoring the form of the breast. It may begin either at the time of mastectomy or at a later date. Achieving an optimal result usually requires more than one surgery, done in stages. The opposite breast may be reshaped to improve the match between the two breasts. Prior radiation may impair or prevent breast reconstruction and must be brought to the attention of the surgeon. You should investigate the extent of financial coverage available through your health insurance while plans for treatment are being formulated.

Internal Prostheses

Internal prostheses are placed in the soft tissue in front of the ribs to replace the volume of removed breast. They are composed of silicone, salt water, or polyurethane and are of the same style as the implants used for cosmetic breast enlargement over the last 25 years. So far, there is no evidence to show that they cause cancer.

Advantages. Internal prostheses may be placed at the time of mastectomy. The overlying skin usually regains much of its sensation and is the same color as the other breast. A one-step procedure may make further surgery unnecessary.

Disadvantages. Some patients develop a thick "peel" (capsule) around the implant which can distort the implant and result in a breast mound which may become firmer. This capsule, which is not a cancer, may have to be treated surgically and, in rare cases, requires the removal of the implant. While an implant does not impair the physician's ability to detect the return of cancer, it may require special techniques for both x-ray examination and any future biopsies.

Flap Procedures (Autogenous Reconstruction Graft)

This operation is accomplished by transferring skin, fat, and muscle to the mastectomy site from a nearby area of the body such as the back, abdomen, or buttock. Depending on the size of tissue transferred and the other breast, an internal prosthesis may also be used. Since the tissue is from the patient's own body, there is no possibility of a rejection of the transplant.

Advantages. Since the tissue is your own, it will usually grow with you (i.e., if you gain or lose weight, it will do the same). Many reconstructions can be done without an implant, so once reconstruction is complete, there is no concern with artificial material in your body.

Disadvantages. Successful grafting requires adequate blood supply to the tissue. If blood flow problems develop, part or all of the tissue may be lost. There may be temporary or permanent weakness in the area from which the tissue was taken. There are additional scars (usually hidden by clothing). This surgery and recovery take longer than placement of an internal prosthesis, and can be considerably more complicated and difficult.

Nipple/Areolar Reconstruction

This is a final option which one may consider after the breast has been reconstructed. There are many techniques used which can be discussed with you surgeon.

Advantages. Offers greater similarity to the other breast, especially under clothing.

Disadvantages. There is often a change in color of the areola and the size of the nipple may decrease. The sensations present in normal nipple/areola are not restored.

Follow-up

The success of cancer treatment depends on early detection, effective treatment, and a careful, consistent follow-up program. Regular visits to your physician and monthly self-examination are essential. Yearly mammograms (breast x-rays) may detect new cancers in the opposite breast, and may reveal a return of the cancer, if it occurs in the remaining breast tissue on the treated side. New methods of detection and treatment are being continually developed and may be used to your advantage.

Many very helpful and thoughtful women who have been through a similar experience can lend you their support and guidance. They can be contacted through your physician, your hospital, your local unit of the American Cancer Society, or the National Cancer Institute's Cancer Information Service.

Summary

The purpose of this brochure is to increase your knowledge of the effective methods of treating breast cancer, and to emphasize the importance of your role in choosing the best method to be used.

There are three basic forms of therapy that are utilized in the management of breast cancer. *Surgical procedures* are undertaken to establish the diagnosis (biopsy), to remove the local disease in the breast (lumpectomy, mastectomy), and to estimate the extent of the disease and treat the remaining cancer if it has spread to the lymph nodes (lymph node dissection). *Radiation therapy* is administered to control local disease in the breast or to treat specific sites of spread. *Chemotherapy and hormone therapy* may be used to treat cancer in the breast, to reduce likelihood of recurrence, and to treat known spread of breast cancer to other body sites. In most situations, effective therapy involves use of more than one form of treatment.

In order to reach a decision of the best treatment method for you, it is important for you to understand the nature of the disease, the extent of your problem, the treatment needed, the method or methods of providing that treatment suitable to your particular situation, and finally the results that reasonably may be expected. This is best done by having a complete evaluation followed by a thorough discussion with your physician(s). The brochure will assist you in participating in these discussions. It provides background information that will prepare you to ask questions about your individual treatment, its advantages, disadvantages, and risks.

Many important details are necessarily left out. You should ask your personal physician for complete and current information. Being well informed and having thoroughly discussed the options with you doctor will make it easier for you to reach an informed decision. Knowledge of all the optional treatments will give you a justified confidence that you have made the best possible choice. This confidence will be a tremendous help to you and your physician as you carry out your treatment and establish your follow-up program.

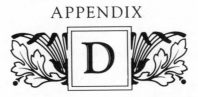

INFORMED CONSENT FOR SILICONE GEL–FILLED BREAST IMPLANTS

The following document is an example of the informed consent information provided by the manufacturers under the guidance of the FDA for women requesting silicone gel–filled breast implants under the ongoing clinical trials for these devices. It informs patients of the procedures required for participation in the study and of the benefits and risks of implants. This document was provided by Mentor Corporation; a similar informed consent document is also supplied by McGhan Medical. All of the information contained in these documents has been developed in conjunction with the FDA.

Consent To Be a Subject in the Mentor H/S Silicone Gel–Filled Mammary Prosthesis Clinical Research Study

Investigator: _____

_____

City   State

Patient's Study No. (SS#): _____

You are being asked to participate in the Mentor H/S Silicone Gel–Filled Mammary Prosthesis Clinical Study. This *informed consent* gives you information about your breast implant procedure and your participation in this study and verifies that you have received it.

To be eligible for participation in this clinical study, *you must be 18 years or older; not have specific connective tissue disorders; be a candidate for breast reconstruction in which saline-filled implants are not suitable; and complete a basic screening by your surgeon.* In addition, ***you must sign this document*** indicating that you have been provided with the required information. You should ask your surgeon to clarify any terms which you do not understand. Additionally, ***your surgeon must provide you with a copy of this document.***

A. PURPOSE AND BACKGROUND OF THE STUDY

Breast implants have been used in over one million women for nearly 30 years. Although there are risks and complications of having breast implants, most women implanted have had satisfactory results. The Food and Drug Administration (FDA) is concerned that there is not enough information about possible health problems from the use of these devices. The FDA has called for detailed scientific studies and has allowed breast implants to be available under these studies while the data are being collected. This study will be used to collect short-term (5-year) data about possible health problems associated with breast implants. This data will be used to help determine if these implants are both safe and effective. If they are proven safe and effective, they will continue to be available. If the data from the studies do not show they are safe and effective, they will not be available in the future.

B. DEVICE DESCRIPTION

The manufacturer of the implants you and your doctor have chosen is Mentor H/S. You may receive one of three different types of silicone gel—filled implants. Two of the types of implants contain both silicone gel and saline solution and the third type contains only silicone. Your plastic surgeon will discuss the various types of implants with you and explain why a particular device may be best suited for you.

C. PROCEDURES

1. You will talk about your procedure and participation in this study with your surgeon in advance and you should take sufficient time to think about participating.
2. If you agree to be in this study, you will first have to be examined to determine if you are a good candidate and if you are eligible. This screening may involve referral to other physicians. Follow-up visits to other physicians may also be required.
3. **Description of operation:** The operation you will have will be performed by a surgeon using accepted standards of practice. The operation may be performed in the physician's office or in a hospital operating room or in an outpatient surgical center. Hospitalization may or may not be required. Your surgeon will explain the particular type of implant that will be used, how and where it will be placed and the type of anesthesia to be used. He/she will also give you an overall description of the operation. This may not

be a one-time operation. Further procedures involving expansion/inflation of your implant or management of complications may be needed.

4. **Surgical consent:** In addition to this Consent Form, you may have signed, or will be asked to sign a surgical consent form which addresses specific risks of the surgical procedure and risks of anesthesia.

5. **Additional follow-up visits/extra appointments with your surgeon:** In addition to normal visits/appointments with your surgeon (i.e., 1-2 weeks, 1 month, 6 months), there may be additional appointments which are required as part of the research. Your participation in the research will be for 5 years. The study schedule requires follow-up visits 12 months, 36 months and 60 months after your surgery. Each visit will take about 30-60 minutes. You are making a commitment to continue in the study for the duration and to complete all of these follow-up visits. If you move within 5 years, arrangements will be made with your surgeon for follow up with someone in your area.

6. **Analysis of removed implant:** If there is a problem resulting in a medical need to remove your breast implant, FDA requires the implant to be sent to Mentor. Mentor will store it and will ask you for permission to analyze it, a process which may alter or destroy it. The results will be sent directly to your surgeon. You will also be asked if you want the results of the analysis sent directly to you, Mentor H/S and the FDA. Mentor H/S and FDA believe there is scientific benefit to testing an explanted implant.

7. **Implant registry:** You will additionally be asked to enroll in a breast implant registry which will allow Mentor H/S to notify you, if necessary, of important new information about your silicone gel–filled breast implant(s). Every effort will be made to keep the information in the registry confidential and will only be provided to the FDA, upon their request. However, under certain circumstances, Congress has the right to get clinical data from the FDA or a court could order disclosure of certain information which could include your clinical study records. You may object to participating in a breast implant registry. If you do object, your doctor will describe in writing how he/ she will inform you of any important new information about your implants that he/she receives.

   _____ *I choose not to participate in this implant registry.* You should also remain in contact with the surgeon to get current important information or, if you leave the surgeon, you should leave an address.

8. **Implant identification:** Your surgeon will provide you with identification information which pertains to your implant(s) after your surgery. This will let you know what type of implant you have. This should be kept with your important papers for future reference.

9. **Second opinions:** If any problems or complications occur during the study, you may be asked or wish to obtain second opinions. You have the right to consult a physician of your choice.

D. BENEFITS OF BREAST IMPLANTS

The major effect of breast implants is to enhance or restore the appearance of a woman's breasts. Breast implant surgery may benefit you by providing a successful surgical breast reconstruction procedure. There may be psychological benefits to having breast reconstruction with silicone gel–filled implants. Women have also reported that breast reconstruction with breast implants has been an aid in their recovery from breast cancer, and has reduced emotional stress by helping to return their body to a more natural appearance as opposed to having nothing done or using an external prosthesis. Each individual woman has her own private sense of how she wishes to look and whether she wishes to go through surgery to achieve this appearance. Several "surveys" have shown that over 90% of women are pleased with the results. However, there are insufficient controlled scientific studies to prove that these results are long lasting. Ongoing studies will help evaluate whether breast implants improve a woman's quality of life.

When compared with other possible surgical treatments (i.e., flap reconstruction, etc.), breast implants have fewer surgical complications; require less surgical procedure time; are less costly; and have a shorter recovery period.

Entering in the study may also benefit other women by providing information about gel breast implants used in reconstruction, including any possible health problems associated with gel breast implants.

E. RISKS

1. **Risks, complications and discomforts of the operation:** Breast surgery requires an incision into the breast under anesthesia. As with any surgical procedure, there are risks such as *infection, delayed wound healing, hematoma formation (a collection of blood inside the body in and around where the incision is made), bleeding and possible reactions from anesthesia.* These complications are uncommon.

   An *infection* can result from any surgery and produce swelling, tenderness, pain and fever. Almost all infections appear within a few days of the operation but on rare occasions may appear at any time after your surgery. If you get a serious infection which doesn't go away with antibiotics, your implant may have to be removed. Small *hematomas* will be absorbed by your body like any bruise but large ones may have to be drained surgically to permit proper healing. Any incision in the skin will leave a scar. Surgical techniques, under most circumstances, can minimize though not eliminate them.

2. **Risks, complications and discomforts of the breast implant(s):** Breast implants have certain specific risks and complications which may include:
   a. *Capsular contracture:* The scar tissue that forms around the implant can tighten and squeeze the implant as a natural response to having any foreign object implanted in the body, making it feel firm. This

firmness can range from slight to hard and the firmest ones can cause varying degrees of discomfort or pain and can also make the detection of breast cancer by mammography more difficult.

If you wish to have them softened, the scar tissue can be released or removed altogether during a surgical procedure called an *open capsulotomy*.

Your surgeon may recommend a technique called *closed capsulotomy* in which he/she will apply forceful external pressure to the breast(s) to "break up" the scar tissue. **This technique is not recommended by the manufacturer,** because it could result in several complications, such as breakage of the implant. However, your surgeon may feel this is the best method for correcting the firmness because if it works it is quick, simple and avoids surgery, although it may be briefly painful. If your surgeon uses this technique, several complications may occur. These include **bleeding, displacement of the implant which may result in asymmetry, distortion and breakage of the implant.**

Your surgeon will explain the possible complications as well as help you determine your choice for correcting capsular contracture.

b. **Calcium deposits:** Any surgery or injury to the breast can produce small spots of calcium in the breast tissue which can be seen on x-rays (mammography). These deposits may not occur until years after implant surgery. They are benign and cause no problems but must be differentiated from the calcium that is often seen in breast cancers. An expert radiologist can usually tell a benign calcium spot from a malignant one but occasionally a biopsy may be necessary to be absolutely sure. Some patients may develop a thin layer of calcium in the scar capsule that surrounds the implant. This is almost always associated with capsular contracture but otherwise causes no known problem.

c. **Rupture/deflation of the implant:** Breast implants may not last a lifetime. The shell of a silicone gel implant can break due to injury or normal wear over time, releasing the silicone gel filling. Two of the types of implants included in this study (Becker device and combination gel-saline device) contain both silicone gel and saline (salt water). If the envelope containing the saline portion breaks, the saline is absorbed harmlessly by the body within hours. As the saline portion of the implant is usually small, the decrease in breast size is minor. Surgical replacement is necessary if you wish to restore your size and shape.

Gel implants can break without any noticeable symptoms. Some women have reported a burning sensation or a change in the feel or shape of the breast. You should see your doctor if you notice these symptoms or if you think for any reason your implant may have broken. While no guaranteed method to detect breakage now exists without surgically opening the pocket containing the implant, mammography, ultrasound and physical examination can usually make the diagnosis.

The gel released as a result of rupture may be contained within the capsule surrounding the implant. If the scar envelope also tears, the gel can travel (migrate) and be squeezed into the breast tissue or into the muscle or fatty tissue next to the breast, abdominal wall or arm. Fortunately this is uncommon. The risks from this escaped gel are unknown. See section on "Unknown Risks."

d. *Gel bleed:* It is known that some very small amounts of silicone "bleeds" through the implant's covering or envelope. Although most of this stays in the implant pocket or is trapped in the surrounding scar, microscopic amounts of this silicone could possibly travel (migrate) to different parts of the body.

Silicone can also be in the body from a variety of sources and it is undetermined whether the silicone from the breast implants poses any risk. See section on "Unknown Risks."

e. *Changes in nipple and breast sensation:* Any surgery on the breast, including a biopsy or breast implant surgery, can result in increased or decreased sensation of the breast and/or the nipple. This change can vary in degree and may be temporary or permanent. It may affect comfort while nursing or sexual response.

f. *Interference with mammography:* An implant can interfere with the detection of early breast cancer because it may "hide" suspicious lesions in the breast during an x-ray exam. It is especially important for women who are at high risk of developing breast cancer to consider this before having implants. The earlier cancer is detected, the better the chance for a cure.

Since the breast is compressed during mammography, it is possible, but rare for an implant to rupture. These problems can be reduced, but not eliminated, by making sure the mammography facility is accredited by the American College of Radiology (ACR) and asking if the personnel at the facility are experienced in performing mammography on women with implants.

Before the mammography exam, you should tell the technologist that you have implants. The technologist should take special care when compressing the breast to avoid implant rupture. Also, an experienced technologist should know how to push the implant away from the breast tissue to get the best possible views of the tissue. Even when this special technique is used, some breast tissue may be missed in the x-ray. Also, women with implants are subject to some additional radiation and higher costs because more x-ray views are needed for women with implants.

The small amount of additional radiation should not deter you from having mammograms when needed. The risk of a missed cancer is far greater than the slight amount of extra x-ray.

g. ***Cosmetic complications:*** You may not be satisfied with the appearance of your implant. ***Incorrect implant size, inappropriate scar location or appearance, and misplacement of implants may interfere with a satisfactory appearance. Asymmetry (unequal breast size or shape) may occur.*** The implanted breast may sag or droop ***(ptosis)*** over time, much like a natural breast. Very rarely the implant may change position or break through the skin, particularly if you have very thin breast tissue covering it. You may be able to feel or see wrinkles in the implant through your skin. If your implant has a valve, you may also be able to feel the implant valve with your hand. Although these complications are not dangerous, you should be aware of these possibilities when considering a breast implant operation as they can detract from the quality of the result.

h. ***Interference with breast feeding:*** Many women with breast implants have nursed their babies successfully. Surgery that removes a great deal of breast tissue, such as mastectomy, could of course interfere with breast feeding. Any breast surgery, including breast implant surgery, could theoretically interfere with your ability to nurse your baby. Further studies will provide more information about this possible risk.

i. ***Granulomas:*** These are non-cancerous lumps that can form when certain body cells surround foreign material, such as silicone. Like any lump, it should be further evaluated to distinguish it from a lump that might be cancerous and may require a biopsy.

j. ***Unknown risks:*** In addition to these known risks, there are unanswered questions about silicone gel—filled breast implants. Both rupture and "*gel bleed*" may result in the silicone going to other parts of the body. The medical complications which may occur as a result of these devices are unknown; however, there may be long-term effects which include:

Connective tissue disorders: There have been a few reports and substantial speculation that there could be an association between certain silicone and certain connective tissue disorders. These are a group of disorders in which the body reacts to its own tissue as though it was foreign material. These disorders can cause long-term, serious, disabling health problems. Symptoms include pain and swelling of joints, tightness, redness or swelling of the skin, swollen glands or lymph nodes, unusual and unexplained fatigue, swelling of the hands and feet and unusual hair loss. Generally, people who have these relatively rare connective tissue disorders experience a combination of these and other symptoms.

Some cases of these disorders have been reported in women with breast implants. Some of these women have reported a reduction in symptoms after their implants were removed. Since connective tissue diseases are rare, they are difficult to research and will require large-scale epidemiologic studies to determine if there is an association with implants. More research needs to be done to determine if women with implants have higher rates of these diseases than women without implants. To explore whether a possible link exists between breast implants and connective tissue disorders, FDA has required manufacturers to sponsor large-scale scientific studies. Final study results are expected no sooner than 1997.

Cancer: There is presently no scientific evidence that links either silicone gel–filled or saline-filled breast implants with cancer. However, the possibility cannot be ruled out. Scientific studies are continuing to determine whether women with implants have a higher rate of cancer than women without implants over a longer term.

Birth defects: Preliminary animal studies show no evidence that birth defects are caused by breast implants. However, to rule out that possibility for humans, further scientific studies are necessary to show whether or not breast implants are associated with birth defects.

Your doctor will discuss any additional information about the risks of silicone gel breast implants and your surgical procedure. You are also encouraged to read the Product Information Data Sheet which your doctor will provide to you, upon request.

3. **Non-medical risks:**

   a. **Costs:** This study may require one or more visits to a rheumatologist or other specialist. There may be an extra charge for these visits. All costs incurred for this study are between you and your physician. This includes costs for any additional procedures or visits to another specialist that may be required for the operation or for participation in the study. Your operation and associated costs may or may not be reimbursed through insurance.

   b. **Insurance:** Breast reconstruction using silicone gel–filled breast implants has been covered under existing insurance policies. Neither Mentor H/S nor FDA knows of any reason why existing coverage policies should not continue. It is, however, your responsibility with your doctor's help, to contact your insurance company and determine the coverage available for this procedure.

   c. **Confidentiality:** Your confidentiality will be protected as much as possible throughout this study. Your medical records will be reviewed by representatives of Mentor H/S and will be made available for review as required by the FDA. Results of data collected will be reported as statistical information only.

Your name, date of birth (DOB) and Social Security number (SSN) will be listed on the clinical study forms. Disclosing your SSN is optional. If you choose not to disclose your SSN an alternative identifier will be assigned.

Under certain circumstances, your clinical records could be obtained by Congress or by a court order. While every effort will be taken to keep this information confidential, under certain circumstances this could mean public disclosure of your surgery and loss of your privacy.

d. **Legal risk:** If your implant needs to be removed, FDA requires the implant be returned to Mentor H/S for evaluation. This could have implications in any legal action involving your implant. Should Mentor H/S wish to do an evaluation of the implant which is removed which could alter or destroy it, you will be contacted first through your surgeon and asked whether you wish to give permission for such an evaluation.

F. ALTERNATIVE PROCEDURES

There are several alternative procedures to breast reconstruction with silicone gel–filled breast implants. These include having nothing done or wearing an external prosthesis inside your brassiere (no surgery required). Breasts can be made by transferring fatty tissues from other parts of the body such as the stomach, buttock or back (flap procedure). Although for many women saline breast implants are an alternative, you have been advised that gel implants will produce a superior result for you than will saline implants.

You may also choose to have your silicone gel breast implant procedure using another physician who is participating in a study using another brand of implant. If you choose to not participate in the study, you may not be provided with silicone gel implants by the manufacturer. Your surgeon should discuss these alternatives with you.

G. COMPENSATION FOR INJURY

Compensation for physical injuries, complications or medical treatment from your participation in this study is not available from Mentor H/S. If a problem occurs, medical treatment will continue to be available. Your surgeon will let you know what to do if you experience any complications while you are in this study.

H. QUESTIONS

During the course of the study, you will be advised by your physician regarding any new information about Mentor H/S breast implants which may become known during the study. You also have the right to ask questions and have them answered.

1. For questions about your procedure, you should contact your surgeon, Dr. _____ at (   ) _____.
2. For questions about the study or any additional information about Mentor H/S breast implants, you may call or write to Mentor H/S at:

   Mentor H/S
   Adjunct Study Coordinator
   5425 Hollister Ave.
   Santa Barbara, CA 93111
   805-681-6000
3. For questions regarding your participation in the study and your rights as a research subject, you may contact an independent reviewer of the research:

   Independent Review Consulting (IRC)
   305 San Anselmo Ave., Ste. 305
   San Anselmo, CA 94960
   800-IRC-3421; FAX 415-485-0328

I. ACKNOWLEDGMENT

I was provided this consent form in advance (a minimum of 3 days prior to surgery, when possible) and met with my surgeon, Dr. _____ on _____ to discuss the information. All my questions have been answered to my satisfaction and I have been provided a copy of this form and Experimental Subject's Bill of Rights (in California only).

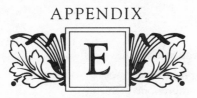

Histopathologic TNM Classification of Breast Carcinoma

The following classification is prepared by the American Joint Committee on Cancer (AJCC) and the International Union Against Cancer (UICC). It describes the tumor, the condition of the lymph nodes, and the presence of metastasis individually and then combines that information to classify breast cancer into four stages.

Primary Tumor (T)

T_x Primary tumor cannot be assessed

T_0 No evidence of primary tumor

T_{is} Carcinoma in situ or Paget's disease of the nipple with no associated tumor

T_1 Tumor 2 cm or less in greatest dimension

T_2 Tumor more than 2 cm but not more than 5 cm in greatest dimension

T_3 Tumor more than 5 cm in greatest dimension

T_4 Tumor of any size with direct extension to chest wall or skin

Regional Lymph Nodes (N)

N_x Regional lymph nodes cannot be assessed
N_0 No regional lymph node metastasis
N_1 Metastasis to ipsilateral axillary lymph nodes
N_2 Metastasis to ipsilateral axillary lymph node(s) fixed to one another or
        other structures
N_3 Metastasis to ipsilateral internal mammary lymph node(s)

Distant Metastasis (M)

M_x Presence of distant metastasis cannot be assessed
M_0 No distant metastasis
M_1 Distant metastasis (includes metastasis to supraclavicular lymph node[s])

AJCC/UICC* Stage Grouping of Primary Tumor Regional Nodes and Distant Metastasis

The descriptions are combined to define four stages:

Stage 0	T_{is}	N_0	M_0
Stage I	T_1	N_0	M_0
Stage IIA	T_0	N_1	M_0
	T_1	N_1	M_0
	T_2	N_0	M_0
Stage IIB	T_2	N_1	M_0
	T_3	N_0	M_0
Stage IIIA	T_0	N_2	M_0
	T_1	N_2	M_0
	T_2	N_2	M_0
	T_3	N_1, N_2	M_0
Stage IIIB	T_4	Any N	M_0
	Any T	N_3	M_0
Stage IV	Any T	Any N	M_1

Histopathologic Type*

The histologic types are as follows:

Ductal
Intraductal (in situ)
Invasive with predominant intraductal
   component
Invasive ductal NOS (not otherwise
   specified)
Comedo
Inflammatory
Medullary with lymphocytic
   infiltrate
Mucinous (colloid)
Papillary
Scirrhous
Tubular
Other

Lobular
In situ
Invasive with predominant in situ
   component
Invasive

Nipple
Paget's disease NOS
Paget's disease with intraductal
   carcinoma
Paget's disease with invasive ductal
   carcinoma
Other

Undifferentiated carcinoma

Histopathologic Grade (G)

GX   Grade cannot be assessed
G1   Well differentiated
G2   Moderately differentiated
G3   Poorly differentiated
G4   Undifferentiated

*World Health Organization (WHO), modified.

GLOSSARY

For a physician reading a medical journal or consulting with another colleague, medical terminology is a familiar part of communication. Consequently, it is natural for doctors to continue using technical language when speaking to patients, not realizing the confusion and anxiety they may cause. For the woman seeking information on breast cancer and breast reconstruction, it is a source of frustration. Before a woman is able to make an intelligent decision about breast reconstruction, she must be able to decipher the terminology. This glossary defines some of the more commonly used medical terms that women need to understand when consulting doctors about breast problems.

A

adjunctive (adjuvant) therapy A secondary treatment in addition to the primary therapy. For example, chemotherapy is often an adjunctive therapy to mastectomy.

adjuvant chemotherapy The use of anticancer drugs after surgery to prevent a recurrence of cancer. For women with breast cancer, the most important indicator for adjuvant chemotherapy is the spread of the cancer to the lymph nodes in the woman's underarm (axillary lymph nodes).

advanced breast cancer Stage of cancer in which the disease has spread from the breast to other body systems by traveling through the bloodstream or lymphatic system.

anterior axillary fold Fold created where the breast and arm meet at the front of the armpit area. The large chest muscle (pectoralis major), which extends from the chest to the upper arm, is the main component of this fold.

areola The circle of pigmented skin on the breast that surrounds the nipple.

aspirate To remove or withdraw fluid or tissue from a cavity by applying suction.

aspiration Withdrawal of fluid or tissue from a cyst or lump through a needle.

atypical hyperplasia Excessive growth of cells, some of which are abnormal.

augmentation mammaplasty (breast augmentation) An operation that enlarges a woman's breast, usually by placing a silicone breast implant behind the breast.

autologous From the same person. An autologous blood transfusion is blood removed and then transfused back to the same person at a later date.

autologous flap breast reconstruction Breast reconstruction with a woman's own natural tissues. Common donor sites for flaps for this operation are the abdomen, back, buttocks, and thigh.

axilla The underarm area behind the anterior axillary fold. It contains the axillary lymph nodes.

axillary dissection Surgical removal of lymph nodes from the armpit. This tissue is then sent to the pathologist to determine if the breast cancer has spread.

axillary lymph nodes Lymph nodes draining the breast found in the armpit area.

B

baseline mammogram A woman's first mammogram, usually done by age 40, and used as a standard for evaluating changes in future mammograms.

benign Opposite of cancerous, or malignant. A benign tumor is a noncancerous growth. It is self-limiting and does not spread to other areas of the body.

bilateral Involving both sides, such as both breasts.

bilateral mastectomy The surgical removal of both breasts.

biopsy Removal of tissue with a needle or scalpel for the purpose of examining it under a microscope to determine whether it is cancerous or benign.

bone marrow Soft inner part of large bones that makes blood cells.

bone scan Test to determine if there is any sign of cancer in the bones.

BRCA1 A breast cancer gene on chromosome 17 (*17q*) that has been linked to familial breast cancer.

breast-conserving surgery and irradiation Treatment option for breast cancer whereby the tumor and axillary lymph nodes are surgically removed. Most of the breast is preserved, and the remaining tissue is then treated by a course of radiation therapy.

breast implant A soft, silicone form that can be placed in the body for simulation of a breast.

breast reconstruction An operation to create or rebuild a natural-looking breast shape after a mastectomy.

breast self-examination (BSE) Monthly self-examination of the breasts in which a woman becomes familiar with the normal look and feel of her breasts.

C

calcifications Small calcium deposits in the breast tissue that can be seen by mammography.

cancer A general term for the more than 100 diseases characterized by abnormal and uncontrolled growth of cells.

cancerophobia An exaggerated fear of cancer.

capsular contracture   A capsule or shell of scar tissue that may form around a woman's breast implant, giving it a feeling of firmness, as her body reacts to the implant.

cathepsin-D   An enzyme present in breast tissue and in other cells that helps break down tissue. Large quantities of this enzyme in breast tissue may indicate a high degree of invasion into surrounding healthy tissue.

catheter   A tube implanted or inserted into the body to inject or withdraw fluid.

chemotherapy   Treatment of cancer with powerful anticancer drugs capable of destroying cancer cells.

clavicle   Collarbone.

clinical trials   Studies designed to evaluate new cancer treatments.

cyst   A sac arising within the body that is filled with liquid or semisolid material.

D

differentiated   Clearly defined. Differentiated tumor cells are similar in appearance to normal cells.

DNA (deoxyribonucleic acid)   Genetic material contained in the nucleus of the cell.

donor site   That part of the body from which tissue is taken and transferred to another part of the body for reconstruction.

drain   Tubes or suction devices inserted after mastectomy or breast reconstruction to drain the fluids that accumulate postoperatively. Drains may be left in place for several days as needed.

duct   In the female breast, milk travels through a system of tubelike ducts from milk glands to milk reservoirs in the nipple area. The duct is the site of most breast cancers.

E

early-stage breast cancer   When cancer is limited to the breast and has not spread to the lymph nodes or other parts of the body. Also called in situ, or localized, breast cancer.

edema   Excess fluid in the body, or a body part, that usually causes puffiness or swelling.

engorgement   An area of the body that is filled and stretched with fluid or distended with blood.

epidermal growth factor receptors   Indirect measurements of the rate of tumor growth. They can be used to predict how a patient will respond to hormone therapy, along with the hormone receptor tests.

***erb B-2/neu* gene (or *HER-2/neu* gene)**   Name of oncogene that is often associated with a poor prognosis. These genes are known to have a high growth rate.

excisional biopsy   Surgical removal of tissue to be examined by opening the skin and removing the suspected tissue.

F

fascia   A sheet or broad band of fibrous or connective tissue that covers muscles and various organs of the body and attaches the breasts and other body structures to underlying muscles.

fat necrosis   Area of dead fat, usually following some form of trauma or surgery. May appear as lumps or thickened areas.

fibroadenoma   A benign, firm, identifiable breast tumor that commonly occurs in the breasts of young women.

fibrocystic breasts   A recurring benign condition characterized by breast tenderness, pain, swelling, and the appearance of cysts or lumps.

fibrous   Gristlelike strands of tough tissue that can grow in the body. In breast reconstruction this usually refers to shell or scar tissue formation sometimes found around implants.

flap   A portion of tissue with its blood supply moved from one part of the body to another. Flaps of muscle, fat, and skin are frequently used to provide additional tissue for reconstructing a woman's breasts. Common donor sites for flap reconstruction are the abdomen (transverse rectus abdominis musculocutaneous, or TRAM, flap), back (latissimus dorsi flap), buttocks (gluteus maximus flap), and thigh.

flow cytometry   Test that measures DNA content in tumors and indicates the aggressiveness of the tumor.

frozen section   A tissue sample removed in a biopsy and quick frozen prior to thin-slicing for microscopic examination.

G

gluteus maximus musculocutaneous flap   Breast reconstruction operation that uses a distant flap of the patient's own tissue (autologous) from the buttock area to build a new breast.

growth rate factors   Important markers used to predict the growth rate of cancerous cells and the likelihood that the cancer will spread.

H

Halsted radical mastectomy   Surgical removal of the breast, skin, pectoralis muscles (both major and minor), all axillary lymph nodes, and fat for local treatment of a breast cancer.

hematoma   A collection of blood that can form in a wound after an injury or operation.

hormone receptor assay   A diagnostic test to determine whether a breast cancer's growth is influenced by hormones or can be treated with hormones.

hormone therapy   Treating cancer by removing or adding hormones to alter the hormonal balance; some breast cancer cells will only grow in the presence of certain hormones.

hyperplasia   Excessive growth of cells.

I

in situ cancer   Localized or noninvasive cancer that has not begun to spread.

incisional biopsy   An operation to remove a portion of tissue that is suspected to be abnormal.

inert   Does not react or cause a reaction.

informed consent   Legal standard that states how much a patient must know about the potential risks and benefits of a therapy before being able to undergo it knowledgeably. Many states have "informed consent" laws regarding breast cancer that require physicians to provide treatment options to patients before any medical treatment is given.

infraclavicular nodes   Lymph nodes lying beneath the collarbone.

inframammary crease   The crease where a lower portion of the breast and chest wall meet.

infusion   Introducing fluids into the veins by slow drip through a tube.

intraductal   Within the duct. Intraductal can describe a benign or malignant process.

intravenous (IV) line   A needle inserted into a vein to administer blood products, nutrients, and medications directly into the blood through a tube.

invasive cancer   Cancer that has spread outside its site of origin to infiltrate and grow in surrounding tissue.

inverted nipple   The turning inward of the nipple. Usually a congenital condition, but if the nipple was projecting and suddenly becomes inverted, it can be a sign of breast cancer.

irradiation   A form of ionizing energy that can destroy or damage cells. Cancer cells tend to be more easily destroyed than the normal cells in the surrounding tissue. For breast cancer treatment, this therapy can be used as an adjunct to breast-conserving surgery to reduce the chance of cancer recurrence.

L

latissimus dorsi muscle   Triangular back muscle that is transferred with some overlying skin as donor flap tissue for reconstructing a breast after mastectomy.

lobular   Having to do with the lobules of the breast.

local treatment of cancer   Treatment only of the tumor in the breast.

localized cancer   A cancer confined to its site of origin.

lump   Mass of tissue found in the breast or other parts of the body; 80% of breast lumps are benign.

lumpectomy   Surgical removal of a cancerous tumor along with a small margin of surrounding tissue.

lymph   Fluid that flows through the body, like blood, but in a separate system of vessels called the lymphatic system. Lymph fluid contains some waste products that are filtered through the lymph nodes and then this tissue fluid is returned to the blood.

lymph nodes   Structures in the lymphatic system that act as filters, catching bacteria and cancer cells, and contribute to the body's immune system, which fights infection and disease.

lymphedema   A condition characterized by the collection of excess fluid in the hand and arm after lymph nodes are removed or blocked.

M

malignant   Cancerous.

mammaplasty   Breast operation to alter breast size.

mammogram   A low-dose breast x-ray film detailing the structure of breast tissue.

mammography   Process of taking breast x-ray films to detect breast cancer at an early stage.

mastectomy   Surgical removal of the breast, usually for treatment of cancer.

mastopexy   Breast lift to tighten the breast by removing skin that the forces of gravity and the effects of aging have caused to sag.

menopause   The cessation of menstruation, usually as a result of aging. The level of female sex hormones is reduced in menopausal women.

metastasis   Spread of cancer from one part of the body to another. It can spread through the lymphatic system, the bloodstream, or across body cavities.

microcalcification   Tiny calcifications in the breast tissue usually seen only on a mammogram. If clusters are present, it may be a sign of ductal carcinoma in situ.

microsurgical breast reconstruction   Method of breast reconstruction whereby a flap of a woman's own tissue is moved from a distant area of the body such as the abdomen, back, thigh, or buttocks to the chest wall area to build a breast. Once this tissue is transferred, the blood vessels are sutured and reattached under the magnification of the operating microscope.

modified radical mastectomy   Surgical removal of the breast, some fat, and most of the lymph nodes in the armpit, leaving the chest wall muscles largely intact.

multicentric   More than one origin. Cancer cells may grow in several locations within the breasts and not be related to each other.

muscle flap   A muscle or portion of muscle that can be transferred with its blood supply to another part of the body for reconstructive purposes.

musculocutaneous (myocutaneous)   Muscle and skin.

N

needle aspiration   Diagnostic method of removing fluid or tissue from a breast tumor or cyst by a fine needle for microscopic examination.

needle biopsy   Removal of a small sample of tissue with a wide-bore needle and suction.

needle localization   Procedure to pinpoint a lump before biopsy.

negative nodes   Lymph nodes that are free of cancer cells.

nipple   The pigmented, central projection on the breast containing the outer openings of the breast ducts.

nulliparous   Never having given birth to a child.

O

oncogenes   Growth-regulating genes that can cause tumors when activated (*onco* comes from Latin root meaning "tumor").

oncologist   Doctor that specializes in treating cancer. (There are medical, surgical, and radiation oncologists.)

oncology   The study and treatment of cancer.

one-step procedure   Breast biopsy and mastectomy performed in a single operation.

P

palliative   Affording relief of symptoms such as pain but not a cure.

palpable   Distinguishable by touch.

palpate   To feel.

palpation   Examining with the hand.

partial or segmental mastectomy   Breast surgery that removes only a portion of the breast, including the cancer and a surrounding margin of breast tissue.

pathologist   A physician who specializes in the diagnosis of disease via the study of cells and tissue.

patient-controlled anesthesia (PCA)   Recent advance in pain control that allows the patient to be in charge of her own pain relief. When pain relief is needed, the patient pushes a button on the PCA machine that delivers a predetermined dose of pain medication.

pectoralis muscles   Muscular tissues attached to the front of the chest wall and extending to the upper arms. These are divided into the pectoralis major and pectoralis minor muscles. The pectoralis muscles usually are removed during a standard radical mastectomy, leaving a large deformity. They are preserved in a modified radical mastectomy.

pedicle   A connection of nourishing blood vessels from the body to a flap of tissue.

permanent section   A tissue sample removed in a biopsy and embedded in wax or paraffin prior to thin-slicing and staining for microscopic examination.

ploidy   A measurement of the amount of DNA in a tumor cell that helps to predict tumor behavior.

positive nodes   Lymph nodes that have been invaded by cancer cells.

predisposition   A latent susceptibility to disease that may be activated under certain conditions.

primary   The first.

prognosis   Forecast as to the expected outcome of disease.

prophylactic mastectomy   Removal of high-risk breast tissue to prevent the development of a cancer. This procedure usually is combined with breast reconstruction.

prosthesis   Any artificial body part. After a breast has been removed because of cancer a breast-shaped form may be worn outside the body. It fits into the woman's brassiere in a specially designed pocket. Prostheses are made of different materials.

ptosis Sagging. Breast ptosis is usually the result of normal aging and the pull of gravity or changes caused by pregnancy or weight loss.

Q

quadrant mastectomy (quadrantectomy) Removal of one fourth of the breast.

R

radiation therapy (radiotherapy, radiation oncology) Treatment of disease by x-rays or other ionized energy.

radical mastectomy Removal of the breast, underlying muscles, and underarm (axillary) lymph nodes.

radiologist A doctor with special training in diagnosing disease by studying x-ray films and other images and using these procedures to facilitate treatment.

radiolucent Allows x-rays to pass through.

radiopaque Blocks x-rays; appears as white on an x-ray film.

radiotherapist Also known as a radiation therapist or radiation oncologist. A physician that specializes in treating cancer patients with radiation therapy.

randomized Chosen at random. In a randomized research study, subjects are chosen to receive a particular treatment by means of a computer programmed to randomly select names.

reconstructive mammaplasty (breast reconstruction) Rebuilding of the breast by plastic surgery techniques.

rectus abdominis muscles The vertical paired muscles on either side of the midline of the abdomen. These muscles can be used as donor tissue for breast reconstruction (*see* TRAM flap breast reconstruction).

recurrence Return of a tumor after the initial treatment of the primary tumor.

reduction mammaplasty An operation for reducing the size of the breasts by removing glandular and fatty tissue.

S

saline solution Saltwater; sometimes used in breast implants.

seroma A fluid mass caused by the localized accumulation of lymph fluid within a body part or area. This condition sometimes occurs after an operation. In breast surgery it may occur after an axillary dissection.

side effects Reactions to drugs or treatments that are usually temporary and reversible.

silicone A chemical polymer that is used to replace numerous body parts. Breast implant envelopes are made of silicone.

silicone gel Silicone produced in a semisolid, semiliquid state, used as a filling in breast implants; similar in consistency to a normal breast.

simple or total mastectomy Removal of the breast only; lymph nodes and pectoralis muscles are preserved.

sloughing   The process in which the body rids itself of dead tissue. Frequently this happens when the tissue being used does not have an adequate blood supply.

S-phase fraction   Measurement of how fast a tumor is growing.

staging   System for classifying cancer according to the size of the tumor, its stage of development, and the extent of its spread.

subcutaneous mastectomy   Preventive mastectomy that removes most of the breast tissue but leaves the nipple intact.

survival rate   The percentage of people who live a period of time after a surgical procedure or the diagnosis of a disease as opposed to the percentage of those who die.

symmetry   Balance. When one side matches the other. One of the chief goals of the patient and plastic surgeon for breast reconstruction.

systemic   Involving the entire body.

systemic treatment   Treatment involving the whole body, usually with drugs.

T

tamoxifen   An anti-estrogen (estrogen blocker) drug commonly used as a hormonal therapy for breast cancer. Tamoxifen is often prescribed as an alternative to chemotherapy in postmenopausal women.

total mastectomy with axillary dissection   A mastectomy in which the breast tissue and most of the axillary lymph nodes are removed. Another name for modified radical mastectomy.

tissue expander   An adjustable implant that can be inflated with saltwater to stretch the tissues at the mastectomy site.

TRAM flap breast reconstruction   Breast reconstruction operation that utilizes a flap of the patient's own lower abdominal tissue (transverse rectus abdominis musculocutaneous flap) to build a breast. The TRAM flap can be a *pedicle flap* in which the tissue is moved while still attached to its blood supply, or it can be a *free flap* in which the flap is totally separated from its donor site and moved to its new location and the vessels are reattached microsurgically.

tumor   An abnormal growth of tissue that can be benign or malignant.

tumor markers   Substances released by the tumor or in response to the presence of a tumor. They are studied as potential diagnostic and prognostic tools.

two-step procedure   Breast biopsy and breast cancer treatment performed as two steps, allowing diagnosis of cancer and treatment to be separated by hours, days, or even longer periods of time.

X

x-ray   High-energy radiation used in high doses to treat cancer or in low doses to diagnose the disease.

BIBLIOGRAPHY

This bibliography contains materials that we found helpful to us in preparing this book. Many of the pamphlets cited are available free through the American Cancer Society (ACS), the National Alliance of Breast Cancer Organizations (NABCO), and the National Cancer Institute (NCI). To allow our readers to explore these topics in whatever depth they feel is appropriate, we have included a mixture of articles and books; some are written for a general audience and others are written for a professional audience. Some books or pamphlets were particularly valuable to us, and these have been indicated by bullets throughout the reference listings.

Breast Examination

- Breast exams: What you should know. Pub No 91-2000, Washington, DC: National Cancer Institute, 1992.

  Examining your breasts: How to do it right. Ladies' Home J 103:59, Aug, 1986.

- Foster RS Jr, Costanza M. Breast self-examination practices and breast cancer survival. Cancer 53:999, 1984.

  How to examine your breasts. Pub No 2088-LE, Atlanta: American Cancer Society, 1990.

  Milan AR. Breast Self-Examination. New York: Liberty Publishing Co, 1980.

- National Alliance of Breast Cancer Organizations (NABCO) fact sheets and news articles (available free of charge from NABCO; see Appendix A):

  An Abnormal Mammogram: What it Means

  New Mammography Guidelines (June 1989)

  Painful Mammography

  Shopping for a Mammogram

- Special touch: A personal plan of action for breast health. Pub No 2095- LE, Atlanta: American Cancer Society, 1991.

Breast Lumps and Their Diagnosis

Black ST. Specter of breast cancer: Don't sit home and be afraid. McCall's, Feb, 1973.

Breast biopsy: What you should know. Pub No 90-657, Washington, DC: National Cancer Institute, 1993.

Breast cancer: Earlier diagnoses and new attitudes. Ladies' Home J 104:112, Oct, 1987.

Castleman M. Early detection: The best defense. Family Circle 105:107, Oct 13, 1992.

Castleman M. What's normal, what's not. Family Circle 105:101, Oct 13, 1992.

Chances are . . . you need a mammogram. Pub No PF4730, Washington, DC: AARP, 1991. (Contact AARP, 601 E St, Washington, DC, 20049.)

Good news about mammograms. US News & World Report 103:17, Sept, 1987.

Good news, better news, best news . . . cancer prevention. Pub No 84-2671, Washington, DC: National Cancer Institute, 1984.

The lessons from Mrs. R's case: Early detection through mammography greatly reduces the risks of breast cancer. Newsweek 110:30, Oct, 1987.

Love SM, Gelman RS, Silen W. Fibrocystic disease of the breast—A nondisease? N Engl J Med 307:1010, 1982.

Mammograms: A must. Weight Watchers 19:10, Oct, 1986.

McGinn KA. Keeping Abreast: Breast Changes That Are Not Cancer. Palo Alto, CA: Bull Publishing Co, 1987.

• Questions and answers about breast lumps. Pub No 90-2401, Washington, DC: National Cancer Institute, 1993.

Questions and answers about choosing a mammography facility. Pub No 91-3228, Washington, DC: National Cancer Institute, 1992.

Strax P. Make Sure You Do Not Have Breast Cancer. New York: St Martin's Press, 1989.

Thompson WR, Bowen JR, Dorman BA, et al. Mammographic localization and biopsy of nonpalpable breast lesions—a 5-year study. Arch Surg 126:730, 1991.

Breast Cancer Risk

Anderson DE. Breast cancer in families. Cancer 40:1855, 1977.

• Baker NC. Relative Risk: Living With a Family History of Breast Cancer. New York: Viking Press, 1991.

Castleman M. Are you at risk for breast cancer? Family Circle 105:103. Oct 13, 1992.

Eades MD. If It Runs in Your Family. Breast Cancer: Reducing Your Risk. New York: Bantam Books, 1991.

• Kelly PT. Understanding Breast Cancer Risk. Philadelphia: Temple University Press, 1991.

King MC. Zeroing in on a breast cancer susceptibility gene. Science 259:622, 1993.

Weber B, Collins F. Genetic counseling: A prefix of what's in store. Science 259:624, 1993.

Breast Cancer Information

After breast cancer: A guide to follow-up care. Pub No 90-2400, Washington, DC: National Cancer Institute, 1987.

Berkel H, Birdsell DC, Jenkins H. Breast augmentation: A risk factor for breast cancer? N Engl J Med 326:1649, 1992.

Black women and breast cancer. Essence Magazine 17:64, June, 1986.

Breast cancer: We're making progress every day. Pub No 86-2409, Washington, DC: National Cancer Institute, 1985.

• The breast cancer digest: A guide to medical care, emotional support and educational programs. Pub No 84-1691, Washington, DC: National Cancer Institute, 1993.

• Cancer facts and figures, 1992. Pub No 5008.92-LE. Atlanta: American Cancer Society, 1992.

Cancer facts for women. Pub No 2007-LE, Atlanta: American Cancer Society, 1992.

Castleman M. Medical breakthrough! The new ways to detect and treat breast cancer. Redbook 169:180, Sept, 1987.

Cooper GM. Elements of Human Cancer. Boston: Jones & Bartlett Publishers, 1992.

Everything doesn't cause cancer, but how can we tell which things cause cancer and which ones don't? Pub No 87-2039, Washington, DC: National Cancer Institute, 1992.

Friedberg EC, Cancer—Encouraging Answers to 25 Questions You Were Always Afraid to Ask. New York: WH Freeman & Co, 1992.

Halbert DS. Your Breast and You: What Every Woman Needs to Know About Breast Diseases, Breast Cancer and Cosmetic Breast Surgery Before She Has a Breast Problem. Abilene, TX: Askon Publishing Co, 1986.

• Harris JR, Hellman S, Henderson IC, et al. Breast Diseases, 2nd ed. Philadelphia: JB Lippincott Co, 1991.

• Harris JR, Lippman ME, Veronesi U, et al. Medical progress: Breast cancer [first of three parts]. N Engl J Med 327:319, 1992.

• Harris JR, Lippman ME, Veronesi U, et al. Medical progress: Breast cancer [second of three parts]. N Engl J Med 327:390, 1992.

• Harris JR, Lippman ME, Veronesi U, et al. Medical progress: Breast cancer [third of three parts]. N Engl J Med 327:473, 1992.

Hirshaut Y, Pressman P. Breast Cancer: The Complete Guide. New York: Bantam Books, 1992.

Journal of the American Medical Women's Association: Special edition on breast cancer. (Contact JAMWA, 801 N Fairfax St, Alexandria, VA, 22314 for a single copy.)

Kessler DA. Breast implants—Protection or paternalism? N Engl J Med 326:1695, 1992.

• Love SM, Lindsey K. Dr. Susan Love's Breast Book. Reading, MA: Addison-Wesley Publishing Co, 1990.

Morra M, Potts E. Breast cancer. Special Health Section No. 44. Good Housekeeping 204:157, May, 1987.

• National Alliance of Breast Cancer Organizations (NABCO) fact sheets and NABCO news articles:
Breast Cancer and the Pill
The Diet–Breast Cancer Link
Hormone Used in Menopause Therapy Linked to Breast Cancer

Seligson M. Breast cancer: Report from the research front. Lear's 5:46, Dec, 1992.

Seltzer VL. Every Woman's Guide to Breast Cancer Prevention, Treatment, and Recovery. New York: Penguin Books, 1988.

Thinking about breast cancer. US News & World Report 102:65, May, 1987.

What you need to know about cancer of the breast. Pub No 91-1556, Washington, DC: National Cancer Institute, 1993.

When cancer recurs: Meeting the challenge again. Pub No 87-2709, Washington, DC: National Cancer Institute, 1993.

When someone in your family has cancer. Pub No 90-2685, Washington, DC: National Cancer Institute, 1992.

Preventive (Prophylactic) Mastectomy for the Woman at Risk

Berman C. Breast surgery to prevent cancer: The big dispute. Good Housekeeping 192:151, March, 1981.

Buchler P. Patient selection for prophylactic mastectomy: Who is at high risk? Plast Reconstr Surg 72:324, 1983.

Clark M, Shapiro D. Breast surgery before cancer. Newsweek 96:100, Dec 1, 1980.

Jarrett JR, Cutler RG, Teal DF. Subcutaneous mastectomy in small, large or ptotic breasts with immediate submuscular placement of implants. Plast Reconstr Surg 62:381, 1978.

Love S. Discussion of patient selection for prophylactic mastectomy: Who is at high risk? Plast Reconstr Surg 72:326, 1983.

• Weber B, Collins F. Genetic counseling: A preview of what's in store. Science 259:624, 1993.

Personal Accounts of Breast Cancer and Reconstruction

• Brinker N. The Race Is Run One Step at a Time: My personal struggle and Every Woman's Guide to Taking Charge of Breast Cancer. New York: Simon & Schuster, 1990.

Ford B. The Times of My Life. New York: Harper & Row, Publishers, 1978.

• Gross A, Ito D. Women Talk About Breast Surgery. New York: Harper Perennial, 1990.

Hargrove A. Getting Better: Conversations With Myself and Other Friends While Healing From Breast Cancer. Minneapolis: CompCare Publishers, 1988.

Kahane DH. No Less a Woman: Ten Women Shatter the Myths About Breast Cancer. New York: Prentice Hall Press, 1990.

Kushner R. My side. Working Woman 8:160, May, 1983.

Lamberg L. Back to business: Surviving the biggest crisis of all. Working Woman 6:85, April, 1981.

Mitchell JS. Winning the Chemo Battle. New York: WW Norton & Co, 1988.

Moss RW. A Real Choice: Seven Women, Aided by an Understanding Doctor, Confront Breast Cancer on Their Own Terms. New York: St Martin's Press, 1984.

Pepper CB. The victors—Patients who conquered cancer. The New York Times, Jan 29, 1984.

Rogers J. One woman's battle against cancer. 50 Plus 26:34, 1986.

Rollin B. First You Cry. Philadelphia: JB Lippincott Co, 1976.

Shapero L, Goodman A. Never Say Die: A Doctor and Patient Talk About Breast Cancer. New York: Appleton-Century-Crofts, 1980.

• Sheehy G. They fought and won: Surviving breast cancer. Family Circle 105:94, Oct 13, 1992.

Simons A. My story: A doctor's personal battle. Family Circle 105:118, Oct 13, 1992.

Wadler J. My Breast: One Woman's Cancer Story. Reading, MA: Addison-Wesley Publishing Co, 1992.

• Zalon J. I Am Whole Again: The Case for Breast Reconstruction After Mastectomy. New York: Random House, 1978.

Breast Cancer Treatment Options

Adjuvant chemotherapy: A breast cancer fact sheet. Pub No 87-2877, Washington, DC: National Cancer Institute, 1993.

Balch CM. Clinical decision making in early breast cancer. Ann Surg 217:207, 1993.

Beadle GF, Silver B, Botnik L, et al. Cosmetic results following primary radiation therapy for early breast cancer. Cancer 54:2911, 1984.

Bedwani R. Management and survival of patients with "minimal" breast cancer. Cancer 47:2769, 1981.

• Bedwinek J. Breast cancer: Primary treatment. In Gilbert H, ed. Modern Radiation Oncology: Classic Literature and Current Management, vol 2. Philadelphia: Harper & Row, 1984.

Bedwinek J. Treatment of stage I and II adenocarcinoma of the breast by tumor excision and irradiation. Int J Radiat Oncol Biol Phys 7:1553, 1981.

• Breast cancer: Understanding treatment options. Pub No 91 86-2675, Washington, DC: National Cancer Institute, 1990.

Breast cancer: When chemotherapy works. Ms Magazine 16:70, Nov, 1987.

• Bruning N. Coping With Chemotherapy. New York: Ballantine, 1992.

• Cancer treatments: Consider the possibilities. Pub No 89-3060, Washington, DC: National Cancer Institute, 1989.

Castleman M. Good news: Treatment breakthroughs. Family Circle 105:114, Oct 13, 1992.

• Chemotherapy and you: A guide to self-help during treatment. Pub No 91-1136, Washington, DC: National Cancer Institute, 1991.

Chemotherapy: Your Weapon Against Cancer. New York: The Chemotherapy Foundation (phone 212-213-9292).

Dowden, RV. Advising the mastectomy patient about reconstruction. Am Fam Physician 19(5):103, 1979.

Fisher B. Five-year results of a randomized clinical trial comparing total mastectomy and segmental mastectomy with or without radiation in the treatment of breast cancer. N Engl J Med 312:665, 1985.

Kuehn P. Breast Care Options for the 1990's. South Windsor, CT: Newmark Publishing Co, 1991.

Kushner R. Alternatives: New Developments in the War on Breast Cancer. Cambridge, MA: Warner Books, 1986.

Lippman ME, ed. National Institutes of Health consensus development conference on adjuvant chemotherapy and endocrine therapy for breast cancer. Washington, DC: US Government Printing Office, 1986.

Lippman ME, Lichter AS, Danforth DS Jr, et al. Diagnosis and Management of Breast Cancer. Philadelphia: WB Saunder Co, 1987.

Mastectomy: A treatment for breast cancer. Pub No 91-658, Washington, DC: National Cancer Institute, 1990.

Mitchell JS. Winning the Chemo Battle. New York: WW Norton & Co, 1988.

Montague EC, Gutierrez AE, Barker JL, et al. Conservation surgery and irradiation for the treatment of favorable breast cancer. Cancer 43:1058, 1979.

More or less? Lumpectomy and radiotherapy found as effective as mastectomy on breast cancer. Sci Am 253:59, Aug, 1985.

• Morra M, Potts E. Choices: Realistic Alternatives in Cancer Treatment. New York: Avon Books, 1987.

• National Alliance of Breast Cancer Organizations (NABCO) fact sheets and NABCO news articles:
  Autologous Bone Marrow Transplantation (ABMT) Information Package
  Metastatic Breast Cancer: Treatment Update
  Participation in Clinical Trials for Breast Cancer
  Some Questions and Answers Re: The Clinical Alert Tamoxifen

• NIH consensus conference statement: Treatment of early stage breast cancer, vol 8, p 6. (Available from the Office of Medical Applications of Research, National Institutes of Health, Bldg 1, Room 260, Bethesda, MD 20892 or NABCO.)

• Nowack EJ, Vikhanski L. The Well-Informed Patient's Guide to Breast Surgery. New York: Dell Publishing, 1992.

• Radiation therapy and you: A guide to self-help during treatment. Pub No 91-2227, Washington, DC: National Cancer Institute, 1990.

• Schain WS, Edwards BE, Garrell CR, et al. Psychosocial and physical outcomes of primary breast cancer therapy: Mastectomy versus excisional biopsy and irradiation. Breast Cancer Res Treat 3:377, 1983.

Spletter MA. A Woman's Choice: New Options in the Treatment of Breast Cancer. Boston: Beacon Press, 1982.

Weitzman S, et al. Confronting Breast Cancer. New York: Vintage Books, 1987.

What are clinical trials all about? A booklet for patients with cancer. Pub No 88-2706, Washington, DC: National Cancer Institute, 1993.

Wohlberg WH. Mastectomy or breast conservation in the management of primary breast cancer: Psychological factors. Oncology 4:101, 1990.

Psychological and Sexual Considerations After Breast Cancer

Brand PC, Van Keep PA. Breast Cancer Psycho-Social Aspects of Early Detection and Treatment. Baltimore: University Park Press, 1978.

Dackman L. Affirmations, Meditations, and Encouragements for Women Living With Breast Cancer. Los Angeles: Lowell House, 1991.

• Dackman L. Up Front: Sex and the Post-Mastectomy Woman. New York: Viking Press, 1990.

• Greenberg M. Invisible Scars: A Guide to Coping With the Emotional Impact of Breast Cancer. New York: Walker & Co, 1988.

Jobin J. How men respond to mastectomy. Woman's Day, Nov, 1977.

Kaye R. Spinning Straw Into Gold: Your Emotional Recovery From Breast Cancer. New York: Simon & Schuster, 1991.

• Morra M, Potts E. Triumph—Getting Back to Normal When You Have Cancer. New York: Avon Books, 1990.

• Murcia A. Man to Man: When the Woman You Love Has Breast Cancer. New York: St Martin's Press, 1989.

Nessim S, Ellis J. Cancervive—The Challenge of Life After Cancer. Boston: Houghton Mifflin Co, 1991.

The psychological impact of cancer. Professional Education Pub No 3009-P.E., Atlanta: American Cancer Society, 1988.

• Royak-Schaler R. Challenging the Breast Cancer Legacy: A Program of Emotional Support and Medical Care for Women at Risk. New York: HarperCollins, 1992.

Schain WS. Psychosocial and interpersonal aspects of breast reconstruction. In Noone RB, ed. Plastic and Reconstructive Surgery of the Breast. CV Mosby Co, 1990.

Schain WS. Sexual and intimate consequences of breast cancer treatments. Cancer J Clinicians 38:154, 1988.

• Schain WS. Sexual problems of patients with cancer. In DeVita VT Jr, Hellman S, Rosenberg SA, eds. Cancer Principles and Practices of Oncology. Philadelphia: JB Lippincott Co, 1982.

• Schain WS, Edwards BE, Garrell CR, et al. Psychosocial and physical outcomes of primary breast cancer therapy: Mastectomy versus excisional biopsy and irradiation. Breast Cancer Res Treat 3:377, 1983.

Schover LR. In Randers-Pehrson M, ed. Sexuality & Cancer: For the Woman Who Has Cancer and Her Partner. Atlanta: American Cancer Society, 1988.

Schover L, Schain WS, Montague DK. Sexual problems of patients with cancer. In DeVita VT Jr, Hellman S, Rosenberg SA, eds. Principles and Practices of Oncology, 3rd ed. Philadelphia: JB Lippincott Co, 1989, pp 2206-2219.

Tarrier N. Living With Breast Cancer and Mastectomy: A Self-Help Guide. Wolfeboro, NH: Longwood Publishing Group, 1987.

• Wellish DK. Psychosocial aspects of mastectomy: II. The man's perspective. Am J Psychiatry 135:543, 1978.

Nutrition, Exercise, and Beauty Aids

Buyer's guide to wigs and hairpieces. (Contact Ruth L. Weintraub Co, Inc, 420 Madison Ave, Ste 406, New York, NY 10017; 212-838-1333.)

Darion E. Exercises for mastectomy patients. McCall's 109:44, April, 1982.

Diet, nutrition & cancer prevention: A guide to food choices. Pub No 87- 2878, Washington, DC: National Cancer Institute, 1993.

• Eating hints: Recipes and tips for better nutrition during cancer treatment. Pub No 91-2079, Washington, DC: National Cancer Institute, 1990.

Eating smart. Pub No 87-2042, Atlanta: American Cancer Society, 1989.

Good news, better news, best news . . . Cancer prevention. Pub No 84-2671, Washington, DC: National Cancer Institute, 1984.

Graham S. Alcohol and breast cancer. N Engl J Med 316:1211, 1987.

• Kalter S. Looking Up: The Complete Guide to Looking and Feeling Good for the Recovering Cancer Patient. New York: McGraw-Hill, 1987.

Kaplan J. Does alcohol increase the risk of breast cancer? Vogue 177:174, Nov, 1987.

Lieberman S, Bruning N. Design Your Own Vitamin and Mineral Program. New York: Avery, 1990.

• Lindsay A, Fink DJ. The American Cancer Society Cookbook. New York: Hearst Books, 1988.

Mendel D. Proper Doctoring. New York: Springer-Verlag, 1984.

Noyes D, Mellody P. Beauty and Cancer. Los Angeles, CA: AC Press, 1988.

• Spear R. Low Fat and Loving It. New York: Warner Books, 1990.

Insurance and Other Resource Information

• Cancer treatments your insurance should cover, Rockville, MD: The Association of Community Cancer Centers (11600 Nebel St, Ste 201, Rockville, MD 20852; 301-984-9496).

Cancer: Your job, insurance and the law. Pub No 4585-PS. Atlanta: American Cancer Society, 1987.

The consumer's guide to disability insurance. Pub No C104, Washington, DC: Health Insurance Association of America, 1991.

The consumer's guide to health insurance. Pub No C103, Washington, DC: Health Insurance Association of America, 1991.

The consumer's guide to long-term care insurance. Pub No C101, Washington, DC: Health Insurance Association of America, 1991.

The consumer's guide to medicare supplement insurance. Pub No C102, Washington, DC: Health Insurance Association of America, 1991.

Rehabilitation and Support

• Charting the Journey: An Almanac of Practical Resources for Cancer Survivors. The National Coalition for Cancer Survivorship. New York: Consumer Reports Books, 1990.

• Fabian C. Recovering From Breast Cancer. New York: HarperCollins, 1992.

Facing forward: A guide for cancer survivors. Pub No 90-2424, Washington, DC: National Cancer Institute, 1990.

McCauley CS. Surviving Breast Cancer. New York: EP Dutton, 1979.

Subak-Sharpe GJ. Overcoming Breast Cancer. New York: Doubleday & Co, 1987.

Taking time: Support for people with cancer and the people who care about them. Pub No 91-2059, Washington, DC: National Cancer Institute, 1992.

Breast Implants

The American disease [editorial]. The Wall Street Journal, Jan 20, 1992.

Angell M. Breast implants—Protection or paternalism? N Engl J Med 326:1695, 1992.

Berket H, Birdsell DC, Jenkins H. Breast augmentation: A risk factor for breast cancer? N Engl J Med 326:1649, 1992.

Brody GS, Conway DP, Deadpen DM, et al. Consensus statement on the relationship of breast implants to connective-tissue disorders. Plast Reconstr Surg 90:1102, 1992.

Bruning N. Breast implants: Everything you need to know. Alamed, CA: Hunter House, 1992.

Burton TMA, Woo J. Lawyers contest implant class action. The Wall Street Journal, March 16, 1992.

Deapen D, Pike MC, Casagrande JT, et al. The relationship between breast cancer and augmentation mammoplasty: An epidemiologic study. Plast Reconstr Surg 77:361, 1986.

Eklund GW, Busby RC, Miller SH, et al. Improved imaging of the augmented breast. AJR 151:469, 1988.

Feder BJ. A war baby, versatile silicone now shows up everywhere. The New York Times, December 29, 1991.

Fisher JC. The silicone controversy—When will science prevail? N Engl J Med 326:1696, 1992.

Fisher JC, Brody GS. Breast implants under siege: An historical commentary. J Long Term Effects Med Implants 1:243, 1992.

Fisher JC, Potchen EJ, Sergent J. Office communication with breast implant patients: Radiologic and rheumatologic concerns. Perspect Plast Surg 6(2):79, 1992.

Glicksman CA, Glicksman AS, Courtiss EH. Breast imaging for plastic surgeons. Plast Reconstr Surg 90:1106, 1992.

Goldrich SN. Restoration drama: A cautionary tale by a woman who had breast implants after mastectomy. Ms Magazine, 16:20, June, 1988.

Gorczyca DP, Sinha S, Ahn CY, et al. Silicone breast implants in vivo: MR imaging. Radiology 185:407, 1992.

Green S. A woman's right to choose breast implants. The Wall Street Journal, Jan 20, 1992.

Gumucio CA, Pin P, Young VL, et al. The effect of breast implants on the radiographic detecting of microcalcification and soft-tissue masses. Plast Reconstr Surg, 84:772, 1989.

Handel N, Wellisch D, Silverstein MJ, et al. Knowledge, concern, and satisfaction among augmentation mammaplasty patients. Ann Plast Surg 30:1, 1993.

Huber P. Gallileo's Revenge: Junk Science in the Courtroom. New York: Basic Books, 1991.

Huber P. A woman's right to choose. Forbes 149:138, Feb 17, 1992.

Implants and the press [editorial]. The Wall Street Journal, Jan 27, 1992.

Kessler DA. The basis of the FDA's decision on breast implants. N Engl J Med 326:1713, 1992.

Nowack EJ, Vikhanski L. The Well-Informed Patient's Guide to Breast Surgery. New York: Dell Publishing, 1992.

Risk assessment of polyurethane breast implants. Department of Health & Human Services, FDA, July 1, 1991.

Schusterman MA, Kroll SS, Reece GP, et al. Incidence of autoimmune disease in patients after breast reconstruction with silicone gel implants versus autogenous tissue. Ann Plast Surg 31:1, 1993.

Science abdicates [editorial]. The Wall Street Journal, Jan 9, 1992.

Silverstein MJ, Gierson ED, Gamagami P, et al. Breast cancer diagnosis and prognosis in women augmented with silicone gel-filled implants. Cancer 66:97, 1990.

Udkoff R, Alim A, Ahn C, et al. MR imaging in the evaluation of breast implants [abstr]. Radiology 181:347, 1991.

Update on silicone gel-filled breast implants. Department of Health and Human Services, FDA, May 25, 1992.

Woods JE, Arnold PE. Fiction obscures the facts of breast implants. The Wall Street Journal, April 7, 1992.

Breast Reconstruction

• Bostwick J III. Plastic and Reconstructive Breast Surgery. St Louis: Quality Medical Publishing, 1990.

• Breast reconstruction after mastectomy. Pub No 4630, Atlanta: American Cancer Society, 1991.

Breast reconstruction following mastectomy. (Contact The American Society of Plastic and Reconstructive Surgeons, 444 East Algonquin Rd, Arlington Heights, IL 60005; 708-228-9900.)

Chen L, Hartrampf CR, Bennett GK. Successful pregnancies following TRAM flap surgery. Plast Reconstr Surg 91:69, 1993.

Goin MK. Discussion: The psychological impact of immediate breast reconstruction for women with early breast cancer. Plast Reconstr Surg 73:627, 1984.

Goin MK, Goin JM. Midlife reactions to mastectomy and subsequent breast reconstruction. Arch Gen Psychiatry 38:225, 1981.

Goin MK, Goin JM. Psychological reactions to prophylactic mastectomy synchronous with contralateral breast reconstruction. Plast Reconstr Surg 70:355, 1982.

Hartrampf CR. Breast reconstruction with a transverse abdominal island flap: A retrospective evaluation. Perspect Plast Surg 1(1):123, 1987.

Hartrampf CR, Scheflan M, Black PW. Breast reconstruction following mastectomy with a transverse abdominal island flap: Anatomical and clinical observations. Plast Reconstr Surg 69:216, 1982.

• Levinson J. Breast reconstruction: A patient's view. Plast Reconstr Surg 73:703, 1984.

Little JW, Spear SL. The finishing touches in nipple-areolar reconstruction. Perspect Plast Surg 2(1):1, 1988.

Nahai F. Breast reconstruction with a free gluteus maximus musculocutaneous flap. Persp Plas Surg 6(2):65, 1993.

• National Alliance of Breast Cancer Organizations (NABCO) fact sheets and articles on breast reconstruction (available free of charge; see Appendix A.)

Noone RB, Murphy JB, Spear SL, et al. A 6-year experience with immediate reconstruction after mastectomy for cancer. Plast Reconstr Surg 76:258, 1985.

• Schain WS. Reconstructive mammoplasty: Reversibility of a trauma. In Western States Conference on Cancer Rehabilitation. Palo Alto, CA: Bull Publishing Co, 1982.

• Schain WS, Edwards BK, Gorrell CR, et al. The sooner the better: A study of psychological factors of women undergoing immediate versus delayed breast reconstruction. Am J Psychiatry 142:40, 1985.

• Schain WS, Jacobs E, Wellisch DK. Psychosocial issues in breast reconstruction: Intrapsychic, interpersonal, and practical concerns. Clin Plast Surg 2:237, 1984.

Snyder M. An Informed Decision: Understanding Breast Reconstruction. New York: M Evans & Co, 1988.

Stevens LA, McGrath MH, Druss RG, et al. The psychological impact of immediate breast reconstruction for women with early breast cancer. Plast Reconstr Surg 73:619, 1984.

Teimourian B, Adham MN. Survey of patients' responses to breast reconstruction. Ann Plast Surg 9:321, 1982.

To be whole again: Mastectomy treated Peggy McCann's cancer, but breast reconstruction made her well. Life 10:78, May, 1987.
* Zalon J. I Am Whole Again: The Case for Breast Reconstruction After Mastectomy. New York: Random House, 1978.

Resources, References, and Additional Reading

Many of the cancer-related pamphlets listed previously are from one of the following three major organizations.

American Cancer Society (ACS). For materials listed contact your local American Cancer Society unit or state chartered division. If the material is not available locally, contact the ACS National Office, 15999 Clifton Road NE, Atlanta, GA 30329; 404-320-3333.

National Cancer Institute (NCI). Order all materials from Public Inquiry Section, Office of Cancer Communications, National Cancer Institute, Bldg 31, Room 10 A 24, Bethesda, MD 20892; 1-800-4CANCER.

National Alliance of Breast Cancer Organizations (NABCO). Order all NABCO fact sheets and NABCO news articles from The National Alliance of Breast Cancer Organizations, 1180 Avenue of the Americas, 2nd floor, New York, NY 10036; 212-719-0154.

References for Locating Articles in the Popular Literature

Articles appearing in the popular literature are listed in the *Readers' Guide to Periodical Literature* or in the *Public Affairs Information Service*, available in most public libraries. Look in the index under the subject in which you are interested or under the author's name.

References for Locating Articles in Health Science Journals

For articles appearing in the scientific literature, check the *Index Medicus*, which is found in medical libraries, most university and college libraries, and some public libraries. This book lists articles appearing in over 2500 science journals. The National Library of Medicine has a series of medical databases called MEDLARS, which are also helpful. These include the following:

MEDLINE   A database with over 4 million citations and abstracts taken from approximately 3200 medical journals published in the United States and throughout the world.

Physician Date Query (PDQ)   A database providing current cancer information. PDQ is discussed in Appendix A.

CANCERLIT   A database containing approximately 550,000 citations and abstracts of articles published since 1978 on all aspects of cancer.

INDEX